LEXI-COMP'S

Pediatric Pharmacology Companion Guide

including

Comparative Charts, Therapy Guidelines, and Supplemental Data

Extracted from the

Pediatric Dosage Handbook
12th Edition

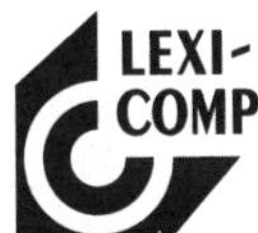

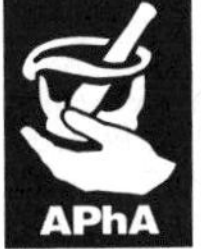

NOTICE

This handbook is intended to serve the user as a handy quick reference and not as a complete drug information resource. It does not include information on every therapeutic agent available. The publication covers commonly used drugs and is specifically designed to present certain important aspects of drug data in a more concise format than is generally found in medical literature or product material supplied by manufacturers.

The nature of drug information is that it is constantly evolving because of ongoing research and clinical experience and is often subject to interpretation. While great care has been taken to ensure the accuracy of the information presented, the reader is advised that the authors, editors, reviewers, contributors, and publishers cannot be responsible for the continued currency of the information or for any errors, omissions, or the application of this information, or for any consequences arising therefrom. Therefore, the author(s) and/or the publisher shall have no liability to any person or entity with regard to claims, loss, or damage caused, or alleged to be caused, directly or indirectly, by the use of information contained herein. Because of the dynamic nature of drug information, readers are advised that decisions regarding drug therapy must be based on the independent judgment of the clinician, changing information about a drug (eg, as reflected in the literature and manufacturer's most current product information), and changing medical practices. The editors are not responsible for any inaccuracy of quotation or for any false or misleading implication that may arise due to the text or formulas as used or due to the quotation of revisions no longer official. Further, the reader/user, herewith, is advised that dosing information is provided only as an indication of the amount of the drug typically given or taken during therapy. Actual dosing amount for any specific drug should be based on an in-depth evaluation of the individual patient's therapy requirement and strong consideration given to such issues as contraindications, warnings, precautions, adverse reactions, along with the interaction of other drugs. The manufacturers most current product information or other standard recognized references should always be consulted for such detailed information prior to drug use.

The editors, authors, and contributors have written this book in their private capacities. No official support or endorsement by any federal agency or pharmaceutical company is intended or inferred.

The publishers have made every effort to trace the copyright holders for borrowed material. If they have inadvertently overlooked any, they will be pleased to make the necessary arrangements at the first opportunity.

If you have any suggestions or questions regarding any information presented in this handbook, please contact our drug information pharmacist at (330) 650-6506.

This manual was produced using the FormuLex™ Program – a complete publishing service of Lexi-Comp, Inc.

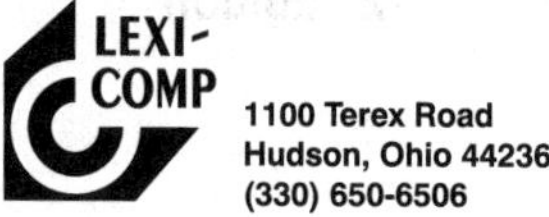

1100 Terex Road
Hudson, Ohio 44236
(330) 650-6506

Website: www.lexi.com
ISBN 1-59195-122-4

TABLE OF CONTENTS

APPENDIX TABLE OF CONTENTS *(Continued)*

CPR PEDIATRIC DRUG DOSAGES

(PALS Medications for Cardiac Arrest and Symptomatic Arrhythmias)

Drug	Dose	Remarks
Adenosine	0.1 mg/kg Repeat dose: 0.2 mg/kg Maximum single dose: 12 mg	Rapid I.V., I.O. bolus Rapid flush to central circulation Monitor ECG during dose
Amiodarone for pulseless VF/VT Amiodarone for perfusing tachycardias	I.V., I.O.: 5 mg/kg Loading dose: I.V., I.O.: 5 mg/kg Maximum dose: 15 mg/kg/day	Rapid I.V. bolus I.V. over 20-60 minutes Routine use in combination with drugs prolonging QT interval is **not** recommended; hypotension is most frequent side effect
Atropine sulfate[1]	I.V.: 0.02 mg/kg (minimum dose = 0.1 mg) Maximum single dose (may repeat once): Children: 0.5 mg Adolescents: 1 mg	May give I.V., I.O., or E.T. Tachycardia and pupil dilation may occur but **not** fixed dilated pupils
Calcium chloride 10% = 100 mg/mL (=27.2 mg/mL elemental Ca)	I.V., I.O.: 20 mg/kg (0.2 mL/kg)	Give slow I.V. push for hypocalcemia, hypermagnesemia, calcium channel blocker toxicity, preferably via central vein; monitor heart rate - bradycardia may occur
Calcium gluconate 10% = 100 mg/mL (=9 mg/mL elemental Ca)	I.V., I.O.: 60-100 mg/kg (0.6-1 mL/kg)	Give slow I.V. push for hypocalcemia, hypermagnesemia, calcium channel blocker toxicity, preferably via central vein
Epinephrine for symptomatic bradycardia[1] Epinephrine for pulseless arrest[1] Epinephrine for **neonatal** resuscitation	I.V., I.O.: 0.01 mg/kg (1:10,000; 0.1 mL/kg) E.T.: 0.1 mg/kg (1:1000; 0.1 mL/kg) First dose: I.V., I.O.: 0.01 mg/kg (1:10,000; 0.1 mL/kg) E.T.: 0.1 mg/kg (1:1000; 0.1 mL/kg) Subsequent doses: Repeat initial dose or may increase up to 10 times (0.1 mg/kg, 1:1000, 0.1 mL/kg) Administer epinephrine every 3-5 minutes I.V., I.O., E.T. doses as high as 0.2 mg/kg of 1:1000 may be effective I.V., E.T.: 0.01-0.03 mg/kg (1:10,000; 0.1-0.3 mL/kg) Repeat every 3-5 minutes as indicated	Tachyarrhythmias, hypertension may occur Data in neonates is not sufficient to recommend higher doses for E.T. route; I.O. route not commonly used in the newly born (umbilical vein is more accessible, smaller bones are fragile, I.O. space is small in premature infants), but may be used in neonate and older infant.

Drug	Dose	Remarks
Glucose (10%, 25%, or 50%)	I.V., I.O.: 0.5-1 g/kg • 1-2 mL/kg 50% • 2-4 mL/kg 25% • 5-10 mL/kg 10%	For suspected hypoglycemia; avoid hyperglycemia
Lidocaine[1] Lidocaine infusion	I.V., I.O., E.T.: 1 mg/kg I.V., I.O. (start after a bolus): 20-50 mcg/kg/min	Rapid bolus 1-2.5 mL/kg/hour of 120 mg/100 mL solution or use "Rule of 6"
Magnesium sulfate (500 mg/mL)	I.V., I.O.: 25-50 mg/kg Maximum dose: 2 g/dose	Rapid I.V. infusion for torsades or suspected hypomagnesemia; 10- to 20-minute infusion for asthma that responds poorly to beta-adrenergic agonists
Naloxone[1]	≤5 years or ≤20 kg: 0.1 mg/kg >5 years or >20 kg: 2 mg	For total reversal of narcotic effect. Use small repeated doses (0.01-0.03 mg/kg) titrated to desired effect
Procainamide for perfusing tachycardias (100 mg/mL and 500 mg/mL)	Loading dose: I.V., I.O.: 15 mg/kg	Infusion over 30-60 minutes; routine use in combination with drugs prolonging QT interval is **not** recommended
Sodium bicarbonate (1 mEq/mL and 0.5 mEq/mL)	I.V., I.O.: 1 mEq/kg/dose	Infuse slowly and only if ventilation is adequate

I.V. = intravenous; I.O. = intraosseous; E.T. = endotracheal

[1]For endotracheal administration, use higher doses (2-10 times the I.V. dose); dilute medication with NS to a volume of 3-5 mL and follow with several positive-pressure ventilations.

Adapted with permission of Lippincott Williams & Wilkins, "Guidelines 2000 for Cardiopulmonary Resuscitation and Emergency Cardiovascular Care. Part 10: Pediatric Advanced Life Support. The American Heart Association in Collaboration With the International Liaison Committee on Resuscitation," *Circulation*, 2000, 102(8 Suppl):I308.

EMERGENCY PEDIATRIC DRIP CALCULATIONS

Note: See JCAHO and the "Rule of Six" below.

Drips

Drug	Dose	Calculation[1]	Rate & Dose
Dobutamine	5-20 mcg/kg/min	6 x body wt (kg) is the mg added to make 100 mL	1 mL/h = 1 mcg/kg/min
Dopamine	2-20 mcg/kg/min	6 x body wt (kg) is the mg added to make 100 mL	1 mL/h = 1 mcg/kg/min
Epinephrine	0.1-1 mcg/kg/min	0.6 x body wt (kg) is the mg added to make 100 mL	1 mL/h = 0.1 mcg/kg/min
Isoproterenol	0.1-1 mcg/kg/min	0.6 x body wt (kg) is the mg added to make 100 mL	1 mL/h = 0.1 mcg/kg/min
Lidocaine	20-50 mcg/kg/min	120 mg in 100 mL of D_5W	1 mL/kg/h = 20 mcg/kg/min

[1]**Note:** Patients ≥40 kg and those requiring fluid restriction may need more concentrated solutions in order to deliver less fluid per hour. In those cases, or as an alternative to the listed calculations above, use the following equation:

$$\text{Rate (mL/h)} = \frac{\text{dose (mcg/kg/min) x weight (kg) x 60 min/h}}{\text{concentration (mcg/mL)}}$$

JCAHO and the "Rule of Six"

In its 2004 National Patient Safety Goals (NPSG), the Joint Commission on Accreditation of Healthcare Organizations (JCAHO) required organizations to "standardize and limit the number of drug concentrations available in the organization" to meet patient safety goal # 3 ("Improve the safety of using high-alert medications"). High-alert medications are drugs that possess a great risk of causing significant injury to patients when they are used in error. Emergency medications (eg, vasopressors) qualify as high-alert drugs.

The above table uses the "Rule of Six" (the equation in the calculation column) to calculate patient-specific I.V. concentrations of dobutamine, dopamine, epinephrine, and isoproterenol, so that 1 mL/hour will deliver a set mcg/kg/minute dose. For example, application of the "Rule of Six" will calculate the mg amount of dobutamine or dopamine to be added to a 100 mL I.V. solution, so that a rate of 1 mL/hour will deliver 1 mcg/kg/minute.

JCAHO has determined that using the "Rule of Six" or other methods to individualize a concentration of a high-alert drug for a specific patient (ie, use of a nonstandardized concentration) is **not** in compliance with the requirement of the above NPSG goal. [Limiting and standardizing the number of drug concentrations (as opposed to using the "Rule of Six") is thought to be safer and less error prone.] Institutions are required to develop a transition plan to use a limited number of standardized concentrations. Full implementation of the plan was originally required by January 1, 2005, but has been extended to December 31, 2008. Hospitals may request permission to continue to use the "Rule of Six" as an alternative approach to the NPSG requirement during some or all of the interim period. However, ongoing evidence of progress toward full implementation by December 31, 2008 is required.

JCAHO's criteria for institutions to participate in the exceptions process during the transition period include:

- "The exception applies only to neonatal or pediatric acute care services.
- All (emergent and nonemergent) admixtures are prepared only by pharmacy staff in a sterile environment.
- Calculations of the drug solutions are validated during the preparation.
- The labeling of solution concentration and drug per milliliter are clear to all caregivers, and the solution concentration (amount of drug per unit volume of solution) is clearly indicated on the label.
- If the 'Rule of Six' is used in a pediatric setting, but standardized drug concentrations are used in other parts of the hospital, guidance aids are made available to caregivers who may not be familiar with one of these systems.
- If the organization has a Neonatal Intensive Care Unit, the pharmacy is open 24 hours a day to support the admixture service.
- Smart pumps are used. (Smart pumps are designed to recognize prescription errors, dose misinterpretations, and keypad programming errors.)" (See JCAHO, 2005).

Some centers use the following pediatric standardized concentrations according to patient weight (see Campbell, 1994).

Standardized Concentrations by Patient Weight

Drug	Patient Weight (kg)	Concentration (mcg/mL)
Dopamine	2-3	200
	4-8	400
	9-15	800
	>15	1600
Epinephrine,	2-3	5
Isoproterenol, or	4-8	10
Norepinephrine	≥9	20

Other centers use the following standardized concentrations depending on both patient weight and dose (Hodding, 2004):

Drug	Standardized Concentrations (mcg/mL)		
Dobutamine	800	1600	3200
Dopamine	800	1600	3200
Epinephrine	8	16	60
Norepinephrine	8	16	60
Isoproterenol	8	16	60

EMERGENCY PEDIATRIC DRIP CALCULATIONS *(Continued)*

When using standardized concentrations, calculate the rate of infusion using the following equation:

$$\text{Rate (mL/h)} = \frac{\text{dose (mcg/kg/min)} \times \text{weight (kg)} \times \text{60 min/h}}{\text{concentration (mcg/mL)}}$$

If a standardized concentration delivers the dose in too low of a volume (eg, <1 mL/hour) then a lower standardized concentration is used. If a standardized concentration delivers the dose in too high of a volume (depending on patient's size and fluid status) then a higher standardized concentration is used. Each center should develop standardized concentrations and guidelines for their own institution.

References

Campbell MM, Taeubel MA, and Kraus DM, "Updated Bedside Charts for Calculating Pediatric Doses of Emergency Medications," *Am J Hosp Pharm*, 1994, 51(17):2147-52.

Hodding JH, Director, Pharmacy Services, Miller Children's Hospital, Long Beach, CA, Personal Correspondence, June 2004.

Joint Commission on Accreditation of Healthcare Organizations, "2004 National Patient Safety Goals, Frequently Asked Questions: Updated 8/30/04," August 30, 2004. Available at http://www.jcaho.org/accredited+organizations/patient+safety/04+npsg/04_npsgs_final2.pdf.

Joint Commission on Accreditation of Healthcare Organizations, "Transition Plan From 'Rule of 6'," JCAHOnline, December 2004/January 2005. Available at http://www.jcaho.org/about+us/news+letters/jcahonline/jo_01_05.htm.

NEONATAL RESUSCITATION ALGORITHM

Algorithm for Resuscitation of the Newly Born Infant

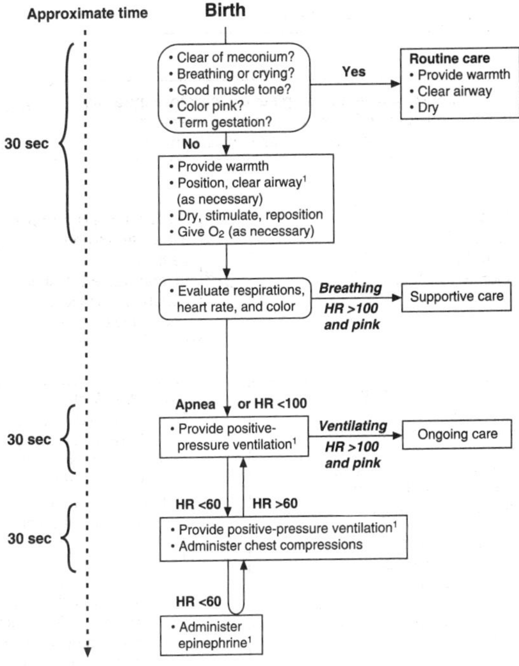

[1]Endotracheal intubation may be considered at several steps.

Epinephrine dose for neonatal resuscitation: I.V., E.T.: 0.01-0.03 mg/kg (1:10,000; 0.1-0.3 mL/kg). Repeat every 3-5 minutes as indicated. Data in neonates is not sufficient to recommend higher doses for E.T. route; I.O. route not commonly used in the newly born (umbilical vein is more accessible, smaller bones are fragile, I.O. space is small in premature infants), but may be used in neonate and older infant.

Adapted with permission of Lippincott Williams & Wilkins, "Guidelines 2000 for Cardiopulmonary Resuscitation and Emergency Cardiovascular Care, Part 11: Neonatal Resuscitation, the American Heart Association in Collaboration With the International Liaison Comittee in Resuscitation," *Circulation*, 2000, 102(8 Suppl):I349.

PEDIATRIC ALS ALGORITHMS

PALS Bradycardia Algorithm

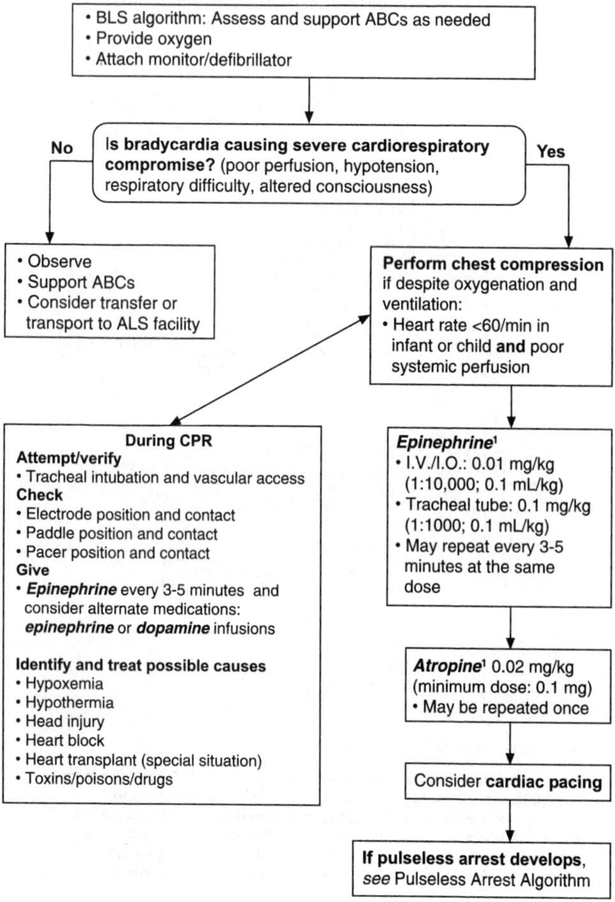

- BLS algorithm: Assess and support ABCs as needed
- Provide oxygen
- Attach monitor/defibrillator

Is bradycardia causing severe cardiorespiratory compromise? (poor perfusion, hypotension, respiratory difficulty, altered consciousness)

No

- Observe
- Support ABCs
- Consider transfer or transport to ALS facility

Yes

Perform chest compression if despite oxygenation and ventilation:
- Heart rate <60/min in infant or child **and** poor systemic perfusion

During CPR

Attempt/verify
- Tracheal intubation and vascular access

Check
- Electrode position and contact
- Paddle position and contact
- Pacer position and contact

Give
- ***Epinephrine*** every 3-5 minutes and consider alternate medications: ***epinephrine*** or ***dopamine*** infusions

Identify and treat possible causes
- Hypoxemia
- Hypothermia
- Head injury
- Heart block
- Heart transplant (special situation)
- Toxins/poisons/drugs

Epinephrine[1]
- I.V./I.O.: 0.01 mg/kg (1:10,000; 0.1 mL/kg)
- Tracheal tube: 0.1 mg/kg (1:1000; 0.1 mL/kg)
- May repeat every 3-5 minutes at the same dose

Atropine[1] 0.02 mg/kg (minimum dose: 0.1 mg)
- May be repeated once

Consider **cardiac pacing**

If pulseless arrest develops, *see* Pulseless Arrest Algorithm

[1]Give atropine first for bradycardia due to suspected increased vagal tone or primary AV block.

Adapted with permission of Lippincott Williams & Wilkins, "Guidelines 2000 for Cardiopulmonary Resuscitation and Emergency Cardiovascular Care, Part 10: Pediatric Advanced Life Support, The American Heart Association in Collaboration With the International Liaison Committee on Resuscitation," *Circulation*, 2000, 102(8 Suppl):I313.

PALS Pulseless Arrest Algorithm

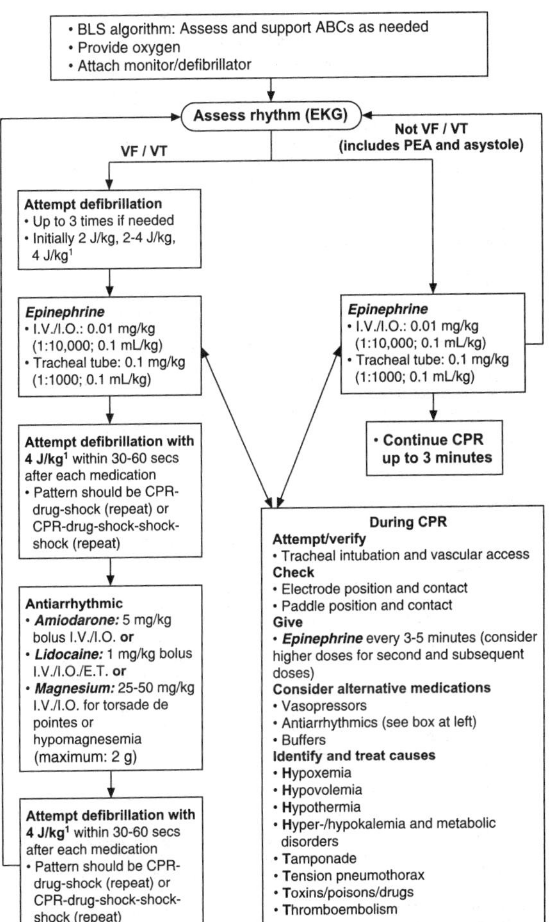

[1]Alternative waveforms and higher doses are Class Indeterminate for children.

Adapted with permission of Lippincott Williams & Wilkins, "Guidelines 2000 for Cardiopulmonary Resuscitation and Emergency Cardiovascular Care, Part 10: Pediatric Advanced Life Support, The American Heart Association in Collaboration With the International Liaison Committee on Resuscitation," *Circulation*, 2000, 102(8 Suppl):I311.

PEDIATRIC ALS ALGORITHMS *(Continued)*

PALS Tachycardia Algorithm for Infants and Children With Rapid Rhythm and Adequate Perfusion

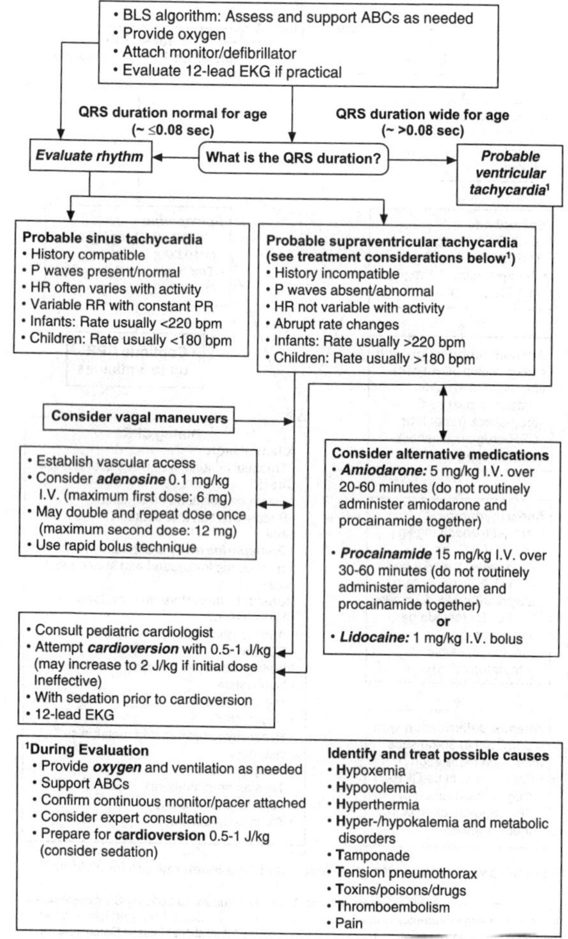

Adapted with permission of Lippincott Williams & Wilkins, "Guidelines 2000 for Cardiopulmonary Resuscitation and Emergency Cardiovascular Care, Part 10: Pediatric Advanced Life Support, The American Heart Association in Collaboration With the International Liaison Committee on Resuscitation," *Circulation*, 2000, 102(8 Suppl):I315.

PALS Tachycardia Algorithm for Infants and Children With Rapid Rhythm and Evidence of Poor Perfusion

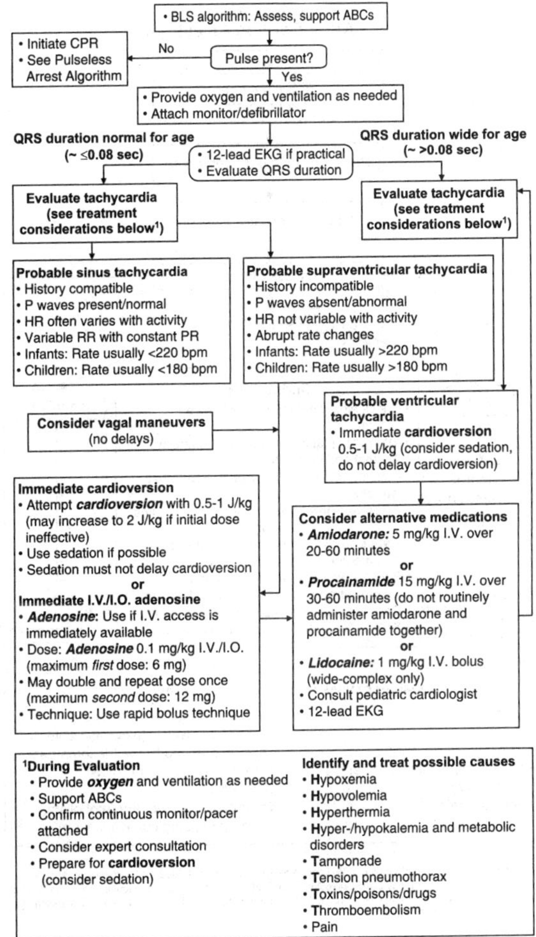

[1]**During Evaluation**
- Provide ***oxygen*** and ventilation as needed
- Support ABCs
- Confirm continuous monitor/pacer attached
- Consider expert consultation
- Prepare for **cardioversion** (consider sedation)

Identify and treat possible causes
- **H**ypoxemia
- **H**ypovolemia
- **H**yperthermia
- **H**yper-/hypokalemia and metabolic disorders
- **T**amponade
- **T**ension pneumothorax
- **T**oxins/poisons/drugs
- **T**hromboembolism
- Pain

Adapted with permission of Lippincott Williams & Wilkins, "Guidelines 2000 for Cardiopulmonar Resuscitation and Emergency Cardiovascular Care, Part 10: Pediatric Advanced Life Support, The American Heart Association in Collaboration With the International Liaison Committee on Resuscitation," *Circulation*, 2000, 102(8 Suppl):I316.

ADULT ACLS ALGORITHMS

ILCOR Universal / International ACLS Algorithm

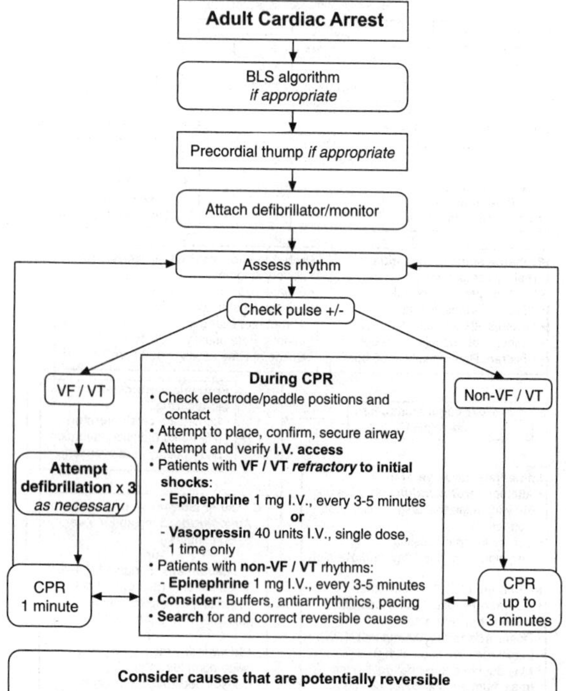

Consider causes that are potentially reversible

- **H**ypovolemia
- **H**ypoxia
- **H**ydrogen ion - acidosis
- **H**yper-/hypokalemia, other metabolic
- **H**ypothermia
- "**T**ablets" (drug OD, accidents)
- **T**amponade, cardiac (pericardiocentesis)
- **T**ension pneumothorax (decompress)
- **T**hrombosis, coronary (ACS); (fibrinolytics)
- **T**hrombosis, pulmonary (embolism, fibrinolytics, surgical evacuation)

Adapted with permission of Lippincott Williams & Wilkins, "Guidelines 2000 for Cardiopulmonary Resuscitation and Emergency Cardiovascular Care, Part 6: Advanced Cardiovascular Life Support, The American Heart Association in Collaboration With the International Liaison Committee on Resuscitation," *Circulation*, 2000, 102(8 Suppl):I143.

Comprehensive ECC Algorithm

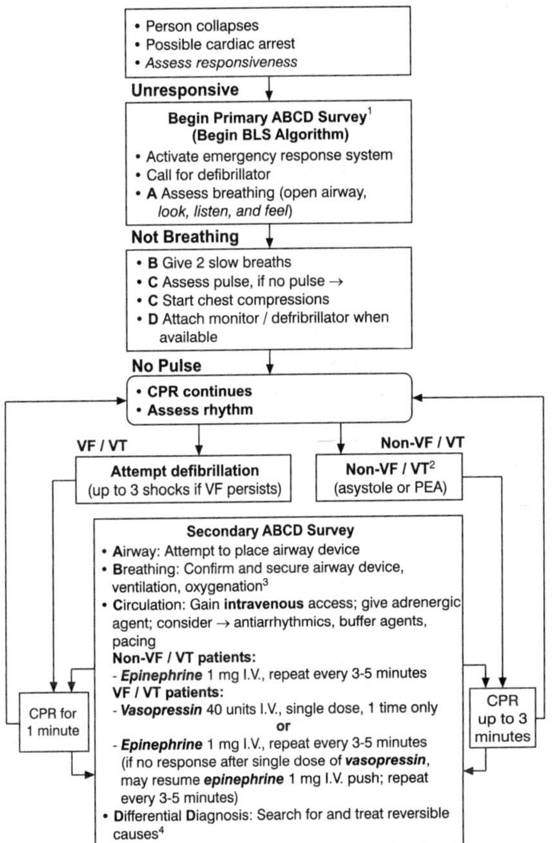

[1]Do not attempt resuscitation if any objective indicators of DNAR status or clinical indicators that resuscitation attempts are not indicated (eg, signs of death).

[2]Recommendation is to consider non-VF / VT rhythms as one rthythm when the patient is in cardiac arrest.

[3]Use 2 methods to confirm tube placement: Primary physical examination criteria plus a secondary device (qualitative and quantitative measures of end-tidal CO_2).

[4]Reversible causes: See ILCOR Universal / International ACLS Algorithm.

Adapted with permission of Lippincott Williams & Wilkins, "Guidelines 2000 for Cardiopulmonary Resuscitation and Emergency Cardiovascular Care, Part 6: Advanced Cardiovascular Life Support, The American Heart Association in Collaboration With the International Liaison Committee on Resuscitation," *Circulation*, 2000, 102(8 Suppl):I144.

ADULT ACLS ALGORITHMS *(Continued)*

Ventricular Fibrillation / Pulseless VT Algorithm

Primary ABCD Survey[1]
Focus: *Basic CPR and defibrillation*

- **Check** responsiveness
- **Activate** emergency response system
- **Call** for defibrillator

A Airway: Open the airway
B Breathing: Provide positive-pressure ventilations
C Circulation: Give chest compressions
D Defibrillation: Assess for and shock VF / pulseless VT, up to 3 times (200 J, 200-300 J, 360 J, or equivalent *biphasic*) if necessary

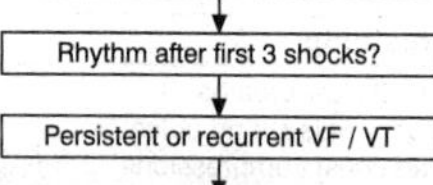

Secondary ABCD Survey
Focus: *More advanced assessments and treatments*

A Airway: Place airway device as soon as possible
B Breathing: Confirm airway device placement by exam plus confirmation device[2]
B Breathing: Secure airway device; purpose-made tube holders preferred[3]
B Breathing: Confirm effective oxygenation and ventilation[4]
C Circulation: Establish I.V. access
C Circulation: Identify rhythm $\rightarrow$ monitor
C Circulation: Administer drugs appropriate for rhythm and condition
D Differential Diagnosis: Search for and treat identified reversible causes

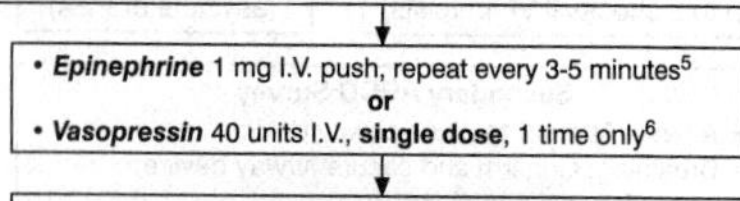

Resume attempts to defibrillate
1 x 360 J (or equivalent *biphasic*) within 30-60 seconds

Consider antiarrhythmics:[7]
Amiodarone (IIb): 300 mg I.V. push. If VF/pulseless VT recurs, consider a second dose of 150 mg (maximum cumulative dose: 2.2 g over 24 hours)
Lidocaine (indeterminate): 1-1.5 mg/kg I.V. push. Consider repeat in 3-5 minutes to maximum cumulative dose of 3 mg/kg
Magnesium sulfate (IIb if hypomagnesemic state): 1-2 g I.V. in polymorphic VT (torsade de pointes) and suspected hypomagnesemic state
Procainamide (IIb for intermittent/recurrent VF / VT): 30 mg/min in refractory VF (maximum total dose: 17 mg/kg) - acceptable but not recommended due to prolonged administration time
Consider buffers

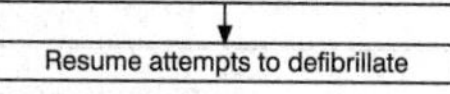

[1]Do not attempt resuscitation if any objective indicators of DNAR status or clinical indicators that resuscitation attempts are not indicated (eg, signs of death).
[2]Consider continuous qualitative end-tidal CO_2 monitor (Class IIa - acceptable, probably effective).
[3]Commercial purpose-made tracheal tube holders recommended (Class IIb - acceptable, possibly effective).
[4]End-tidal CO_2 monitor and oxygen saturation monitor.
[5]If this fails, higher doses of epinephrine (up to 0.2 mg/kg) are acceptable (growing evidence of potential harm).
[6]No evidence about value of repeat vasopressin doses.
[7]Numbers in parentheses represent strength of recommendation (Class IIb - acceptable, possibly effective).

Adapted with permission of Lippincott Williams & Wilkins, "Guidelines 2000 for Cardiopulmonary Resuscitation and Emergency Cardiovascular Care, Part 6: Advanced Cardiovascular Life Support, The American Heart Association in Collaboration With the International Liaison Committee on Resuscitation," *Circulation*, 2000, 102(8 Suppl):I147.

Pulseless Electrical Activity Algorithm

(PEA = rhythm on monitor, without detectable pulse)

Primary ABCD Survey[1]
Focus: *Basic CPR and defibrillation*

- **Check** responsiveness
- **Activate** emergency response system
- **Call** for defibrillator

A Airway: Open the airway
B Breathing: Provide positive-pressure ventilations
C Circulation: Give chest compressions
D Defibrillation: Assess for and shock VF / pulseless VT

↓

Secondary ABCD Survey
Focus: *More advanced assessments and treatments*

A Airway: Place airway device as soon as possible
B Breathing: Confirm airway device placement by exam plus confirmation device[2]
B Breathing: Secure airway device; purpose-made tube holders preferred[3]
B Breathing: Confirm effective oxygenation and ventilation[4]
C Circulation: Establish I.V. access
C Circulation: Identify rhythm → monitor
C Circulation: Administer drugs appropriate for rhythm and condition
C Circulation: Assess for occult blood flow ("pseudo-EMT")
D Differential Diagnosis: Search for and treat identified reversible causes

↓

Review for most frequent causes[5]

- **H**ypovolemia
- **H**ypoxia
- **H**ydrogen ion - acidosis
- **H**yper-/hypokalemia
- **H**ypothermia
- "**T**ablets" (drug OD, accidents)
- **T**amponade, cardiac
- **T**ension pneumothorax
- **T**hrombosis, coronary (ACS)
- **T**hrombosis, pulmonary (embolism)

↓

- ***Epinephrine*** 1 mg I.V. push, repeat every 3-5 minutes[6]

↓

- ***Atropine*** 1 mg I.V. (if PEA rate is **slow**), repeat every 3-5 minutes as needed, to a total dose of 0.04 mg/kg

[1]Do not attempt resuscitation if any objective indicators of DNAR status or clinical indicators that resuscitation attempts are not indicated (eg, signs of death).
[2]Consider continuous qualitative end-tidal CO_2 monitor (Class IIa - acceptable, probably effective).
[3]Commercial purpose-made tracheal tube holders recommended (Class IIb - acceptable, possibly effective).
[4]End-tidal CO_2 monitor and oxygen saturation monitor.
[5]Sodium bicarbonate 1 mEq/kg recommended in the following:
Class I: If patient has known, preexisting hyperkalemia
Class IIa: Known, preexisting bicarbonate-responsive acidosis, in tricyclic antidepressant overdose, or to alkalinize the urine in aspirin or other drug overdoses
Class IIb: In intubated and ventilated patients with long arrest interval, or on return of circulation after a long arrest interval
Note: Ineffective or harmful in hypercarbic acidosis (Class III)
[6]If this fails, higher doses of epinephrine (up to 0.2 mg/kg) are acceptable (growing evidence of potential harm).

Adapted with permission of Lippincott Williams & Wilkins, "Guidelines 2000 for Cardiopulmonary Resuscitation and Emergency Cardiovascular Care, Part 6: Advanced Cardiovascular Life Support, The American Heart Association in Collaboration With the International Liaison Committee on Resuscitation," *Circulation*, 2000, 102(8 Suppl):I151.

ADULT ACLS ALGORITHMS *(Continued)*

Asystole: The Silent Heart Algorithm

Primary ABCD Survey[1]
Focus: *Basic CPR and defibrillation*

- **Check** responsiveness
- **Activate** emergency response system
- **Call** for defibrillator

A Airway: Open the airway
B Breathing: Provide positive-pressure ventilations
C Circulation: Give chest compressions
C Confirm true asystole
D Defibrillation: Assess for VF / pulseless VT; shock if indicated

Rapid scene survey: Any evidence personnel should **not** attempt resuscitation?

↓

Secondary ABCD Survey[2,3]
Focus: *More advanced assessments and treatments*

A Airway: Place airway device as soon as possible
B Breathing: Confirm airway device placement by exam plus confirmation device
B Breathing: Secure airway device; purpose-made tube holders preferred[4]
B Breathing: Confirm effective oxygenation and ventilation[5]
C Circulation: Confirm true asystole
C Circulation: Establish I.V. access
C Circulation: Identify rhythm → monitor
C Circulation: Administer drugs appropriate for rhythm and condition
C Circulation: Give medications appropriate for rhythm and condition
D Differential Diagnosis: Search for and treat identified reversible causes

↓

Transcutaneous pacing
If considered, perform immediately

↓

- ***Epinephrine*** 1 mg I.V. push, repeat every 3-5 minutes[6]

↓

- ***Atropine*** 1 mg I.V., repeat every 3-5 minutes up to a total of 0.04 mg/kg

↓

Asystole persists
Withhold or cease resuscitation efforts?

- Consider quality of resuscitation?
- Atypical clinical features present?
- Support for cease-efforts protocols in place?

[1] Do not attempt resuscitation if any objective indicators of DNAR status or clinical indicators that resuscitation attempts are not indicated (eg, signs of death).
[2] Confirm true asystole.
[3] Sodium bicarbonate 1 mEq/kg indicated for patients with tracheal intubation plus long arrest intervals, on return of spontaneous circulation if long arrest interval, tricyclic antidepressant overdose, to alkalinize urine (eg, ASA overdose). **Note:** Ineffective or harmful in hypercarbic acidosis.
[4] Commercial purpose-made tracheal tube holders recommended (Class IIb - acceptable, possibly effective).
[5] End-tidal CO_2 monitor and oxygen saturation monitor
[6] If this fails, higher doses of epinephrine (up to 0.2 mg/kg) are acceptable (growing evidence of potential harm).

Adapted with permission of Lippincott Williams & Wilkins, "Guidelines 2000 for Cardiopulmonary Resuscitation and Emergency Cardiovascular Care, Part 6: Advanced Cardiovascular Life Support, The American Heart Association in Collaboration With the International Liaison Committee on Resuscitation," *Circulation*, 2000, 102(8 Suppl):I153.

Bradycardia Algorithm

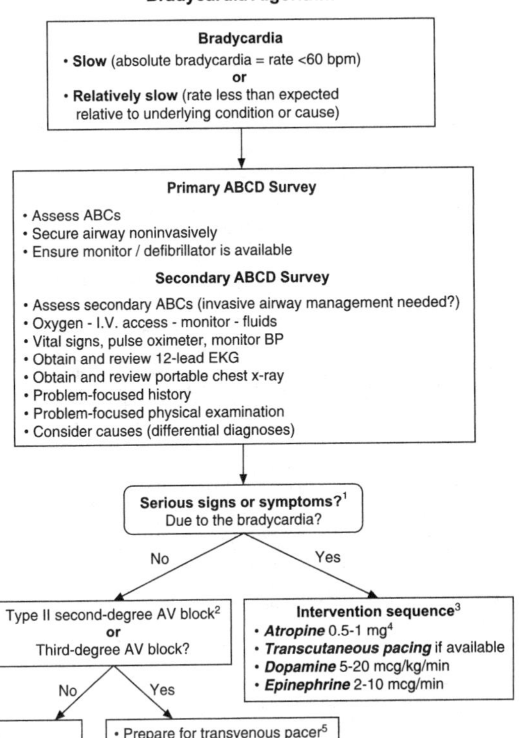

[1]Signs/symptoms must be attributable to slow rate. Manifestations include chest pain, shortness of breath, decreased LOC, hypotension, shock, CHF, pulmonary congestion.

[2]Never treat combination of third-degree heart block and ventricular escape beats with lidocaine (or any agent which suppresses ventricular escape rhythms).

[3]Do not delay transcutaneous pacing in symptomatic patients while waiting for I.V. access or for atropine to take effect; denervated transplanted hearts will not respond to atropine - go directly to catecholamine infusion or pacing.

[4]Atropine should be repeated every 3-5 minutes up to 0.03-0.04 mg/kg total dose; use every 3 minutes in severe clinical conditions.

[5]Verify patient tolerance and mechanical capture. Use analgesia and sedation as needed.

Adapted with permission of Lippincott Williams & Wilkins, "Guidelines 2000 for Cardiopulmonary Resuscitation and Emergency Cardiovascular Care, Part 6: Advanced Cardiovascular Life Support, The American Heart Association in Collaboration With the International Liaison Committee on Resuscitation," *Circulation*, 2000, 102(8 Suppl):I156.

ADULT ACLS ALGORITHMS *(Continued)*

Tachycardia Overview Algorithm

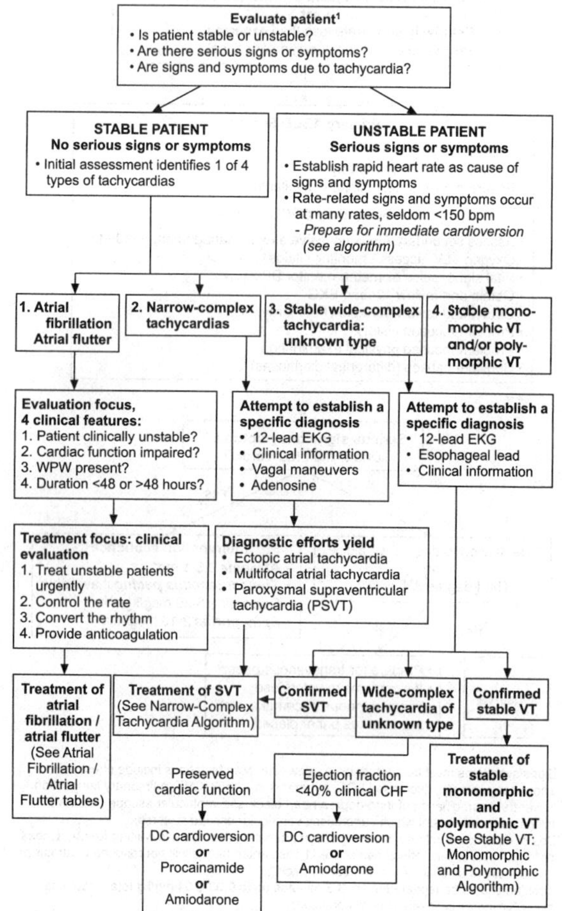

[1]Unstable condition must be related to the tachycardia. Signs and symptoms may include chest pain, shortness of breath, decreased LOC, hypotension, shock, pulmonary congestion, CHF, and AMI.

Adapted with permission of Lippincott Williams & Wilkins, "Guidelines 2000 for Cardiopulmonary Resuscitation and Emergency Cardiovascular Care, Part 6: Advanced Cardiovascular Life Support, The American Heart Association in Collaboration With the International Liaison Committee on Resuscitation," *Circulation*, 2000, 102(8 Suppl):I159.

Narrow-Complex Supraventricular Tachycardia Algorithm

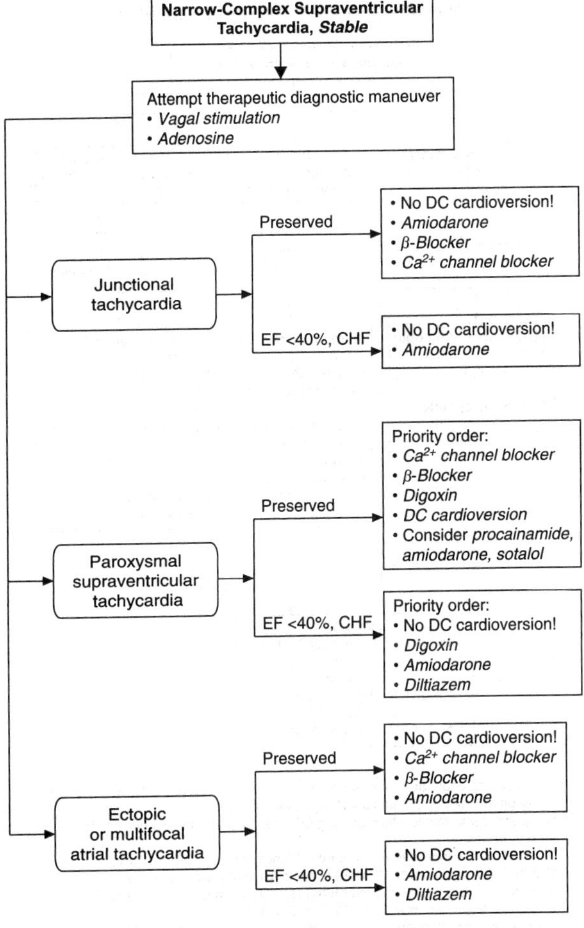

Adapted with permission of Lippincott Williams & Wilkins, "Guidelines 2000 for Cardiopulmonary Resuscitation and Emergency Cardiovascular Care, Part 6: Advanced Cardiovascular Life Support, The American Heart Association in Collaboration With the International Liaison Committee on Resuscitation," *Circulation*, 2000, 102(8 Suppl):I162.

ADULT ACLS ALGORITHMS *(Continued)*

Stable Ventricular Tachycardia (Monomorphic or Polymorphic) Algorithm

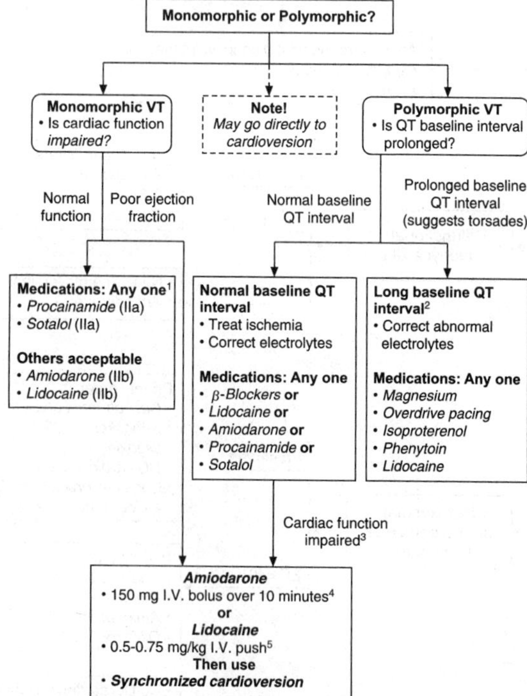

[1]Use just one agent at a time. **Note:** Numbers in parentheses represent strength of recommendation, not antiarrhythmic classification.

[2]Stop/avoid treatments which prolong QT. Identify and treat any electrolyte abnormalities.

[3]Clinical signs suggestive of impaired LV function (EF <40% or CHF).

[4]Repeat 150 mg I.V. over 10 minutes every 10-15 minutes as needed. Alternative infusion: 360 mg over 6 hours, then 540 mg over the remaining 18 hours. Maximum total dose: 2.2 g in 24 hours.

[5]Repeat every 5-10 minutes, then infuse 1-4 mg/min. Maximum total dose: 3 mg/kg (or 300 mg) over 1 hour.

Note: Class IIa recommendation: Acceptable, probably effective;
Class IIb: Acceptable, possibly effective.

Adapted with permission of Lippincott Williams & Wilkins, "Guidelines 2000 for Cardiopulmonary Resuscitation and Emergency Cardiovascular Care, Part 6: Advanced Cardiovascular Life Support, The American Heart Association in Collaboration With the International Liaison Committee on Resuscitation," *Circulation*, 2000, 102(8 Suppl):I163.

Synchronized Cardioversion Algorithm

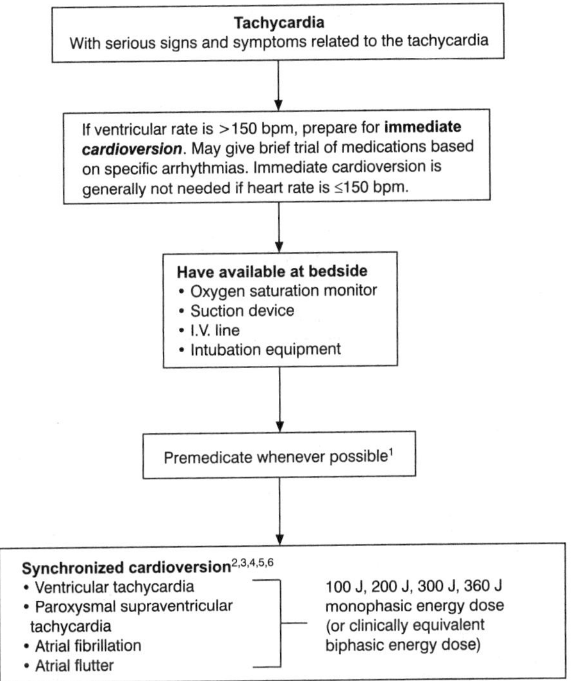

[1]Effective regimens have included a sedative (eg, ***diazepam***, ***midazolam***, ***barbiturates***, ***etomidate***, ***ketamine***, ***methohexital***) with or without an analgesic agent (eg, ***fentanyl***, ***morphine***, ***meperidine***). Many experts recommend anesthesia if service is readily available.

[2]Both monophasic and biphasic waveforms are acceptable if documented as clinically equivalent to reports of monophasic shock success.

[3]Note possible need to resynchronize after each cardioversion.

[4]If delays in synchronization occur and clinical condition is critical, go immediately to unsynchronized shocks.

[5]Treat polymorphic ventricular tachycardia (irregular form and rate) like ventricular fibrillation: see ventricular fibrillation/pulseless ventricular tachycardia algorithm.

[6]Paroxysmal supraventricular tachycardia and atrial flutter often respond to lower energy levels (start with 50 J).

Adapted with permission of Lippincott Williams & Wilkins, "Guidelines 2000 for Cardiopulmonary Resuscitation and Emergency Cardiovascular Care, Part 6: Advanced Cardiovascular Life Support, The American Heart Association in Collaboration With the International Liaison Committee on Resuscitation," *Circulation*, 2000, 102(8 Suppl):I164.

ATRIAL FIBRILLATION / ATRIAL FLUTTER

Atrial Fibrillation / Atrial Flutter in Normal Cardiac Function — Control of Rate and Rhythm

Control Rate		Convert Rhythm	
Heart Function Preserved	**Impaired Heart Function EF <40% or CHF**	**Duration <48 Hours**	**Duration >48 Hours or Unknown**
Note: AF >48-hours duration: Use agents to convert rhythm with extreme caution in patient not receiving adequate anticoagulation because of possible embolic complications Use only one of the following agents[1]: • Calcium channel blocker (Class I) • Beta blocker (Class I) • Other drugs (class IIb recommendations) eg, digoxin, amiodarone	Not applicable	**Consider:** • DC cardioversion Use only one of the following agents[1]: • Amiodarone (Class IIa) • Ibutilide (Class IIa) • Flecainide (Class IIa) • Propafenone (Class IIa) • Procainamide (Class IIa) • Other drugs (class IIb recommendations) eg, sotalol, disopyramide	**NO DC CARDIOVERSION!** **Note:** Conversion of AF to NSR with drugs or shock may cause embolization of atrial thrombi unless patient has adequate anticoagulation. Use antiarrhythmic agents with extreme caution (see Note above) if AF is >48-hours duration **OR** ***Delayed cardioversion*** Anticoagulation for 3 weeks at proper levels • Cardioversion, ***then*** • Anticoagulation for 4 more weeks **OR** ***Early cardioversion*** • Begin I.V. heparin at once • TEE to exclude atrial clot, ***then*** • Cardioversion within 24 hours, ***then*** • Anticoagulation for 4 more weeks

Legend: AF: Atrial fibrillation; Class I: Acceptable, definitely effective; Class IIa: Acceptable, probably effective; Class IIb: Acceptable, possibly effective; Class III: Not indicated, may be harmful; EF: Ejection fraction; NSR: Normal sinus rhythm; TEE: Transesophageal echocardiogram

[1]Occasionally, two of the named antiarrhythmic agents may be used, but use of these agents in combination may have proarrhythmic potential; classes listed represent the *Class of Recommendation* rather than the Vaughn-Williams classification of antiarrhythmics.

Adapted with permission from Lippincott Williams & Wilkins, "Guidelines 2000 for Cardiopulmonary Resuscitation and Emergency Cardiovascular Care. Part 6: Advanced Cardiovascular Life Support. The American Heart Association in Collaboration With the International Liaison Committee on Resuscitation," *Circulation,* 2000, 102(8 Suppl), I160-1.

Atrial Fibrillation / Atrial Flutter in Impaired Heart Function (EF <40% or CHF) — Control of Rate and Rhythm

Control Rate		Convert Rhythm	
Heart Function Preserved	**Impaired Heart Function EF <40% or CHF**	**Duration <48 Hours**	**Duration >48 Hours or Unknown**
Not applicable	**Note:** AF >48-hours duration: Use agents to convert rhythm with extreme caution in patient not receiving adequate anticoagulation because of possible embolic complications Use only one of the following agents[1]: • Digoxin (Class IIb) • Diltiazem (Class IIb) • Amiodarone (Class IIb)	**Consider:** • DC cardioversion **OR** • Amiodarone (Class IIb)	• **Anticoagulation** (as described in "Control of Rate and Rhythm - Normal Cardiac Function"), followed by • **DC Cardioversion**

Legend: AF: Atrial fibrillation; Class I: Acceptable, definitely effective; Class IIa: Acceptable, probably effective; Class IIb: Acceptable, possibly effective; Class III: Not indicated, may be harmful; EF: Ejection fraction; NSR: Normal sinus rhythm; TEE: Transesophageal echocardiogram

[1]Occasionally, two of the named antiarrhythmic agents may be used, but use of these agents in combination may have proarrhythmic potential; classes listed represent the *Class of Recommendation* rather than the Vaughn-Williams classification of antiarrhythmics.

Adapted with permission from Lippincott Williams & Wilkins, "Guidelines 2000 for Cardiopulmonary Resuscitation and Emergency Cardiovascular Care. Part 6: Advanced Cardiovascular Life Support. The American Heart Association in Collaboration With the International Liaison Committee on Resuscitation," *Circulation*, 2000, 102(8 Suppl), I160-1.

ATRIAL FIBRILLATION / ATRIAL FLUTTER *(Continued)*

Atrial Fibrillation / Atrial Flutter in Wolff-Parkinson-White Syndrome — Control of Rate and Rhythm

Control Rate		Convert Rhythm	
Heart Function Preserved	**Impaired Heart Function EF <40% or CHF**	**Duration <48 Hours**	**Duration >48 Hours or Unknown**
Note: AF >48-hours duration: Use agents to convert rhythm with extreme caution in patient not receiving adequate anticoagulation because of possible embolic complications • DC Cardioversion **OR** • **Primary antiarrhythmic agents** Use only one of the following agents[1]: • Amiodarone (Class IIb) • Flecainide (Class IIb) • Procainamide (Class IIb) • Propafenone (Class IIb) • Sotalol (Class IIb) • **Class III (can be harmful)** • Adenosine • Beta-blockers • Calcium channel blockers • Digoxin	**Note:** AF >48-hours duration: Use agents to convert rhythm with extreme caution in patient not receiving adequate anticoagulation because of possible embolic complications • DC Cardioversion **OR** • Amiodarone (Class IIb)	• DC Cardioversion **OR** • **Primary antiarrhythmic agents** Use only one of the following agents[1]: • Amiodarone (Class IIb) • Flecainide (Class IIb) • Procainamide (Class IIb) • Propafenone (Class IIb) • Sotalol (Class IIb) • **Class III (can be harmful)** • Adenosine • Beta-blockers • Calcium channel blockers • Digoxin	• **Anticoagulation** (as described in "Control of Rate and Rhythm - Normal Cardiac Function"), followed by • **DC Cardioversion**

Legend: AF: Atrial fibrillation; Class I: Acceptable, definitely effective; Class IIa: Acceptable, probably effective; Class IIb: Acceptable, possibly effective; Class III: Not indicated, may be harmful; EF: Ejection fraction; NSR: Normal sinus rhythm; TEE: Transesophageal echocardiogram

[1]Occasionally, two of the named antiarrhythmic agents may be used, but use of these agents in combination may have proarrhythmic potential; classes listed represent the *Class of Recommendation* rather than the Vaughn-Williams classification of antiarrhythmics.

Adapted with permission from Lippincott Williams & Wilkins, "Guidelines 2000 for Cardiopulmonary Resuscitation and Emergency Cardiovascular Care. Part 6: Advanced Cardiovascular Life Support. The American Heart Association in Collaboration With the International Liaison Committee on Resuscitation," *Circulation,* 2000, 102(8 Suppl), I160-1.

NORMAL HEART RATES

Age	Mean Heart Rate (beats/minute)	Heart Rate Range (2nd – 98th percentile)
<1 d	123	93-154
1-2 d	123	91-159
3-6 d	129	91-166
1-3 wk	148	107-182
1-2 mo	149	121-179
3-5 mo	141	106-186
6-11 mo	134	109-169
1-2 y	119	89-151
3-4 y	108	73-137
5-7 y	100	65-133
8-11 y	91	62-130
12-15 y	85	60-119

Adapted from *The Harriet Lane Handbook*, 12th ed, Greene MG, ed, St Louis, MO: Mosby Yearbook, 1991.

Normal QRS Axes (in degrees)

Age	Mean	Range
1 wk – 1 mo	+110	+30 to +180
1–3 mo	+70	+10 to +125
3 mo – 3 y	+60	+10 to +110
>3 y	+60	+20 to +120
Adults	+50	–30 to +105

NORMAL HEART RATES *(Continued)*

INTERVALS AND SEGMENTS OF AN ECG CYCLE

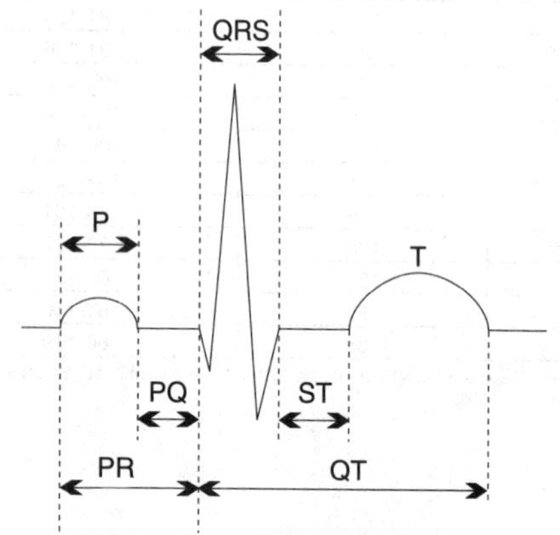

HEXAXIAL REFERENCE SYSTEM

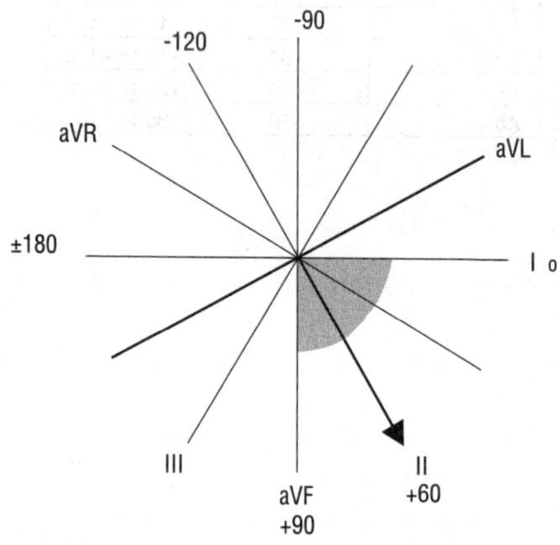

MEASURING PEDIATRIC BLOOD PRESSURE

Figure 1. Determination of Proper Cuff Size, Step 1

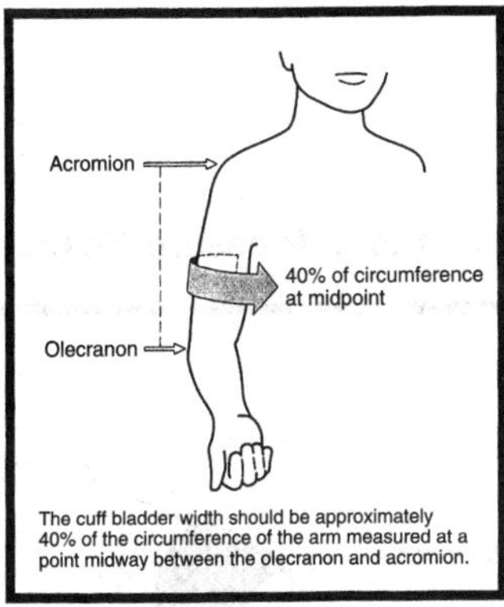

The cuff bladder width should be approximately 40% of the circumference of the arm measured at a point midway between the olecranon and acromion.

Figure 2. Determination of Proper Cuff Size, Step 2

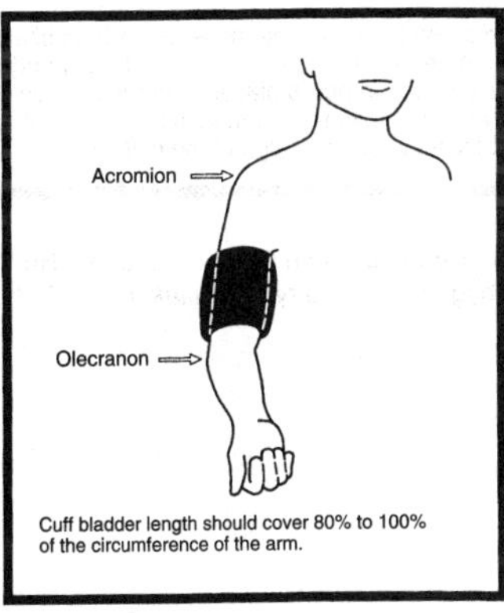

Cuff bladder length should cover 80% to 100% of the circumference of the arm.

MEASURING PEDIATRIC BLOOD PRESSURE *(Continued)*

Figure 3. Blood Pressure Measurement

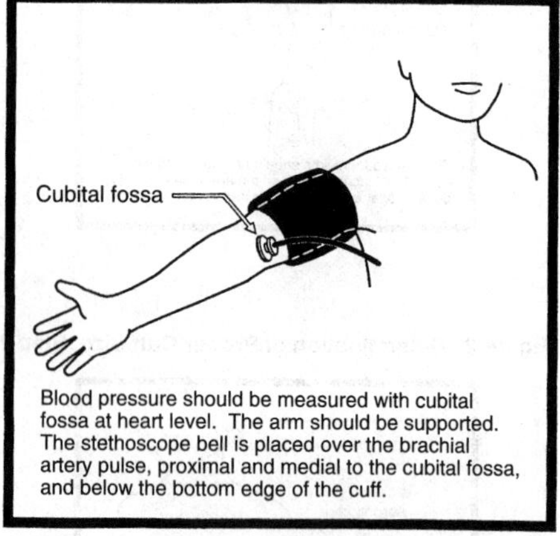

Blood pressure should be measured with cubital fossa at heart level. The arm should be supported. The stethoscope bell is placed over the brachial artery pulse, proximal and medial to the cubital fossa, and below the bottom edge of the cuff.

Used with permission: Perloff D, Grim C, Flack J, et al, "Human Blood Pressure Determination by Sphygmomanometry," *Circulation*, 1993, 88:2460-7.

HYPERTENSION, CLASSIFICATION BY AGE GROUP[1]

Age Group	Significant Hypertension (mm Hg)	Severe Hypertension (mm Hg)
Newborn (7 d)		
systolic BP	≥96	≥106
Newborn (8-30 d)		
systolic BP	≥104	≥110
Infant (<2 y)		
systolic BP	≥112	≥118
diastolic BP	≥74	≥82
Children (3-5 y)		
systolic BP	≥116	≥124
diastolic BP	≥76	≥84
Children (6-9 y)		
systolic BP	≥122	≥130
diastolic BP	≥78	≥86
Children (10-12 y)		
systolic BP	≥126	≥134
diastolic BP	≥82	≥90
Adolescents (13-15 y)		
systolic BP	≥136	≥144
diastolic BP	≥86	≥92
Adolescents (16-18 y)		
systolic BP	≥142	≥150
diastolic BP	≥92	≥98

Adapted from Horan MJ, *Pediatrics*, 1987, 79:1-25.

[1]See also Blood Pressure Measurement, Age Specific Percentiles, and 90th and 95th Percentiles of Blood Pressure by Percentiles of Height.

BLOOD PRESSURE IN PREMATURE INFANTS, NORMAL

(Birth weight 600-1750 g)[1]

Day	600-999 g		1000-1249 g	
	S (± 2SD)	D (± 2SD)	S (± 2SD)	D (± 2SD)
1	37.9 (17.4)	23.2 (10.3)	44 (22.8)	22.5 (13.5)
3	44.9 (15.7)	30.6 (12.3)	48 (15.4)	36.5 (9.6)
7	50 (14.8)	30.4 (12.4)	57 (14)	42.5 (16.5)
14	50.2 (14.8)	37.4 (12)	53 (30)	
28	61 (23.5)	45.8 (27.4)	57 (30)	
Day	**1250-1499 g**		**1500-1750 g**	
	S (± 2SD)	D (± 2SD)	S (± 2SD)	D (± 2SD)
1	48 (18)	27 (12.4)	47 (15.8)	26 (15.6)
3	59 (21.1)	40 (13.7)	51 (18.2)	35 (10)
7	68 (14.8)	40 (11.3)	66 (23)	41 (24)
14	64 (21.2)	36 (24.2)	76 (34.8)	42 (20.3)
28	69 (31.4)	44 (26.2)	73 (5.6)	50 (9.9)

[1]Blood pressure was obtained by the Dinamap method.

S = systolic; D = diastolic; SD = standard deviation.

Modified from Ingelfinger JR, Powers L, and Epstein MF, "Blood Pressure Norms in Low-Weight Infants: Birth Through Four Weeks", *Pediatr Res*, 1983, 17:319A.

BLOOD PRESSURE MEASUREMENTS, AGE-SPECIFIC PERCENTILES

Blood Pressure Measurements: Ages 0-12 Months, BOYS

Korotkoff phase IV (K4) used for diastolic BP. Reproduced with permission from Horan MJ, *Pediatrics*, 1987, 79:11-25.

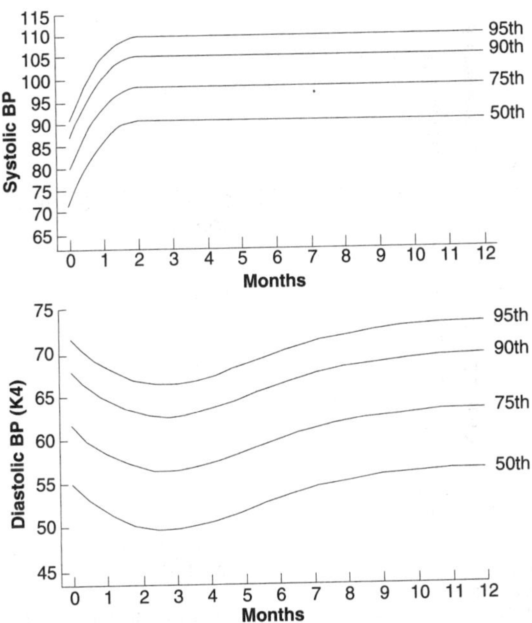

90th Percentile													
Systolic BP	87	101	106	106	106	105	105	105	105	105	105	105	105
Diastolic BP	68	65	63	63	63	65	66	67	68	68	69	69	69
Height cm	51	59	63	66	68	70	72	73	74	76	77	78	80
Weight kg	4	4	5	5	6	7	8	9	9	10	10	11	11

BLOOD PRESSURE MEASUREMENTS, AGE-SPECIFIC PERCENTILES *(Continued)*

Blood Pressure Measurements: Ages 0-12 Months, GIRLS

Korotkoff phase IV (K4) used for diastolic BP. Reproduced with permission from Horan MJ, *Pediatrics*, 1987, 79:11-25.

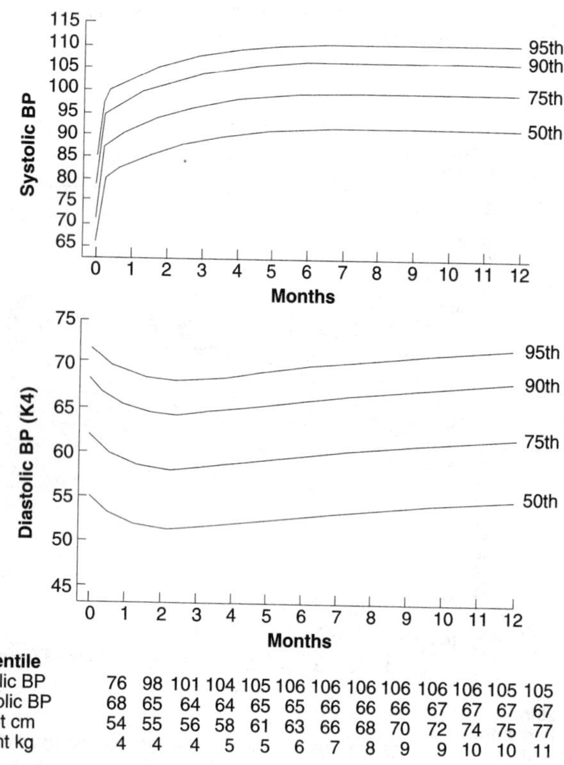

90th Percentile													
Systolic BP	76	98	101	104	105	106	106	106	106	106	106	105	105
Diastolic BP	68	65	64	64	65	65	66	66	66	67	67	67	67
Height cm	54	55	56	58	61	63	66	68	70	72	74	75	77
Weight kg	4	4	4	5	5	6	7	8	9	9	10	10	11

Blood Pressure Levels for BOYS by Age and Height Percentile

Age (y)	BP Percentile[1]	Systolic BP (mm Hg)							Diastolic BP (mm Hg)[2]						
		Height Percentile[3]													
		5%	10%	25%	50%	75%	90%	95%	5%	10%	25%	50%	75%	90%	95%
1	50th	80	81	83	85	87	88	89	34	35	36	37	38	39	39
	90th	94	95	97	99	100	102	103	49	50	51	52	53	53	54
	95th	98	99	101	103	104	106	106	54	54	55	56	57	58	58
	99th	105	106	108	110	112	113	114	61	62	63	64	65	66	66
2	50th	84	85	87	88	90	92	92	39	40	41	42	43	44	44
	90th	97	99	100	102	104	105	106	54	55	56	57	58	58	59
	95th	101	102	104	106	108	109	110	59	59	60	61	62	63	63
	99th	109	110	111	113	115	117	117	66	67	68	69	70	71	71
3	50th	86	87	89	91	93	94	95	44	44	45	46	47	48	48
	90th	100	101	103	105	107	108	109	59	59	60	61	62	63	63
	95th	104	105	107	109	110	112	113	63	63	64	65	66	67	67
	99th	111	112	114	116	118	119	120	71	71	72	73	74	75	75
4	50th	88	89	91	93	95	96	97	47	48	49	50	51	51	52
	90th	102	103	105	107	109	110	111	62	63	64	65	66	66	67
	95th	106	107	109	111	112	114	115	66	67	68	69	70	71	71
	99th	113	114	116	118	120	121	122	74	75	76	77	78	78	79
5	50th	90	91	93	95	96	98	98	50	51	52	53	54	55	55
	90th	104	105	106	108	110	111	112	65	66	67	68	69	69	70
	95th	108	109	110	112	114	115	116	69	70	71	72	73	74	74
	99th	115	116	118	120	121	123	123	77	78	79	80	81	81	82
6	50th	91	92	94	96	98	99	100	53	53	54	55	56	57	57
	90th	105	106	108	110	111	113	113	68	68	69	70	71	72	72
	95th	109	110	112	114	115	117	117	72	72	73	74	75	76	76
	99th	116	117	119	121	123	124	125	80	80	81	82	83	84	84

BLOOD PRESSURE MEASUREMENTS, AGE-SPECIFIC PERCENTILES *(Continued)*

Blood Pressure Levels for BOYS by Age and Height Percentile *(continued)*

Age (y)	BP Percentile[1]	Systolic BP (mm Hg)							Diastolic BP (mm Hg)[2]						
		Height Percentile[3]													
		5%	10%	25%	50%	75%	90%	95%	5%	10%	25%	50%	75%	90%	95%
7	50th	92	94	95	97	99	100	101	55	55	56	57	58	59	59
	90th	106	107	109	111	113	114	115	70	70	71	72	73	74	74
	95th	110	111	113	115	117	118	119	74	74	75	76	77	78	78
	99th	117	118	120	122	124	125	126	82	82	83	84	85	86	86
8	50th	94	95	97	99	100	102	102	56	57	58	59	60	60	61
	90th	107	109	110	112	114	115	116	71	72	72	73	74	75	76
	95th	111	112	114	116	118	119	120	75	76	77	78	79	79	80
	99th	119	120	122	123	125	127	127	83	84	85	86	87	87	88
9	50th	95	96	98	100	102	103	104	57	58	59	60	61	61	62
	90th	109	110	112	114	115	117	118	72	73	74	75	76	76	77
	95th	113	114	116	118	119	121	121	76	77	78	79	80	81	81
	99th	120	121	123	125	127	128	129	84	85	86	87	88	88	89
10	50th	97	98	100	102	103	105	106	58	59	60	61	61	62	63
	90th	111	112	114	115	117	119	119	73	73	74	75	76	77	78
	95th	115	116	117	119	121	122	123	77	78	79	80	81	81	82
	99th	122	123	125	127	128	130	130	85	86	86	88	88	89	90
11	50th	99	100	102	104	105	107	107	59	59	60	61	62	63	63
	90th	113	114	115	117	119	120	121	74	74	75	76	77	78	78
	95th	117	118	119	121	123	124	125	78	78	79	80	81	82	82
	99th	124	125	127	129	130	132	132	86	86	87	88	89	90	90
12	50th	101	102	104	106	108	109	110	59	60	61	62	63	63	64
	90th	115	116	118	120	121	123	123	74	75	75	76	77	78	79
	95th	119	120	122	123	125	127	127	78	79	80	81	82	82	83
	99th	126	127	129	131	133	134	135	86	87	88	89	90	90	91

Blood Pressure Levels for BOYS by Age and Height Percentile *(continued)*

Age (y)	BP Percentile[1]	Systolic BP (mm Hg)							Diastolic BP (mm Hg)[2]						
		Height Percentile[3]													
		5%	10%	25%	50%	75%	90%	95%	5%	10%	25%	50%	75%	90%	95%
13	50th	104	105	106	108	110	111	112	60	60	61	62	63	64	64
	90th	117	118	120	122	124	125	126	75	75	76	77	78	79	79
	95th	121	122	124	126	128	129	130	79	79	80	81	82	83	83
	99th	128	130	131	133	135	136	137	87	87	88	89	90	91	91
14	50th	106	107	109	111	113	114	115	60	61	62	63	64	65	65
	90th	120	121	123	125	126	128	128	75	76	77	78	79	79	80
	95th	124	125	127	128	130	132	132	80	80	81	82	83	84	84
	99th	131	132	134	136	138	139	140	87	88	89	90	91	92	92
15	50th	109	110	112	113	115	117	117	61	62	63	64	65	66	66
	90th	122	124	125	127	129	130	131	76	77	78	79	80	80	81
	95th	126	127	129	131	133	134	135	81	81	82	83	84	85	85
	99th	134	135	136	138	140	142	142	88	89	90	91	92	93	93
16	50th	111	112	114	116	118	119	120	63	63	64	65	66	67	67
	90th	125	126	128	130	131	133	134	78	78	79	80	81	82	82
	95th	129	130	132	134	135	137	137	82	83	83	84	85	86	87
	99th	136	137	139	141	143	144	145	90	90	91	92	93	94	94
17	50th	114	115	116	118	120	121	122	65	66	66	67	68	69	70
	90th	127	128	130	132	134	135	136	80	80	81	82	83	84	84
	95th	131	132	134	136	138	139	140	84	85	86	87	87	88	89
	99th	139	140	141	143	145	146	147	92	93	93	94	95	96	97

[1]Blood pressure percentile determined by a single measurement.

[2]Korotkoff phase V (K5) used for diastolic BP.

[3]Height percentile determined by standard growth curves.

Source: National High Blood Pressure Education Program Working Group on High Blood Pressure in Children and Adolescents, "The Fourth Report on the Diagnosis, Evaluation, and Treatment of High Blood Pressure in Children and Adolescents," *Pediatrics*, 2004, 114(2 Suppl 4th Report):555-76.

BLOOD PRESSURE MEASUREMENTS, AGE-SPECIFIC PERCENTILES *(Continued)*

Blood Pressure Levels for GIRLS by Age and Height Percentile

Age (y)	BP Percentile[1]	Systolic BP (mm Hg)							Diastolic BP (mm Hg)[2]						
		Height Percentile[3]													
		5%	10%	25%	50%	75%	90%	95%	5%	10%	25%	50%	75%	90%	95%
1	50th	83	84	85	86	88	89	90	38	39	39	40	41	41	42
	90th	97	97	98	100	101	102	103	52	53	53	54	55	55	56
	95th	100	101	102	104	105	106	107	56	57	57	58	59	59	60
	99th	108	108	109	111	112	113	114	64	64	65	65	66	67	67
2	50th	85	85	87	88	89	91	91	43	44	44	45	46	46	47
	90th	98	99	100	101	103	104	105	57	58	58	59	60	61	61
	95th	102	103	104	105	107	108	109	61	62	62	63	64	65	65
	99th	109	110	111	112	114	115	116	69	69	70	70	71	72	72
3	50th	86	87	88	89	91	92	93	47	48	48	49	50	50	51
	90th	100	100	102	103	104	106	106	61	62	62	63	64	64	65
	95th	104	104	105	107	108	109	110	65	66	66	67	68	68	69
	99th	111	111	113	114	115	116	117	73	73	74	74	75	76	76
4	50th	88	88	90	91	92	94	94	50	50	51	52	52	53	54
	90th	101	102	103	104	106	107	108	64	64	65	66	67	67	68
	95th	105	106	107	108	110	111	112	68	68	69	70	71	71	72
	99th	112	113	114	115	117	118	119	76	76	76	77	78	79	79
5	50th	89	90	91	93	94	95	96	52	53	53	54	55	55	56
	90th	103	103	105	106	107	109	109	66	67	67	68	69	69	70
	95th	107	107	108	110	111	112	113	70	71	71	72	73	73	74
	99th	114	114	116	117	118	120	120	78	78	79	79	80	81	81
6	50th	91	92	93	94	96	97	98	54	54	55	56	56	57	58
	90th	104	105	106	108	109	110	111	68	68	69	70	70	71	72
	95th	108	109	110	111	113	114	115	72	72	73	74	74	75	76
	99th	115	116	117	119	120	121	122	80	80	80	81	82	83	83

Blood Pressure Levels for GIRLS by Age and Height Percentile *(continued)*

Age (y)	BP Percentile[1]	Systolic BP (mm Hg)							Diastolic BP (mm Hg)[2]						
		Height Percentile[3]													
		5%	10%	25%	50%	75%	90%	95%	5%	10%	25%	50%	75%	90%	95%
7	50th	93	93	95	96	97	99	99	55	56	56	57	58	58	59
	90th	106	107	108	109	111	112	113	69	70	70	71	72	72	73
	95th	110	111	112	113	115	116	116	73	74	74	75	76	76	77
	99th	117	118	119	120	122	123	124	81	81	82	82	83	84	84
8	50th	95	95	96	98	99	100	101	57	57	57	58	59	60	60
	90th	108	109	110	111	113	114	114	71	71	71	72	73	74	74
	95th	112	112	114	115	116	118	118	75	75	75	76	77	78	78
	99th	119	120	121	122	123	125	125	82	82	83	83	84	85	86
9	50th	96	97	98	100	101	102	103	58	58	58	59	60	61	61
	90th	110	110	112	113	114	116	116	72	72	72	73	74	75	75
	95th	114	114	115	117	118	119	120	76	76	76	77	78	79	79
	99th	121	121	123	124	125	127	127	83	83	84	84	85	86	87
10	50th	98	99	100	102	103	104	105	59	59	59	60	61	62	62
	90th	112	112	114	115	116	118	118	73	73	73	74	75	76	76
	95th	116	116	117	119	120	121	122	77	77	77	78	79	80	80
	99th	123	123	125	126	127	129	129	84	84	85	86	86	87	88
11	50th	100	101	102	103	105	106	107	60	60	60	61	62	63	63
	90th	114	114	116	117	118	119	120	74	74	74	75	76	77	77
	95th	118	118	119	121	122	123	124	78	78	78	79	80	81	81
	99th	125	125	126	128	129	130	131	85	85	86	87	87	88	89
12	50th	102	103	104	105	107	108	109	61	61	61	62	63	64	64
	90th	116	116	117	119	120	121	122	75	75	75	76	77	78	78
	95th	119	120	121	123	124	125	126	79	79	79	80	81	82	82
	99th	127	127	128	130	131	132	133	86	86	87	88	88	89	90

BLOOD PRESSURE MEASUREMENTS, AGE-SPECIFIC PERCENTILES *(Continued)*

Blood Pressure Levels for GIRLS by Age and Height Percentile *(continued)*

Age (y)	BP Percentile[1]	Systolic BP (mm Hg)							Diastolic BP (mm Hg)[2]						
		Height Percentile[3]													
		5%	10%	25%	50%	75%	90%	95%	5%	10%	25%	50%	75%	90%	95%
13	50th	104	105	106	107	109	110	110	62	62	62	63	64	65	65
	90th	117	118	119	121	122	123	124	76	76	76	77	78	79	79
	95th	121	122	123	124	126	127	128	80	80	80	81	82	83	83
	99th	128	129	130	132	133	134	135	87	87	88	89	89	90	91
14	50th	106	106	107	109	110	111	112	63	63	63	64	65	66	66
	90th	119	120	121	122	124	125	125	77	77	77	78	79	80	80
	95th	123	123	125	126	127	129	129	81	81	81	82	83	84	84
	99th	130	131	132	133	135	136	136	88	88	89	90	90	91	92
15	50th	107	108	109	110	111	113	113	64	64	64	65	66	67	67
	90th	120	121	122	123	125	126	127	78	78	78	79	80	81	81
	95th	124	125	126	127	129	130	131	82	82	82	83	84	85	85
	99th	131	132	133	134	136	137	138	89	89	90	91	91	92	93
16	50th	108	108	110	111	112	114	114	64	64	65	66	66	67	68
	90th	121	122	123	124	126	127	128	78	78	79	80	81	81	82
	95th	125	126	127	128	130	131	132	82	82	83	84	85	85	86
	99th	132	133	134	135	137	138	139	90	90	90	91	92	93	93
17	50th	108	109	110	111	113	114	115	64	65	65	66	67	67	68
	90th	122	122	123	125	126	127	128	78	79	79	80	81	81	82
	95th	125	126	127	129	130	131	132	82	83	83	84	85	85	86
	99th	133	133	134	136	137	138	139	90	90	91	91	92	93	93

[1]Blood pressure percentile determined by a single measurement.

[2]Korotkoff phase V (K5) used for diastolic BP.

[3]Height percentile determined by standard growth curves.

Source: National High Blood Pressure Education Program Working Group on High Blood Pressure in Children and Adolescents, "The Fourth Report on the Diagnosis, Evaluation, and Treatment of High Blood Pressure in Children and Adolescents," *Pediatrics*, 2004, 114(2 Suppl 4th Report):555-76.

ANTIHYPERTENSIVE AGENTS BY CLASS

Alpha Adrenergic (Alpha 1 and Alpha 2) Antagonists
- Phenoxybenzamine
- Phentolamine

Alpha 1 Antagonists
- Prazosin

Alpha 2 Agonists
- Clonidine
- Methyldopa

Beta Antagonists
- Atenolol
- Esmolol
- Metoprolol
- Nadolol
- Propranolol
- Timolol

Mixed Alpha / Beta Antagonists
- Labetalol

Angiotensin Converting Enzyme Inhibitors
- Captopril
- Enalapril/Enalaprilat
- Lisinopril

Calcium Channel Blockers
- Amlodipine
- Diltiazem
- Nifedipine
- Verapamil

Diuretics
- Amiloride
- Bumetanide
- Chlorothiazide
- Furosemide
- Hydrochlorothiazide
- Mannitol
- Metolazone
- Spironolactone
- Torsemide
- Triamterene

Ganglionic Blockers
- Trimethaphan

Nitrates
- Isosorbide dinitrate
- Nitroglycerin

Vasodilators (Direct-acting)
- Diazoxide
- Hydralazine
- Minoxidil
- Nitroprusside

ANTIDEPRESSANT AGENTS

Comparison of Usual Adult Dosage and Mechanism of Action

Drug	Usual Adult Dosage (mg/d)[1]	Reuptake Inhibition	
		Norepinephrine	Serotonin
First-Generation Antidepressants *Tricyclic Antidepressants*			
Amitriptyline (Elavil® [DSC])	100-300	Moderate	High
Clomipramine (Anafranil®)[2]	100-250	Moderate	High
Desipramine (Norpramin®)	100-300	High	Low
Doxepin (Sinequan®)	100-300	Low	Moderate
Imipramine (Tofranil®, Tofranil-PM®)	100-300	Moderate	Moderate
Nortriptyline (Aventyl® [DSC], Pamelor®)	50-150	Moderate	Low
Protriptyline (Vivactil®)	15-60	Moderate	Low
Trimipramine (Surmontil®)	100-300	Low	Low
Monoamine Oxidase Inhibitors			
Isocarboxazid (Marplan®)	10-30	—	—
Phenelzine (Nardil®)	15-90	—	—
Tranylcypromine (Parnate®)	10-60	—	—
Second-Generation Antidepressants *Older Second-Generation Antidepressants*			
Amoxapine	100-400	Moderate	Low
Maprotiline (Ludiomil® [DSC])	100-225	Moderate	Low
Trazodone (Desyrel®)	150-600	Very low	Moderate
Newer Second-Generation Antidepressants			
Bupropion (Wellbutrin®, Wellbutrin SR®, Wellbutrin XL™, Zyban®)	300-450[3]	Very low[4]	Very low[4]
Third-Generation Antidepressants *Selective Serotonin Reuptake Inhibitors*			
Citalopram (Celexa™)	20-60	Very low	Very high
Escitalopram (Lexapro™)	10-20	Very low	Very high
Fluoxetine (Prozac®, Prozac® Weekly™, Sarafem™)	20-80	Very low	High
Fluvoxamine (Luvox® [DSC])[2]	100-300	Very low	Very high
Paroxetine (Paxil®, Paxil CR™)	20-50	Very low	Very high
Sertraline (Zoloft®)	50-200	Very low	Very high
Serotonin / Norepinephrine Reuptake Inhibitors			
Duloxetine (Cymbalta®)	40-60	Very high	Very high
Venlafaxine (Effexor®, Effexor® XR)	75-375	Very high	Very high
Atypical Antidepressants with 5HT2 Receptor Antagonist Properties			
Mirtazapine (Remeron®, Remeron SolTab®)[5]	15-45	Very low	Very low
Nefazodone (Serzone® [DSC])[5]	300-600	Very low	High

[1]Initial adult doses are lower. See individual monograph or product information for details.

[2]Not approved by FDA for depression. Approved for OCD.

[3]To minimize seizure risk for adults, do not to exceed immediate release 150 mg/dose or sustained release 200 mg/dose.

[4]Norepinephrine and serotonin reuptake inhibition is minimal, but inhibits dopamine reuptake.

[5]These agents work primarily through antagonizing the postsynaptic 5-HT_2 receptor.

Comparison of Adverse Effects

Drug	Adverse Effects					
	ACH	Drowsiness	Orthostatic Hypotension	Conduction Abnormalities	GI Distress	Weight Gain
First-Generation Antidepressants *Tricyclic Antidepressants*						
Amitriptyline (Elavil® [DSC])	4+	4+	3+	3+	1+	4+
Clomipramine (Anafranil®)[1]	4+	4+	2+	3+	1+	4+
Desipramine (Norpramin®)	1+	2+	2+	2+	0	1+
Doxepin (Sinequan®)	3+	4+	2+	2+	0	4+
Imipramine (Tofranil®, Tofranil-PM®)	3+	3+	4+	3+	1+	4+
Nortriptyline (Aventyl® [DSC], Pamelor®)	2+	2+	1+	2+	0	1+
Protriptyline (Vivactil®)	2+	1+	2+	3+	1+	1+
Trimipramine (Surmontil®)	4+	4+	3+	3+	0	4+
Monoamine Oxidase Inhibitors						
Isocarboxazid (Marplan®)	2+	2+	2+	1+	1+	2+
Phenelzine (Nardil®)	2+	2+	2+	0	1+	3+
Tranylcypromine (Parnate®)	2+	1+	2+	1+	1+	2+
Second-Generation Antidepressants *Older Second-Generation Antidepressants*						
Amoxapine	2+	2+	2+	2+	0	2+
Maprotiline (Ludiomil® [DSC])	2+	3+	2+	2+	0	2+
Trazodone (Desyrel®)	0	4+	3+	1+	1+	2+
Newer Second-Generation Antidepressants						
Bupropion (Wellbutrin®, Wellbutrin SR®, Wellbutrin XL™, Zyban®)	0	0	0	1+/0	1+	0

ANTIDEPRESSANT AGENTS *(Continued)*

Comparison of Adverse Effects *(continued)*

Drug	Adverse Effects					
	ACH	Drowsiness	Orthostatic Hypotension	Conduction Abnormalities	GI Distress	Weight Gain
Third-Generation Antidepressants *Selective Serotonin Reuptake Inhibitors*						
Citalopram (Celexa™)	0	0	0	0	3+[2]	1+
Escitalopram (Lexapro™)	0	0	0	0	3+	1+
Fluoxetine (Prozac®, Prozac® Weekly™, Sarafem™)	0	0	0	0	3+[2]	1+
Fluvoxamine (Luvox® [DSC])[1]	0	0	0	0	3+[2]	1+
Paroxetine (Paxil®, Paxil CR™)	1+	1+	0	0	3+[2]	2+
Sertraline (Zoloft®)	0	0	0	0	3+[2]	1+
Serotonin / Norepinephrine Reuptake Inhibitors						
Duloxetine (Cymbalta®)	1+	1+	0	1+	3+[2]	0
Venlafaxine (Effexor®, Effexor® XR)[3]	1+	1+	0	1+	3+[2]	0
Atypical Antidepressants with 5HT2 Receptor Antagonist Properties						
Mirtazapine (Remeron®, Remeron SolTab®)	1+	3+	1+	1+	0	3+
Nefazodone (Serzone® [DSC])	1+	1+	2+	1+	1+	0

Key: ACH = anticholinergic effects (dry mouth, blurred vision, urinary retention, constipation); 0-4+ = absent or rare – relatively common.

[1]Not approved by FDA for depression. Approved for OCD.

[2]Nausea is usually mild and transient.

[3]Comparative studies evaluating the adverse effects of venlafaxine in relation to other antidepressants have not been performed.

CORTICOSTEROIDS, SYSTEMIC

Relative Potencies and Equivalent Doses of Corticosteroids

(Glucocorticoid potency compared to hydrocortisone "mg" for "mg" basis)

Compound	Gluco-corticoid Potency	Mineralo-corticoid Potency	Equivalent Dose (mg)	Duration[1] of Action
Cortisone	0.8	++	25	S
Tablet: 5 mg				
Dexamethasone (Decadron®, Dexasone® [DSC], DexPak®, TaperPak®, Solurex® [DSC], Solurex L.A.® [DSC])	25-30	0	0.75	L
Elixir: 0.5 mg/5 mL				
Injection, solution: 4 mg/mL				
Injection, suspension: 8 mg/mL [DSC]				
Intensol: 1 mg/mL				
Solution: 0.5 mg/5 mL				
Tablet: 0.25 mg, 0.5 mg, 0.75 mg, 1 mg, 1.5 mg, 2 mg, 4 mg, 6 mg				
Fludrocortisone (Florinef®)	10	+++++		I
Tablet: 0.1 mg				
Hydrocortisone (A-hydroCort®, Cortef®, Hydrocortone® [DSC], Solu-Cortef®)	1	++	20	S
Injection: 100 mg, 250 mg, 500 mg, 1 g				
Injection: 50 mg/mL				
Tablet: 5 mg, 10 mg, 20 mg				
MethylPREDNISolone (A-Methapred®, Depo-Medrol®, Medrol®, Solu-Medrol®)	5	0	4	I
Injection: 40 mg, 125 mg, 500 mg, 1 g, 2 g				
Injection, suspension: 20 mg/mL, 40 mg/mL, 80 mg/mL				
Tablet: 2 mg, 4 mg, 8 mg, 16 mg, 32 mg				
PrednisoLONE (Orapred®, Pediapred®, Prelone®)	4	+	5	I
Solution: 5 mg/5 mL, 15 mg/5 mL				
Syrup: 5 mg/5 mL, 15 mg/5 mL				
Tablet: 5 mg				
PredniSONE (Deltasone®, Prednisone Intensol™, Sterapred®, Sterapred® DS)	4	+	5	I
Intensol: 5 mg/mL				
Solution: 5 mg/5 mL				
Tablet: 1 mg, 2.5 mg, 5 mg, 10 mg, 20 mg, 50 mg				

[1]S = Short, 8-12 hours biologic activity.

I = Intermediate, 12-36 hours biologic activity.

L = Long, 36-54 hours biologic activity.

Reference

Adapted and updated from Knoben JE, and Anderson PO, *Handbook of Clinical Drug Data*, 6th ed, Drug Intelligence Pub, Inc, 1988.

CORTICOSTEROIDS, TOPICAL: GUIDELINES FOR SELECTION AND USE

The quantity prescribed and the frequency of refills should be monitored to reduce the risk of adrenal suppression. In general, short courses of high-potency agents are preferable to prolonged use of low potency. After control is achieved, control should be maintained with a low potency preparation.

1. Low-to-medium potency agents are usually effective for treating thin, acute, inflammatory skin lesions; whereas, high or super-potent agents are often required for treating chronic, hyperkeratotic, or lichenified lesions.

2. Since the stratum corneum is thin on the face and intertriginous areas, low-potency agents are preferred but a higher potency agent may be used for 2 weeks.

3. Because the palms and soles shave a thick stratum corneum, high or super-potent agents are frequently required.

4. **Low potency agents are preferred for infants** and the elderly. Infants have a high body surface area to weight ratio; elderly patients have thin, fragile skin.

5. The vehicle in which the topical corticosteroid is formulated influences the absorption and potency of the drug. Ointment bases are preferred for thick, lichenified lesions; they enhance penetration of the drug. Creams are preferred for acute and subacute dermatoses; they may be used on moist skin areas or intertriginous areas. Solutions, gels, and sprays are preferred for the scalp or for areas where a nonoil-based vehicle is needed.

6. In general, super-potent agents should not be used for longer than 3 weeks unless the lesion is limited to a small body area. Medium-to-high potency agents usually cause only rare adverse effects when treatment is limited to 3 months or less, and use on the face and intertriginous areas are avoided. If long-term treatment is needed, intermittent vs continued treatment is recommended.

7. Most preparations are applied once or twice daily. More frequent application may be necessary for the palms or soles because the preparation is easily removed by normal activity and penetration is poor due to a thick stratum corneum. Every-other-day or weekend-only application may be effective for treating some chronic conditions.

Corticosteroids, Topical

The following topical corticosteroid preparations are grouped according to relative anti-inflammatory activity. Preparations in each group are approximately equivalent.

	Steroid	Vehicle
Very High Potency		
0.05%	Augmented betamethasone dipropionate	Ointment
0.05%	Clobetasol propionate	Cream, ointment
0.05%	Diflorasone diacetate	Ointment
0.05%	Halobetasol propionate	Cream, ointment
High Potency		
0.1%	Amcinonide	Cream, ointment, lotion
0.05%	Betamethasone dipropionate, augmented	Cream
0.05%	Betamethasone dipropionate	Cream, ointment
0.1%	Betamethasone valerate	Ointment
0.05%	Desoximetasone	Gel
0.25%	Desoximetasone	Cream, ointment
0.05%	Diflorasone diacetate	Cream, ointment
0.05%	Fluocinonide	Cream, ointment, gel
0.1%	Halcinonide	Cream, ointment
0.5%	Triamcinolone acetonide	Cream, ointment
Intermediate Potency		
0.05%	Betamethasone dipropionate	Lotion
0.1%	Betamethasone valerate	Cream
0.1%	Clocortolone pivalate	Cream
0.05%	Desoximetasone	Cream
0.025%	Fluocinolone acetonide	Cream, ointment
0.05%	Flurandrenolide	Cream, ointment, lotion, tape
0.005%	Fluticasone propionate	Ointment
0.05%	Fluticasone propionate	Cream
0.1%	Hydrocortisone butyrate[1]	Ointment, solution
0.2%	Hydrocortisone valerate[1]	Cream, ointment
0.1%	Mometasone furoate[1]	Cream, ointment, lotion
0.1%	Prednicarbate	Cream, ointment
0.025%	Triamcinolone acetonide	Cream, ointment, lotion
0.1%	Triamcinolone acetonide	Cream, ointment, lotion
Low Potency		
0.05%	Alclometasone dipropionate[1]	Cream, ointment
0.05%	Desonide	Cream
0.01%	Fluocinolone acetonide	Cream, solution
0.5%	Hydrocortisone[1]	Cream, ointment, lotion
0.5%	Hydrocortisone acetate[1]	Cream, ointment
1%	Hydrocortisone acetate[1]	Cream, ointment
1%	Hydrocortisone	Cream, ointment, lotion, solution
2.5%	Hydrocortisone	Cream, ointment, lotion

[1]Not fluorinated.

MULTIVITAMIN PRODUCTS

MULTIVITAMIN PRODUCTS (PARENTERAL)

Product	A (int. units)	B_1 (mg)	B_2 (mg)	B_6 (mg)	B_{12} (mcg)	C (mg)	D (int. units)	E (int. units)	K (mcg)	Additional Information
Formulations for Neonates, Infants, and Children <11 Years of Age										
Infuvite® Pediatric (per 5 mL)	2300	1.2	1.4	1	1	80	400	7	200	Supplied as one 4 mL vial and one 1 mL vial Biotin 20 mcg, folic acid 140 mcg, niacinamide 17 mg, dexpanthenol 5 mg
M.V.I.® Pediatric	2300	1.2	1.4	1	1	80	400	7	200	Biotin 20 mcg, folic acid 140 mcg, niacinamide 17 mg, dexpanthenol 5 mg
Formulations for Children ≥11 Years to Adults										
Infuvite® Adult (per 10 mL)	3300	6	3.6	6	5	200	200	10	150	Supplied as two 5 mL vials Biotin 60 mcg, folic acid 600 mcg, niacinamide 40 mg, dexpanthenol 15 mg
M.V.I.®-12 (per 10 mL)	3300	3	3.6	4	12.5	100	200	10	–	Supplied as two 5 mL vials or a single 2-chambered 10 mL vial Biotin 60 mcg, folic acid 400 mcg, niacinamide 40 mg, dexpanthenol 15 mg

Legend: int. = international.

MULTIVITAMIN PRODUCTS (ORAL / ENTERAL)
Neonatal and Infant Formulations

Product	A (int. units)	B_1 (mg)	B_2 (mg)	B_6 (mg)	B_{12} (mcg)	C (mg)	D (int. units)	E (int. units)	Additional Information
Drops									
ADEKs (per mL) [OTC]	1500	0.5	0.6	0.6	4	45	400	40	Beta carotene 1 mg, biotin 15 mcg, niacin 6 mg, vitamin K 0.1 mg, Zn 5 mg; alcohol free, dye free (60 mL)
Poly-Vi-Sol® (per mL) [OTC]	1500	0.5	0.6	0.4	2	35	400	5	Niacin 8 mg (50 mL)
Poly-Vi-Sol® With Iron (per mL) [OTC]	1500	0.5	0.6	0.4		35	400	5	Fe 10 mg, niacin 8 mg (50 mL)
Tri-Vi-Sol® (per mL) [OTC]	1500					35	400		Fruit flavor (50 mL)
Tri-Vi-Sol® With Iron (per mL) [OTC]	1500					35	400		Fe 10 mg; fruit flavor (50 mL)
Vi-Daylin® (per mL) [OTC]	1500	0.5	0.6	0.4	1.5	35	400	5	Niacin 8 mg; alcohol <0.5%, sugar free, fruit flavor (50 mL)
Vi-Daylin® + Iron (per mL) [OTC]	1500	0.5	0.6	0.4		35	400	5	Fe 10 mg, niacin 8 mg; alcohol <0.5%, sugar free, fruit flavor (50 mL)
Vi-Daylin® ADC (per mL) [OTC]	1500					35	400		Alcohol <0.5%, sugar free, fruit flavor (50 mL)
Vi-Daylin® ADC + Iron (per mL) [OTC]	1500					35	400		Fe 10 mg; benzoic acid, sugar free, fruit flavor (50 mL)

Legend: Ca = elemental calcium, Cr = chromium, Cu = copper, Fe = elemental iron, int. = international, Mg = magnesium, Mn = manganese, Mo = molybdenum, Zn = zinc.

MULTIVITAMIN PRODUCTS *(Continued)*

MULTIVITAMIN PRODUCTS (ORAL / ENTERAL)
Fluoride-Containing Neonatal and Infant Multivitamin Formulations

Product	A (int. units)	B_1 (mg)	B_2 (mg)	B_6 (mg)	B_{12} (mcg)	C (mg)	D (int. units)	E (int. units)	Additional Information
Drops									
Poly-Vi-Flor® 0.25 mg (per mL)	1500	0.5	0.6	0.4	2	35	400	5	**Fluoride 0.25 mg**, niacin 8 mg; fruit flavor (50 mL)
Poly-Vi-Flor® 0.5 mg (per mL)	1500	0.5	0.6	0.4	2	35	400	5	**Fluoride 0.5 mg**, niacin 8 mg; fruit flavor (50 mL)
Poly-Vi-Flor® With Iron 0.25 mg (per mL)	1500	0.5	0.6	0.4		35	400	5	**Fluoride 0.25 mg**, Fe 10 mg, niacin 8 mg; fruit flavor (50 mL)
Soluvite-F® (per 0.6 mL)	1500					35	400		**Fluoride 0.25 mg**; alcohol free, dye free, orange flavor (57 mL)
Tri-Vi-Flor® 0.25 mg (per mL)	1500					35	400		**Fluoride 0.25 mg**; fruit flavor (50 mL)
Tri-Vi-Flor® With Iron 0.25 mg (per mL)	1500					35	400		**Fluoride 0.25 mg**, Fe 10 mg; fruit flavor (50 mL)
Vi-Daylin®/F (per mL)	1500	0.5	0.6	0.4		35	400	5	**Fluoride 0.25 mg**, niacin 8 mg; alcohol <0.1%, benzoic acid, sugar free, fruit flavor (50 mL)
Vi-Daylin®/F + Iron (per mL)	1500	0.5	0.6	0.4		35	400	5	**Fluoride 0.25 mg**, Fe 10 mg, niacin 8 mg; alcohol <0.1%, benzoic acid, sugar free, fruit flavor (50 mL)
Vi-Daylin®/F ADC (per mL)	1500					35	400		**Fluoride 0.25 mg**; sugar free, fruit flavor (50 mL)
Vi-Daylin®/F ADC + Iron (per mL)	1500					35	400		**Fluoride 0.25 mg**, Fe 10 mg; sugar free, fruit flavor (50 mL)

Legend: Ca = elemental calcium, Cr = chromium, Cu = copper, elemental Fe = iron, int. = international, Mg = magnesium, Mn = manganese, Mo = molybdenum, Zn = zinc.

Pediatric Multivitamin Formulations

Product	A (int. units)	B_1 (mg)	B_2 (mg)	B_6 (mg)	B_{12} (mcg)	C (mg)	D (int. units)	E (int. units)	Additional Information
Tablet, Chewable									
ADEKs® [OTC]	4000	1.2	1.3	1.5	12	60	400	150	Beta carotene 3 mg, biotin 50 mcg, folic acid 0.2 mg, niacin 10 mg, pantothenic acid 10 mg, vitamin K 150 mcg, Zn 7.5 mg; dye free
Centrum® Kids Rugrats™ Extra C [OTC]	5000	1.5	1.7	1	5	250	400	15	Ca 108 mg, Cu 0.5 mg, folic acid 0.3 mg, niacin 13.5 mg, phosphorus 50 mg, sodium 15 mg, Zn 4 mg; cherry, fruit punch, and orange flavors
Centrum® Kids Rugrats™ Extra Calcium [OTC]	5000	1.5	1.7	1	5	60	400	15	Ca 200 mg, Cu 0.5 mg, folic acid 0.3 mg, niacin 13.5 mg, phosphorus 50 mg, Zn 4 mg; cherry, fruit punch, and orange flavors
Centrum® Kids Rugrats™ Complete [OTC]	5000	1.5	1.7	2	6	60	400	30	Biotin 45 mcg, Ca 108 mg, Cr 20 mcg, Cu 2 mg, Fe 18 mg, folic acid 0.4 mg, iodine 150 mcg, Mg 40 mg, Mn 1 mg, Mo 20 mcg, niacin 20 mg, pantothenic acid 10 mg, phosphorus 50 mg, vitamin K 10 mg, Zn 15 mg; cherry, fruit punch, and orange flavors
Flintstones® Original [OTC]	2500	1.05	1.2	1.05	4.5	60	400	15	Folic acid 0.3 mg, niacin 13.5 mg
Flintstones® Complete [OTC]	5000	1.5	1.7	2	6	60	400	30	Biotin 40 mcg, Ca 100 mg, Cu 2 mg, Fe 18 mg, folic acid 0.4 mg, iodine 150 mcg, Mg 20 mg, niacin 20 mg, pantothenic acid 10 mg, phosphorus 100 mg, Zn 15 mg; **phenylalanine 4.56 mg**[1]; cherry, grape, and orange flavors
Flintstones® Plus Calcium [OTC]	2500	1.05	1.2	1.05	4.5	60	400	15	Ca 200 mg, folic acid 0.3 mg, niacin 13.5 mg; **phenylalanine <4 mg**[1]; cherry, grape, and orange flavors
Flintstones® Plus Extra C [OTC]	2500	1.05	1.2	1.05	4.5	250	400	15	Folic acid 0.3 mg, niacin 13.5 mg; grape, orange, peach-apricot, raspberry, and strawberry flavors

MULTIVITAMIN PRODUCTS *(Continued)*

Pediatric Multivitamin Formulations *(continued)*

Product	A (int. units)	B_1 (mg)	B_2 (mg)	B_6 (mg)	B_{12} (mcg)	C (mg)	D (int. units)	E (int. units)	Additional Information
Flintstones® Plus Iron [OTC]	2500	1.05	1.2	1.05	4.5	60	400	15	Fe 15 mg, folic acid 0.3 mg, niacin 13.5 mg; grape, orange, peach-apricot, raspberry, and strawberry flavors
My First Flintstones® [OTC]	2500	1.05	1.2	1.05	4.5	60	400	15	Folic acid 0.3 mg, niacin 13.5 mg; cherry, grape, and orange flavors
One-A-Day® Kids Bugs Bunny and Friends Complete [OTC]	5000	1.5	1.7	2	6	60	400	30	Biotin 40 mcg, Ca 100 mg, Cu 2 mg, Fe 18 mg, folic acid 0.4 mg, iodine 150 mcg, Mg 20 mg, niacin 20 mg, pantothenic acid 10 mg, phosphorus 100 mg, Zn 15 mg; sugar free, fruity flavors
One-A-Day® Kids Bugs Bunny and Friends Plus Extra C [OTC]	2500	1.05	1.2	1.05	4.5	250	400	15	Folic acid 0.3 mg, niacin 13.5 mg, **phenylalanine**[1]; sugar free, fruity flavors
One-A-Day® Kids Extreme Sports [OTC]	5000	1.5	1.2	2	6	60	400	30	Biotin 40 mcg, Ca 100 mg, Cu 2 mg, Fe 18 mg, folic acid 0.4 mg, iodine 150 mcg, Mg 20 mg, niacin 20 mg, pantothenic acid 10 mg, phosphorus 100 mg, Zn 15 mg
One-A-Day® Kids Scooby-Doo! Complete [OTC]	5000	1.5	1.7	2	6	60	400	30	Biotin 40 mcg, Ca 100 mg, Cu 2 mg, Fe 18 mg, folic acid 0.4 mg, iodine 150 mcg, Mg 20 mg, niacin 20 mg, pantothenic acid 10 mg, phosphorus 100 mg, Zn 15 mg; fruity flavors
One-A-Day® Kids Scooby-Doo! Plus Calcium [OTC]	2500	1.05	1.2	1.05	4.5	60	400	15	Ca 200 mg, folic acid 0.3 mg, niacin 13.5 mg; fruity flavors

Legend: Ca = elemental calcium, Cr = chromium, Cu = copper, Fe = elemental iron, int. = international, Mg = magnesium, Mn = manganese, Mo = molybdenum Zn = zinc.

[1]Contains phenylalanine; use with caution in phenylketonurics

Adolescent and Adult Multivitamin Formulations

Product	A (int. units)	B_1 (mg)	B_2 (mg)	B_6 (mg)	B_{12} (mcg)	C (mg)	D (int. units)	E (int. units)	Additional Information
Liquid									
Centrum® (per 15 mL) [OTC]	2500	1.5	1.7	2	6	60	400	30	Biotin 300 mcg, Cr 25 mcg, Fe 9 mg, iodine 150 mcg, Mn 2 mg, Mo 25 mg, niacin 20 mg, pantothenic acid 10 mg, Zn 3 mg; alcohol 5.4%, sodium benzoate (240 mL)
Iberet® (per 5 mL) [OTC]		1.2	1.35	0.925	5.63	33.8			Fe 23.6 mg, niacin 6.8 mg, pantothenic acid 2.4 mg; alcohol (240 mL)
Iberet®-500 (per 5 mL) [OTC]		1.2	1.35	0.925	5.63	125			Fe 23.6 mg, niacin 6.8 mg, pantothenic acid 2.4 mg; alcohol (240 mL)
Vi-Daylin® (per 5 mL) [OTC]	2500	1.05	1.2	1.05	4.5	60	400	15	Niacin 13.5 mg; alcohol <0.5%, benzoic acid; lemon/orange flavor (240 mL, 480 mL)
Vi-Daylin® + Iron (per 5 mL) [OTC]	2500	1.05	1.2	1.05	4.5	60	400	15	Fe 10 mg, niacin 13.5 mg; alcohol <0.5%, benzoic acid; lemon/orange flavor (240 mL, 480 mL)
Caplet									
Theragran-M® Advanced Formula [OTC]	5000	3	3.4	6	12	90	400	60	Biotin 30 mcg, boron 150 mcg, Ca 40 mg, chloride 7.5 mg, Cr 50 mcg, Cu 2 mg, Fe 9 mg, folic acid 0.4 mg, iodine 150 mcg, Mg 100 mg, Mn 2 mg, Mo 75 mcg, niacin 20 mg, nickel 5 mcg, pantothenic acid 10 mg, phosphorus 31 mg, potassium 7.5 mg, Se 70 mcg, silicon 2 mg, tin 10 mcg, vanadium 10 mcg, vitamin K 28 mcg, Zn 15 mg
Capsule									
Vitacon Forte	8000	10	5	2	10	150		50	Folic acid 1 mg, Mg 70 mg, Mn 4 mg, niacinamide 25 mg, Zn 80 mg
Vicon Plus® [OTC]	3400	9.3	4.6	1.5		140		45	Mg 5 mg, Mn 1 mg, niacin 24 mg, pantothenic acid 11 mg, Zn 10 mg

MULTIVITAMIN PRODUCTS *(Continued)*

Adolescent and Adult Multivitamin Formulations *(continued)*

Product	A (int. units)	B_1 (mg)	B_2 (mg)	B_6 (mg)	B_{12} (mcg)	C (mg)	D (int. units)	E (int. units)	Additional Information
Tablet									
Centrum® [OTC]	5000	1.5	1.7	2	6	60	400	30	Biotin 30 mcg, boron 150 mcg, Ca 162 mg, chloride 72 mg, Cr 120 mcg, Cu 2 mg, Fe 18 mg, folic acid 0.4 mg, iodine 150 mcg, lutein 250 mcg, Mg 100 mg, Mn 2 mg, Mo 75 mcg, niacin 20 mg, nickel 5 mcg, pantothenic acid 10 mg, phosphorus 109 mg, potassium 80 mg, Se 20 mcg, silicon 2 mg, tin 10 mcg, vanadium 10 mcg, vitamin K 25 mcg, Zn 15 mg
Centrum® Performance™ [OTC]	5000	4.5	5.1	6	18	120	400	60	Biotin 40 mcg, boron 60 mcg, chloride 72 mg, folic acid 0.4 mg, Ca 100 mg, Cr 120 mcg, Cu 2 mg, Fe 18 mg, ginkgo biloba leaf 60 mg, ginseng root 50 mg, iodine 150 mcg, Mg 40 mg, Mn 4 mg, Mo 75 mcg, niacin 40 mg, nickel 5 mcg, pantothenic acid 10 mg, phosphorus 48 mg, potassium 80 mg, Se 70 mcg, silicon 4 mg, tin 10 mcg, vanadium 10 mcg, vitamin K 25 mcg, Zn 15 mg
Iberet®-500 [OTC]		4.96	5.4	3.7	22.5	500			Fe 95 mg (controlled release), niacin 27.2 mg, pantothenic acid 8.28 mg, sodium 65 mg
Iberet-Folic-500® [OTC]		6	6	5	25	500			Fe 105 mg (controlled release), folic acid 0.8 mg, niacinamde 30 mg, pantothenic acid 10 mg
One-A-Day® Active Formula [OTC]	5000	4.5	5.1	6	18	120	400	60	American ginseng 55 mg, biotin 40 mcg, boron 150 mcg, Ca 110 mg, chloride 180 mg, Cr 100 mcg, Cu 2 mg, Fe 9 mg, folic acid 0.4 mg, iodine 150 mcg, Mg 40 mg, Mn 2 mg, Mo 25 mcg, niacin 40 mg, nickel 5 mcg, pantothenic acid 10 mg, phosphorus 48 mg, potassium 200 mg, Se 45 mcg, silicon 6 mg, tin 10 mcg, vanadium 10 mcg, vitamin K 25 mcg, Zn 15 mg

Adolescent and Adult Multivitamin Formulations *(continued)*

Product	A (int. units)	B_1 (mg)	B_2 (mg)	B_6 (mg)	B_{12} (mcg)	C (mg)	D (int. units)	E (int. units)	Additional Information
One-A-Day® Essential Formula [OTC]	5000	1.5	1.7	2	6	60	400	30	Folic acid 0.4 mg, niacin 20 mg, pantothenic acid 10 mg
One-A-Day® Maximum Formula [OTC]	5000	1.5	1.7	2	6	60	400	30	Biotin 30 mcg, boron 150 mcg, Ca 162 mg, chloride 72 mg, Cr 65 mcg, Cu 2 mg, Fe 18 mg, folic acid 0.4 mg, iodine 150 mcg, Mg 100 mg, Mn 3.5 mg, Mo 160 mcg, niacin 20 mg, nickel 5 mcg, pantothenic acid 10 mg, phosphorus 109 mg, potassium 80 mg, Se 20 mcg, silicon 2 mg, tin 10 mcg, vanadium 10 mcg, vitamin K 25 mcg, Zn 15 mg
One-A-Day® Today [OTC]	3000	1.1	1.7	3	18	75	400	33	Biotin 30 mcg, Ca 240 mg, Cr 120 mcg, Cu 2 mg, folic acid 0.4 mg, Mg 120 mg, Mn 2 mg, niacin 14 mg, pantothenic acid 5 mg, potassium 100 mg, Se 70 mcg, soy extract 10 mg, vitamin K 20 mcg, Zn 15 mg
Tablet, Chewable									
Centrum® [OTC]	5000	1.5	1.7	2	6	60	400	30	Biotin 45 mcg, Ca 108 mg, Cr 20 mcg, Cu 2 mg, Fe 18 mg, folic acid 0.4 mg, iodine 150 mcg, Mg 40 mg, Mn 1 mg, Mo 20 mcg, niacin 20 mg, pantothenic acid 10 mg, Zn 15 mg

Legend: Ca = calcium, Cr = chromium, Cu = copper, Fe = iron, int. = international, Mg = magnesium, Mn = manganese, Mo = molybdenum, Se = selenium, Zn = zinc.

MULTIVITAMIN PRODUCTS *(Continued)*

Vitamin B Complex Formulations
Adolescent and Adult

Product	B_1 (mg)	B_2 (mg)	B_6 (mg)	B_{12} (mcg)	C (mg)	E (int. units)	Additional Information
Caplet							
Allbee® with C [OTC]	15	10.2	5		300		Niacinamide 50 mg, pantothenic acid 10 mg
Allbee® C-800 [OTC]	15	17	25	12	800	45	Niacinamide 100 mg, pantothenic acid 25 mg
Allbee® C-800 + Iron [OTC]	15	17	25	12	800	45	Fe 27 mg, folic acid 0.4 mcg, niacinamide 100 mg, pantothenic acid 25 mg
Liquid							
Apatate® (per 5 mL) [OTC]	15		0.5	25			Cherry flavor (120 mL)
Gevrabon® (per 30 mL) [OTC]	5	2.5	1	1			Choline 10 mg, Fe 15 mg, iodine 100 mcg, Mg 2 mg, Mn 2 mg, niacinamide 60 mg, pantothenic acid 10 mg, Zn 2 mg; alcohol, benzoic acid; sherry wine flavor (480 mL)
Softgel							
Nephrocaps®	1.5	1.7	10	6	100		Biotin 150 mcg, folic acid 1 mcg, niacinamide 20 mg, pantothenic acid 5 mg
Tablet							
Nephro-Vite®	1.5	1.7	10	6	60		Biotin 300 mcg, folic acid 0.8 mcg, niacinamide 20 mg, pantothenic acid 10 mg
Nephro-Vite® Rx	1.5	1.7	10	6	60		Biotin 300 mcg, folic acid 1 mcg, niacinamide 20 mg, pantothenic acid 10 mg
Stresstabs® B-Complex [OTC]	10	10	5	12	500	30	Biotin 45 mcg, folic acid 0.4 mcg, niacinamide 100 mg, pantothenic acid 20 mg
Stresstabs® B-Complex + Iron [OTC]	10	10	5	12	500	30	Biotin 45 mcg, Fe 18 mg, folic acid 0.4 mcg, niacinamide 100 mg, pantothenic acid 20 mg
Stresstabs® B-Complex + Zinc [OTC]	10	10	5	12	500	30	Biotin 45 mcg, Cu 3 mg, folic acid 0.4 mcg, niacinamide 100 mg, pantothenic acid 20 mg, Zn 23.9 mg
Surbex-T® [OTC]	15	10	5	10	500		Ca 20 mg, niacinamide 100 mg
Z-Bec® [OTC]	15	10.2	10	6	600	45	Niacinamide 100 mg, pantothenic acid 25 mg, Zn 22.5 mg
Tablet, Chewable							
Apatate® [OTC]	15		0.5	25			Cherry flavor

Legend: Ca = calcium, Cu = copper, Fe = iron, int. = international, Mg = magnesium, Mn = manganese, Zn = zinc.

NARCOTIC ANALGESICS COMPARISON

Drug	Onset (min)	Duration (h)	Equianalgesic I.M. Dose (mg)	Equianalgesic P.O. Dose[1] (mg)	Parenteral Oral Ratio	Partial Antagonist
Alfentanil	I.V.: Immediate	<0.25-0.33	ND	—	—	No
Codeine	I.M.: 10-30 P.O.: 30-60	I.M.: 4-6	120	200	1/2-2/3	No
Fentanyl	I.M.: 7-15 I.V.: Immediate	I.M.: 1-2 I.V.: 0.5-1	0.1-0.2	—	—	No
Hydrocodone	P.O. 10-20	P.O.: 3-6	—	ND	ND	No
Hydromorphone	P.O.: 15-30	P.O.: 4-5	1.5	7.5	1/5	No
Meperidine	P.O., I.M., SubQ: 10-15 I.V.: ≤5	P.O., I.M., SubQ: 2-4 I.V.: 2-3	75-100	300	1/3-1/2	No
Methadone	P.O.: 30-60 I.V.: 10-20	Acute: 4-6 Chronic: >8	Acute: 10 Chronic: 2-4	Acute: 20 Chronic: 2-4	1/2; ratio decreases to 1/1 upon chronic dosing	No
Morphine	P.O.: 15-60 I.V.: ≤5	P.O., I.V., I.M., SubQ: 3-5 Extended release tablets: 8-12	10	Acute: 60 Chronic: 30	1/6; ratio decreases to 1/1.5-2.5 upon chronic dosing	No
Oxycodone	P.O.: 15-30	P.O.: Immediate release: 4-5 controlled release: 12	—	30	—	No
Pentazocine	P.O., I.M., SubQ: 15-30 I.V.: ≤2-3	P.O.: 4-5 I.V., I.M., SubQ: 2-3	50	150	1/3	Yes
Propoxyphene	P.O.: 30-60	P.O.: 4-6	—	HCl salt: 130 Napsylate salt: 200	—	No

[1]Based on acute, short-term use. Chronic administration may alter pharmacokinetics and change parental oral ratio.

ND = no data.

Note: Values are based on adult studies. Duration may be shorter in children due to faster elimination (in general) compared to adults.

OTC COUGH AND COLD PREPARATIONS, PEDIATRIC

Commonly Used Pediatric OTC Cough and Cold Preparations

Brand Name	Type of Preparation
Actifed® Cold & Allergy	Antihistamine/Decongestant
Actifed® Cold & Sinus	Antihistamine/Decongestant
Alavert™	Antihistamine
Alavert™ Allergy and Sinus	Antihistamine/Decongestant
Benadryl® Allergy, Children's	Antihistamine
Benadryl® Allergy & Sinus Children's Elixir	Antihistamine/Decongestant
Benadryl® Allergy & Cold Fastmelt	Antihistamine/Decongestant
Benylin® Pediatric	Antitussive
Benylin® Expectorant	Antitussive/Expectorant
Claritin®	Antihistamine
Claritin-D®	Antihistamine/Decongestant
Chlor-Trimeton®	Antihistamine
Dimetane® DX	Antihistamine/Decongestant/Expectorant
Dimetapp® Children's ND Non-Drowsy Allergy	Antihistamine
Dimetapp® Cold & Cough, Children's	Antihistamine/Antitussive/Decongestant
Dimetapp® Cold & Congestion	Antitussive/Decongestant/Expectorant
Dimetapp® Cold & Allergy	Antihistamine/Decongestant
Dimetapp® Elixir Cold & Allergy, Children's	Antihistamine/Decongestant
Dimetapp® Infant Drops	Decongestant
Dimetapp® Infant Drops Decongestant & Cough	Antitussive/Decongestant
Neo-Synephrine® 12-Hour Children's Nose Drops	Decongestant
Neo-Synephrine® Nose Drops/Nasal Spray	Decongestant
Organidin® NR	Expectorant
PediaCare® Cold & Allergy	Antihistamine/Decongestant
PediaCare® Decongestant Plus Cough Infant Drops	Antitussive/Decongestant
PediaCare® Infant Decongestant Drops	Decongestant
PediaCare® Multisymptom Cold	Antihistamine/Antitussive/Decongestant
PediaCare® "Night Rest" Cough & Cold	Antihistamine/Antitussive/Decongestant
Robitussin® Allergy & Cough	Antihistamine/Antitussive/Decongestant
Robitussin® Cold & Flu	Antitussive/Decongestant/Expectorant
Robitussin® Cough & Cold Infant Drops	Antitussive/Decongestant/Expectorant
Robitussin® DM	Antitussive/Expectorant
Robitussin® DM Drops	Antitussive/Expectorant
Robitussin® Flu	Antihistamine/Antitussive/Decongestant

Commonly Used Pediatric OTC Cough and Cold Preparations (continued)

Brand Name	Type of Preparation
Robitussin® Pediatric Cough Syrup	Antitussive
Robitussin® Pediatric Cough & Cold Syrup	Antitussive/Decongestant
Robitussin® Pediatric Night Relief	Antihistamine/Antitussive/Decongestant
Sudafed® Cold & Cough, Children's	Antitussive/Decongestant
Sudafed® Nasal Decongestant	Decongestant
Sudafed® Nasal Decongestant, Children's	Decongestant
Sudafed® Sinus & Allergy	Antihistamine/Decongestant
Simply Cough™	Antitussive
Simply Stuffy™	Decongestant
Triaminic® Cold & Cough	Antihistamine/Antitussive/Decongestant
Triaminic® Cold & Cough Soft Chews	Antihistamine/Antitussive/Decongestant
Triaminic Cold & Allergy Syrup® (orange)	Antihistamine/Decongestant
Triaminic® Cold, Cough, & Fever	Antihistamine/Antitussive/Decongestant
Triaminic® Cough & Sore Throat (dark red)	Antitussive/Decongestant
Tylenol® Cold, Children's	Antihistamine/Decongestant
Tylenol® Cold Concentrated Drops, Infants	Decongestant
Tylenol® Cold Plus Cough, Children's	Antihistamine/Antitussive/Decongestant
Tylenol® Cold Plus Cough Concentrated Drops, Infants	Antitussive/Decongestant
Tylenol® Flu, Children's	Antihistamine/Antitussive/Decongestant
Tylenol® Sinus, Children's	Decongestant
Vicks® Nyquil®, Children's	Antihistamine/Antitussive/Decongestant
Vicks® 44e® Cough & Chest Congestion Relief, Pediatric	Antitussive/Expectorant
Vicks® 44m® Cough & Cold Relief, Pediatric	Antihistamine/Antitussive/Decongestant

OTC COUGH AND COLD PREPARATIONS, PEDIATRIC *(Continued)*

Content of Commonly Used Pediatric Cough and Cold Preparations

The following chart lists the contents of the more common OTC cough and cold preparations. Products are grouped by preparation type. For specific recommendations, see individual drug monographs.

Brand Name	Generic(s)	Strength	Other Information
	Decongestants		
Dimetapp® Infant Drops	Pseudoephedrine	7.5 mg/0.8 mL	–
Neo-Synephrine® 12-Hour Children's Nose Drops	Oxymetazoline	0.05%	
Neo-Synephrine® Nose Drops/Nasal Spray	Phenylephrine	0.25% 0.25%-0.5%	≤6 y must be diluted prior to use (see Phenylephrine) >6 to 12 y use 0.25%
PediaCare® Decongestant Infant Drops	Pseudoephedrine	7.5 mg/0.8 mL	–
Simply Stuffy™	Pseudoephedrine	15 mg/5 mL	–
Sudafed® Nasal Decongestant	Pseudoephedrine	15 mg/5 mL 30 mg/5 mL 15 mg/tab 30 mg/tab 60 mg/tab 120 mg/tab or cap (timed release) 240 mg/tab (timed release)	–
Tylenol® Cold Concentrated Drops, Infants	Pseudoephedrine	15 mg/1.6 mL	Acetaminophen 160 mg/1.6 mL
Tylenol® Sinus, Children's	Pseudoephedrine	15 mg/5 mL 7.5 mg/tab	Acetaminophen 160 mg/5 mL 80 mg/tab
	Antihistamines		
Alavert™	Loratidine	10 mg (rapidly disintegrating)	Tablet contains phenylalanine
Benadryl® Allergy Children's	Diphenhydramine	12.5 mg/chew tab 12.5 mg/5 mL	Tablet contains aspartame
Claritin®	Loratidine	5 mg/5 mL 10 mg/tab	–
Chlor-Trimeton®	Chlorpheniramine	4 mg/tab 8 mg/tab 12 mg/tab	–
Dimetapp® Children's ND Non-Drowsy Allergy	Loratidine	10 mg/tab 5 mg/5 mL	Contains phenylalanine
	Expectorants		
Mucinex®	Guaifenesin	600 mg/tab (extended release)	–
Organidin® NR, Robitussin®	Guaifenesin	100 mg/5 mL	–
	Antitussives		
Benylin® Pediatric Syrup	Dextromethorphan	7.5 mg/5 mL	–
Robitussin® Pediatric Cough Syrup	Dextromethorphan HBr	7.5 mg/5 mL	–
Simply Cough™	Dextromethorphan	5 mg/5 mL	–
	Antihistamine / Decongestants		
Actifed® Cold & Allergy	Triprolidine Pseudoephedrine	1.25 mg/5 mL 2.5 mg/tab 30 mg/5 mL 60 mg/tab	–

Brand Name	Generic(s)	Strength	Other Information
Actifed® Cold & Sinus	Chlorpheniramine Pseudoephedrine	2 mg/tab 30 mg/tab	Acetaminophen 500 mg/tab
Alavert™ Allergy and Sinus	Loratidine Pseudoephedrine	5 mg/tab 120 mg/tab (extended release)	–
Benadryl® Allergy & Cold Fastmelt	Diphenhydramine citrate Pseudoephedrine	19 mg/tab 30 mg/tab	Citrate salt equivalent to 12.5 mg diphenhydramine HCl Phenylalanine 4.6 mg/tab
Benadryl® Allergy & Sinus, Children's	Diphenhydramine Pseudoephedrine	12.5 mg/5 mL 30 mg/5 mL	–
Claritin-D®	Loratidine Pseudoephedrine	10 mg/tab 240 mg/tab (extended release)	–
Dimetapp® Cold & Allergy	Chlorpheniramine Phenylephrine	2 mg/tab 5 mg/tab	Acetaminophen 325 mg/tab
Dimetapp® Elixir Cold & Allergy, Children's	Brompheniramine Pseudoephedrine	1 mg/5 mL 15 mg/5 mL	–
PediaCare® Cold & Allergy	Chlorpheniramine Pseudoephedrine	1 mg/5 mL 15 mg/5 mL	–
Sudafed® Sinus & Allergy	Chlorpheniramine Pseudoephedrine	4 mg/tab 60 mg/tab	–
Rondec®	Brompheniramine Pseudoephedrine	4 mg/5 mL 45 mg/5 mL	–
Triaminic® Cold & Allergy (orange)	Chlorpheniramine Pseudoephedrine	1 mg/5 mL 15 mg/5 mL	–
Tylenol® Cold, Children's	Chlorpheniramine Pseudoephedrine	1 mg/5 mL 0.5 mg/tab 15 mg/5 mL 7.5 mg/tab	Acetaminophen 160 mg/5 mL 80 mg/tab
Antitussive / Decongestant			
Dimetapp® Infant Drops Decongestant & Cough	Dextromethorphan Pseudoephedrine	2.5 mg/0.8 mL 7.5 mg/0.8 mL	–
Dimetapp® Long-Acting Cough & Cold	Dextromethorphan Pseudoephedrine	7.5 mg/5 mL 15 mg/5 mL	–
PediaCare® Decongestant Plus Cough, Infant Drops	Dextromethorphan Pseudoephedrine	2.5 mg/0.8 mL 7.5 mg/0.8 mL	–
Robitussin® Pediatric Cough & Cold Syrup	Dextromethorphan Pseudoephedrine	7.5 mg/5 mL 15 mg/5 mL	–
Sudafed® Cold & Cough, Children's	Dextromethorphan Pseudoephedrine	5 mg/5 mL 15 mg/5 mL	–
Triaminic® Cough & Sore Throat	Dextromethorphan Pseudoephedrine	7.5 mg/5 mL 15 mg/5 mL	Acetaminophen 160 mg
Tylenol® Cold Plus Cough Concentrated Drops, Infants	Dextromethorphan Pseudoephedrine	5 mg/1.6 mL 15 mg/1.6 mL	Acetaminophen 160 mg/1.6 mL
Antitussive / Expectorant			
Benylin® Expectorant	Dextromethorphan Guaifenesin	5 mg/5 mL 100 mg/5 mL	–
Robitussin® DM	Dextromethorphan Guaifenesin	10 mg/5 mL 100 mg/5 mL	1.4% alcohol
Robitussin® DM Drops	Dextromethorphan Guaifenesin	5 mg/2.5 mL 100 mg/2.5 mL	–
Vicks® 44e® Cough & Chest Congestion Relief, Pediatric	Dextromethorphan Guaifenesin	3.3 mg/5 mL 33 mg/5 mL	–
Antihistamine / Antitussive / Decongestant			
Children's Dimetapp® DM Cold & Cough	Brompheniramine Dextromethorphan Pseudoephedrine	1 mg/5 mL 5 mg/5 mL 15 mg/5 mL	–

OTC COUGH AND COLD PREPARATIONS, PEDIATRIC *(Continued)*

Brand Name	Generic(s)	Strength	Other Information
PediaCare® Multisymptom Cold	Chlorpheniramine Dextromethorphan Pseudoephedrine	1 mg/5 mL 5 mg/5 mL 15 mg/5 mL	–
PediaCare® "Night Rest" Cough & Cold	Chlorpheniramine Dextromethorphan Pseudoephedrine	1 mg/5 mL 7.5 mg/5 mL 15 mg/5 mL	–
Robitussin® Allergy & Cough	Brompheniramine Dextromethorphan Pseudoephedrine	2 mg/5 mL 10 mg/5 mL 30 mg/5 mL	–
Robitussin® Flu	Chlorpheniramine Dextromethorphan Pseudoephedrine	1 mg/5 mL 5 mg/5 mL 15 mg/5 mL	Acetaminophen 160 mg
Robitussin® Pediatric Night Relief	Chlorpheniramine Dextromethorphan Pseudoephedrine	1 mg/5 mL 7.5 mg/5 mL 15 mg/5 mL	–
Triaminic® Cold & Cough	Chlorpheniramine Dextromethorphan Pseudoephedrine	1 mg/5 mL 5 mg/5 mL 15 mg/5 mL	–
Triaminic® Cold & Cough Soft Chews	Chlorpheniramine Dextromethorphan Pseudoephedrine	1 mg/chew tab 5 mg/chew tab 15 mg/chew tab	–
Triaminic® Cold, Cough, & Fever	Chlorpheniramine Dextromethorphan Pseudoephedrine	1 mg/5 mL 7.5 mg/5 mL 15 mg/5 mL	Acetaminophen 160 mg
Tylenol® Cold Plus Cough, Children's	Chlorpheniramine Dextromethorphan Pseudoephedrine	1 mg/5 mL 5 mg/5 mL 15 mg/5 mL	Acetaminophen 160 mg/5 mL
	Chlorpheniramine Dextromethorphan Pseudoephedrine	0.5 mg/tab 2.5 mg/tab 7.5 mg/tab	Acetaminophen 80 mg/tab
Tylenol® Flu, Children's	Chlorpheniramine Dextromethorphan Pseudoephedrine	1 mg/5 mL 7.5 mg/5 mL 15 mg/5 mL	Acetaminophen 160 mg
Vicks® Nyquil®, Children's	Chlorpheniramine Dextromethorphan Pseudoephedrine	0.67 mg/5 mL 5 mg/5 mL 10 mg/5 mL	–
Vicks® 44m® Cough & Cold Relief, Pediatric	Chlorpheniramine Dextromethorphan Pseudoephedrine	0.67 mg/5 mL 5 mg/5 mL 10 mg/5 mL	–
Antitussive / Decongestant / Expectorant			
Dimetane® DX	Brompheniramine Dextromethorphan Pseudoephedrine	2 mg/5 mL 10 mg/5 mL 30 mg/5 mL	0.95% alcohol
Dimetapp® Cold & Congestion	Dextromethorphan Pseudoephedrine Guaifenesin	10 mg/caplet 30 mg/caplet 200 mg/caplet	–
Robitussin® Cold & Cold Infant Drops	Dextromethorphan Pseudoephedrine Guaifenesin	5 mg/2.5 mL 15 mg/2.5 mL 100 mg/2.5 mL	–
Robitussin® Cold & Flu Caplets or Softgels	Dextromethorphan Pseudoephedrine Guaifenesin	10 mg/caplet/softgel 30 mg/caplet/softgel 200 mg/caplet/softgel	–

CONVERSIONS

Apothecary-Metric Exact Equivalents

1 gram (g)	=	15.43 grains	0.1 mg	=	1/600 gr
1 milliliter (mL)	=	16.23 minims	0.12 mg	=	1/500 gr
1 minim	=	0.06 mL	0.15 mg	=	1/400 gr
1 grain (gr)	=	64.8 milligrams	0.2 mg	=	1/300 gr
1 fluid ounce (fl. oz)	=	29.57 mL	0.3 mg	=	1/200 gr
1 pint (pt)	=	473.2 mL	0.4 mg	=	1/150 gr
1 ounce (oz)	=	28.35 grams	0.5 mg	=	1/120 gr
1 pound (lb)	=	453.6 grams	0.6 mg	=	1/100 gr
1 kilogram (kg)	=	2.2 pounds	0.8 mg	=	1/80 gr
1 quart (qt)	=	946.4 mL	1 mg	=	1/65 gr

Apothecary-Metric Approximate Equivalents[1]

Liquids			Solids		
1 teaspoonful	=	5 mL	1/4 grain	=	15 mg
1 tablespoonful	=	15 mL	1/2 grain	=	30 mg
			1 grain	=	60 mg
			1 1/2 grain	=	100 mg
			5 grains	=	300 mg
			10 grains	=	600 mg

[1]Use exact equivalents for compounding and calculations requiring a high degree of accuracy.

Pounds-Kilograms Conversion

1 pound = 0.45359 kilograms
1 kilogram = 2.2 pounds

Temperature Conversion

Celsius to Fahrenheit = (°C x 9/5) + 32 = °F
Fahrenheit to Celsius = (°F - 32) x 5/9 = °C

CYTOCHROME P450 ENZYMES: SUBSTRATES, INHIBITORS, AND INDUCERS

INTRODUCTION

Most drugs are eliminated from the body, at least in part, by being chemically altered to less lipid-soluble products (ie, metabolized), and thus are more likely to be excreted via the kidneys or the bile. Phase I metabolism includes drug hydrolysis, oxidation, and reduction, and results in drugs that are more polar in their chemical structure, while Phase II metabolism involves the attachment of an additional molecule onto the drug (or partially metabolized drug) in order to create an inactive and/or more water soluble compound. Phase II processes include (primarily) glucuronidation, sulfation, glutathione conjugation, acetylation, and methylation.

Virtually any of the Phase I and II enzymes can be inhibited by some xenobiotic or drug. Some of the Phase I and II enzymes can be induced. Inhibition of the activity of metabolic enzymes will result in increased concentrations of the substrate (drug), whereas induction of the activity of metabolic enzymes will result in decreased concentrations of the substrate. For example, the well-documented enzyme-inducing effects of phenobarbital may include a combination of Phase I and II enzymes. Phase II glucuronidation may be increased via induced UDP-glucuronosyltransferase (UGT) activity, whereas Phase I oxidation may be increased via induced cytochrome P450 (CYP) activity. However, for most drugs, the primary route of metabolism (and the primary focus of drug-drug interaction) is Phase I oxidation, and specifically, metabolism.

CYP enzymes may be responsible for the metabolism (at least partial metabolism) of approximately 75% of all drugs, with the CYP3A subfamily responsible for nearly half of this activity. Found throughout plant, animal, and bacterial species, CYP enzymes represent a superfamily of xenobiotic metabolizing proteins. There have been several hundred CYP enzymes identified in nature, each of which has been assigned to a family (1, 2, 3, etc), subfamily (A, B, C, etc), and given a specific enzyme number (1, 2, 3, etc) according to the similarity in amino acid sequence that it shares with other enzymes. Of these many enzymes, only a few are found in humans, and even fewer appear to be involved in the metabolism of xenobiotics (eg, drugs). The key human enzyme subfamilies include CYP1A, CYP2A, CYP2B, CYP2C, CYP2D, CYP2E, and CYP3A.

CYP enzymes are found in the endoplasmic reticulum of cells in a variety of human tissues (eg, skin, kidneys, brain, lungs), but their predominant sites of concentration and activity are the liver and intestine. Though the abundance of CYP enzymes throughout the body is relatively equally distributed among the various subfamilies, the relative contribution to drug metabolism is (in decreasing order of magnitude) CYP3A4 (nearly 50%), CYP2D6 (nearly 25%), CYP2C8/9 (nearly 15%), then CYP1A2, CYP2C19, CYP2A6, and CYP2E1. Owing to their potential for numerous drug-drug interactions, those drugs that are identified in preclinical studies as substrates of CYP3A enzymes are often given a lower priority for continued research and development in favor of drugs that appear to be less affected by (or less likely to affect) this enzyme subfamily.

Each enzyme subfamily possesses unique selectivity toward potential substrates. For example, CYP1A2 preferentially binds medium-sized, planar, lipophilic molecules, while CYP2D6 preferentially binds molecules that possess a basic nitrogen atom. Some CYP subfamilies exhibit polymorphism (ie, multiple allelic variants that manifest differing catalytic properties). The best described polymorphisms involve CYP2C9, CYP2C19, and CYP2D6. Individuals possessing "wild type" gene alleles exhibit normal functioning CYP capacity. Others, however, possess allelic variants that leave the person with a subnormal level of catalytic potential (so called "poor metabolizers"). Poor metabolizers would be more likely to experience toxicity from drugs metabolized by the affected enzymes (or less effects if the enzyme is responsible for converting a prodrug to it's active form as in the case of codeine). The percentage of people classified as poor metabolizers varies by enzyme and population group. As an example, approximately 7% of Caucasians and only about 1% of Orientals appear to be CYP2D6 poor metabolizers.

CYP enzymes can be both inhibited and induced by other drugs, leading to increased or decreased serum concentrations (along with the associated effects), respectively. Induction occurs when a drug causes an increase in the amount of smooth endoplasmic reticulum, secondary to increasing the amount of the affected CYP enzymes in the tissues. This "revving up" of the CYP enzyme system may take several days to reach peak activity, and likewise, may take several days, even months, to return to normal following discontinuation of the inducing agent.

CYP inhibition occurs via several potential mechanisms. Most commonly, a CYP inhibitor competitively (and reversibly) binds to the active site on the enzyme, thus preventing the substrate from binding to the same site, and preventing the substrate from being metabolized. The affinity of an inhibitor for an enzyme may be expressed by an inhibition constant (Ki) or IC50 (defined as the concentration of the inhibitor required to cause 50% inhibition under a given set of conditions). In addition to reversible competition for an enzyme site, drugs may inhibit enzyme activity by binding to sites on the enzyme other than that to which the substrate would bind, and thereby cause a change in the functionality or physical structure of the enzyme. A drug may also bind to the enzyme in an irreversible (ie, "suicide") fashion. In such a case, it is not the concentration of drug at the enzyme site that is important (constantly binding and releasing), but the number of molecules available for binding (once bound, always bound).

Although an inhibitor or inducer may be known to affect a variety of CYP subfamilies, it may only inhibit one or two in a clinically important fashion. Likewise, although a substrate is known to be at least partially metabolized by a variety of CYP enzymes, only one or two enzymes may contribute significantly enough to its overall metabolism to warrant concern when used with potential inducers or inhibitors. Therefore, when attempting to predict the level of risk of using two drugs that may affect each other via altered CYP function, it is important to identify the relative effectiveness of the inhibiting/inducing drug on the CYP subfamilies that significantly contribute to the metabolism of the substrate. The contribution of a specific CYP pathway to substrate metabolism should be considered not only in light of other known CYP pathways, but also other nonoxidative pathways for substrate metabolism (eg, glucuronidation) and transporter proteins (eg, P-glycoprotein) that may affect the presentation of a substrate to a metabolic pathway.

HOW TO USE THE TABLES

The following CYP SUBSTRATES, INHIBITORS, and INDUCERS tables provide a clinically relevant perspective on drugs that are affected by, or affect, cytochrome P450 (CYP) enzymes. Not all human, drug-metabolizing CYP enzymes are specifically (or separately) included in the tables. Some enzymes have been excluded because they do not appear to significantly contribute to the metabolism of marketed drugs (eg, CYP2C18). Others have been combined in recognition of the difficulty in distinguishing their metabolic activity one from another, or the clinical practicality of doing so (eg, CYP2C8/9, CYP3A4). In the case of CYP3A4, the industry routinely uses this single enzyme designation to represent all enzymes in the CYP3A subfamily. CYP3A7 is present in fetal livers. It is effectively absent from adult livers. CYP3A4 (adult) and CYP3A7 (fetal) appear to share similar properties in their respective hosts. The impact of CYP3A7 in fetal and neonatal drug interactions has not been investigated.

The **CYP Substrates table** contains a list of drugs reported to be metabolized, at least in part, by one or more CYP enzymes. An enzyme that appears to play a

CYTOCHROME P450 ENZYMES: SUBSTRATES, INHIBITORS, AND INDUCERS *(Continued)*

clinically significant (major) role in a drug's metabolism is indicated by "●", and an enzyme whose role appears to be clinically insignificant (minor) is indicated by "○". A clinically significant designation is the result of a two-phase review. The first phase considered the contribution of each CYP enzyme to the overall metabolism of the drug. The enzyme pathway was considered potentially clinically relevant if it was responsible for at least 30% of the metabolism of the drug. If so, the drug was subjected to a second phase. The second phase considered the clinical relevance of a substrate's concentration being increased twofold, or decreased by one-half (such as might be observed if combined with an effective CYP inhibitor or inducer, respectively). If either of these changes was considered to present a clinically significant concern, the CYP pathway for the drug was designated "major." If neither change would appear to present a clinically significant concern, or if the CYP enzyme was responsible for a smaller portion of the overall metabolism (ie, <30%), the pathway was designated "minor."

The **CYP Inhibitors table** contains a list of drugs that are reported to inhibit one or more CYP enzymes. Enzymes that are strongly inhibited by a drug are indicated by "●". Enzymes that are moderately inhibited are indicated by "◑". Enzymes that are weakly inhibited are indicated by "○". The designations are the result of a review of published clinical reports, available Ki data, and assessments published by other experts in the field. As it pertains to Ki values set in a ratio with achievable serum drug concentrations ([I]) under normal dosing conditions, the following parameters were employed: [I]/Ki ≥1 = strong; [I]/Ki 0.1-1 = moderate; [I]/Ki <0.1 = weak.

The **CYP Inducers table** contains a list of drugs that are reported to induce one or more CYP enzymes. Enzymes that appear to be effectively induced by a drug are indicated by "●", and enzymes that do not appear to be effectively induced are indicated by "○". The designations are the result of a review of published clinical reports and assessments published by experts in the field.

In general, clinically significant interactions are more likely to occur between substrates and either inhibitors or inducers of the same enzyme(s), all of which have been indicated by "●". However, these assessments possess a degree of subjectivity, at times based on limited indications regarding the significance of CYP effects of particular agents. An attempt has been made to balance a conservative, clinically-sensitive presentation of the data with a desire to avoid the numbing effect of a "beware of everything" approach. Even so, other potential interactions (ie, those involving enzymes indicated by "○") may warrant consideration in some cases. It is important to note that information related to CYP metabolism of drugs is expanding at a rapid pace, and thus, the contents of this table should only be considered to represent a "snapshot" of the information available at the time of publication.

Selected Readings

Bjornsson TD, Callaghan JT, Einolf HJ, et al, "The Conduct of *in vitro* and *in vivo* Drug-Drug Interaction Studies: A PhRMA Perspective," *J Clin Pharmacol*, 2003, 43(5):443-69.

Drug-Drug Interactions, Rodrigues AD, ed, New York, NY: Marcel Dekker, Inc, 2002.

Levy RH, Thummel KE, Trager WF, et al, eds, *Metabolic Drug Interactions*, Philadelphia, PA: Lippincott Williams & Wilkins, 2000.

Michalets EL, "Update: Clinically Significant Cytochrome P-450 Drug Interactions," *Pharmacotherapy*, 1998, 18(1):84-112.

Thummel KE and Wilkinson GR, "*In vitro* and *in vivo* Drug Interactions Involving Human CYP3A," *Annu Rev Pharmacol Toxicol*, 1998, 38:389-430.

Zhang Y and Benet LZ, "The Gut as a Barrier to Drug Absorption: Combined Role of Cytochrome P450 3A and P-Glycoprotein," *Clin Pharmacokinet*, 2001, 40(3):159-68.

Selected Websites

http://www.gentest.com
http://www.imm.ki.se/CYPalleles
http://medicine.iupui.edu/flockhart
http://www.mhc.com/Cytochromes

CYP Substrates

● = major substrate
○ = minor substrate

Drug	1A2	2A6	2B6	2C8/9	2C19	2D6	2E1	3A4
Acetaminophen	○	○		○		○	○	○
Albendazole	○							○
Albuterol								●
Alfentanil								●
Almotriptan						○		○
Alosetron	●			○				○
Alprazolam								●
Aminophylline	●						○	○
Amiodarone	○			●	○	○		●
Amitriptyline	○		○	○	○	●		○
Amlodipine								●
Amoxapine						●		
Amphetamine						○		
Amprenavir				○				●
Aprepitant	○				○			●
Argatroban								○
Aripiprazole						●		●
Aspirin				○				
Atazanavir								●
Atomoxetine					○	●		
Atorvastatin								●
Azelastine	○				○	○		○
Azithromycin								○
Benzphetamine			○					●
Benztropine						○		
Betaxolol	●					●		
Bexarotene								○
Bezafibrate								○
Bisoprolol						○		●
Bortezomib	○			○	○	○		●
Bosentan				●				●
Brinzolamide								○
Bromazepam								●
Bromocriptine								●
Budesonide								●
Bupivacaine	○				○	○		○
Buprenorphine								●
BuPROPion	○	○	●	○		○	○	○
BusPIRone						○		●
Busulfan								●
Caffeine	●			○		○	○	○
Candesartan				○				
Capsaicin							○	

CYTOCHROME P450 ENZYMES: SUBSTRATES, INHIBITORS, AND INDUCERS *(Continued)*

CYP Substrates *(continued)*

Drug	1A2	2A6	2B6	2C8/9	2C19	2D6	2E1	3A4
Captopril						●		
Carbamazepine				○				●
Carisoprodol					●			
Carteolol						○		
Carvedilol	○			●		●	○	○
Celecoxib				○				○
Cerivastatin								●
Cetirizine								○
Cevimeline						○		○
Chlordiazepoxide								●
Chloroquine						●		●
Chlorpheniramine						○		●
ChlorproMAZINE	○					●		○
ChlorproPAMIDE				○				
Chlorzoxazone	○	○				○	●	○
Cilostazol	○				○	○		●
Cinacalcet	○					○		○
Cisapride	○	○	○	○	○			●
Citalopram					●	○		●
Clarithromycin								●
Clobazam					●			●
Clofibrate								○
ClomiPRAMINE	●				●	●		○
Clonazepam								●
Clopidogrel	○							○
Clorazepate								●
Clozapine	●	○		○	○	○		○
Cocaine								●
Codeine[1]						●		○
Colchicine								●
Cyclobenzaprine	●					○		○
Cyclophosphamide[2]		○	●	○	○			●
CycloSPORINE								●
Dacarbazine	●						●	
Dantrolene								●
Dapsone				○	○		○	●
Delavirdine						○		●
Desipramine	○					●		
Desogestrel					●			
Dexamethasone								○
Dexmedetomidine		●						
Dextroamphetamine						●		
Dextromethorphan		○		○	○	●	○	○
Diazepam	○		○	○	●			●
Diclofenac	○		○	○	○	○		○
Digitoxin								●
Digoxin								○
Dihydrocodeine[1]						●		

CYP Substrates *(continued)*

Drug	1A2	2A6	2B6	2C8/9	2C19	2D6	2E1	3A4
Dihydroergotamine								●
Diltiazem				○		○		●
Dirithromycin								○
Disopyramide								●
Disulfiram	○	○	○			○	○	○
Docetaxel								●
Dofetilide								○
Dolasetron				○				○
Domperidone								○
Donepezil						○		○
Dorzolamide				○				○
Doxepin	●					●		●
DOXOrubicin						●		●
Doxycycline								●
Drospirenone								○
Duloxetine	●					●		
Dutasteride								○
Efavirenz			●					●
Eletriptan								●
Enalapril								●
Enflurane							●	
Eplerenone								●
Ergoloid mesylates								●
Ergonovine								●
Ergotamine								●
Erythromycin			○					●
Escitalopram					●			●
Esomeprazole					●			○
Estazolam								○
Estradiol	●	○	○	○	○	○	○	●
Estrogens, conjugated A/synthetic	●	○	○	○	○	○	○	●
Estrogens, conjugated equine	●	○	○	○	○	○	○	●
Estrogens, conjugated esterified	●		○	○			○	●
Estrone	●		○	○			○	●
Estropipate	●		○	○			○	●
Ethinyl estradiol				○				●
Ethosuximide								●
Etonogestrel								○
Etoposide	○						○	●
Exemestane								●
Felbamate							○	●
Felodipine								●
Fenofibrate								○
Fentanyl								●
Fexofenadine								○
Finasteride								○
Flecainide	○					●		
Fluoxetine	○		○	●	○	●	○	○
Fluphenazine						●		

CYTOCHROME P450 ENZYMES: SUBSTRATES, INHIBITORS, AND INDUCERS *(Continued)*

CYP Substrates *(continued)*

Drug	1A2	2A6	2B6	2C8/9	2C19	2D6	2E1	3A4
Flurazepam								●
Flurbiprofen				○				
Flutamide	●							●
Fluticasone								●
Fluvastatin				○		○		○
Fluvoxamine	●					●		
Formoterol		○		○	○	○		
Fosamprenavir (as amprenavir)				○				●
Fosphenytoin (as phenytoin)				●	●			○
Frovatriptan	○							
Fulvestrant								○
Galantamine						○		○
Gefitinib								●
Gemfibrozil								○
Glimepiride				●				
GlipiZIDE				●				
Granisetron								○
Guanabenz	●							
Halazepam								○
Halofantrine				○		○		●
Haloperidol	○					●		●
Halothane		○	○	○		○	●	○
Hydrocodone[1]						●		
Hydrocortisone								○
Ibuprofen				○	○			
Ifosfamide[3]		○	○	○	○			●
Imatinib	○			○	○	○		●
Imipramine	○		○		●	●		○
Imiquimod	○							○
Indinavir						○		●
Indomethacin				○	○			
Irbesartan				○				
Irinotecan			●					●
Isoflurane							●	
Isoniazid							●	
Isosorbide								●
Isosorbide dinitrate								●
Isosorbide mononitrate								●
Isradipine								●
Itraconazole								●
Ivermectin								○
Ketamine			●	●				●
Ketoconazole								●
Labetalol						●		
Lansoprazole				○	●			●
Letrozole		○						●
Levobupivacaine	○							○

CYP Substrates *(continued)*

Drug	1A2	2A6	2B6	2C8/9	2C19	2D6	2E1	3A4
Levonorgestrel								●
Lidocaine	○	○	○	○		●		●
Lomustine						●		
Lopinavir								○
Loratadine						○		○
Losartan				●				●
Lovastatin								●
Maprotiline						●		
MedroxyPROGESTERone								●
Mefenamic acid				○				
Mefloquine								●
Meloxicam				○				○
Mephenytoin			○	●	●			
Mephobarbital			○	○	●			
Mestranol[4]				●				●
Methadone				○	○	○		●
Methamphetamine						●		
Methoxsalen		○						
Methsuximide					●			
Methylergonovine								●
Methylphenidate						●		
MethylPREDNISolone								○
Metoclopramide	○					○		
Metoprolol					○	●		
Mexiletine	●					●		
Miconazole								●
Midazolam			○					●
Mifepristone								○
Miglustat								●
Mirtazapine	●			○		●		●
Moclobemide					●	●		
Modafinil								●
Mometasone furoate								○
Montelukast				●				●
Moricizine								●
Morphine sulfate						○		
Naproxen	○			○				
Nateglinide				●				●
Nefazodone						●		●
Nelfinavir				○	●	○		●
Nevirapine			○			○		●
NiCARdipine	○			○		○	○	●
Nicotine	○	○	○	○	○	○	○	○
NIFEdipine						○		●
Nilutamide					●			
Nimodipine								●
Nisoldipine								●
Nitrendipine								●
Norelgestromin								○
Norethindrone								●
Norgestrel								●

CYTOCHROME P450 ENZYMES: SUBSTRATES, INHIBITORS, AND INDUCERS *(Continued)*

CYP Substrates *(continued)*

Drug	1A2	2A6	2B6	2C8/9	2C19	2D6	2E1	3A4
Nortriptyline	○				○	●		○
Olanzapine	○					○		
Omeprazole		○		○	●	○		○
Ondansetron	○			○		○	○	●
Orphenadrine	○		○			○		○
Oxybutynin								○
Oxycodone[1]						●		
Paclitaxel				●				●
Palonosetron	○					○		○
Pantoprazole					●			○
Paroxetine						●		
Pentamidine					●			
Pergolide								●
Perphenazine	○			○	○	●		○
Phencyclidine								●
Phenobarbital				○	●		○	
Phenytoin				●	●			○
Pimecrolimus								○
Pimozide	●							●
Pindolol						●		
Pioglitazone				●				●
Pipecuronium				○				
Pipotiazine						●		●
Piroxicam				○				
Pravastatin								○
Prazepam								○
PrednisoLONE								○
PredniSONE								○
Primaquine								●
Procainamide						●		
Progesterone	○	○		○	●	○		●
Proguanil	○				○			○
Promethazine			●			●		
Propafenone	○					●		○
Propofol	○	○	●	●	○	○	○	○
Propranolol	●				○	●		○
Protriptyline						●		
Quazepam								○
Quetiapine						○		●
Quinidine				○			○	●
Quinine	○				○			○
Rabeprazole					●			●
Ranitidine	○				○	○		
Repaglinide				●				●
Rifabutin	●							●
Rifampin		●		●				●
Riluzole	●							
Risperidone						●		○

CYP Substrates *(continued)*

Drug	1A2	2A6	2B6	2C8/9	2C19	2D6	2E1	3A4
Ritonavir	○		○			○		●
Rofecoxib				○				
Ropinirole	●							○
Ropivacaine	○		○			○		○
Rosiglitazone				●				
Rosuvastatin				○				○
Saquinavir						○		●
Selegiline	○	○	●	●		○		○
Sertraline			○	○	●	●		○
Sevoflurane		○	○				●	○
Sibutramine								●
Sildenafil				○				●
Simvastatin								●
Sirolimus								●
Spiramycin								●
Sufentanil								●
SulfaDIAZINE				●			○	○
Sulfamethoxazole				●				○
Sulfinpyrazone				●				○
SulfiSOXAZOLE				●				
Suprofen				○				
Tacrine	●							
Tacrolimus								●
Tamoxifen		○	○	●		●	○	●
Tamsulosin						●		●
Telithromycin	○							●
Temazepam			○	○	○			○
Teniposide								●
Terbinafine	○			○	○			○
Testosterone			○	○	○			○
Tetracycline								●
Theophylline	●			○		○	●	●
Thiabendazole	○							
Thioridazine					○	●		
Thiothixene	●							
Tiagabine								●
Ticlopidine								●
Timolol						●		
Tinidazole								○
Tiotropium						○		○
Tizanidine	●							○
TOLBUTamide				●	○			
Tolcapone		○						○
Tolterodine				○	○	●		●
Toremifene	○							●
Torsemide				●				
Tramadol[1]						●		○
Trazodone						○		●
Tretinoin		○	○	○				
Triazolam								●
Trifluoperazine	●							

CYTOCHROME P450 ENZYMES: SUBSTRATES, INHIBITORS, AND INDUCERS *(Continued)*

CYP Substrates *(continued)*

Drug	1A2	2A6	2B6	2C8/9	2C19	2D6	2E1	3A4
Trimethadione				○	○		●	○
Trimethoprim				●				●
Trimipramine					●	●		●
Troleandomycin								●
Valdecoxib				○				○
Valproic acid		○	○	○	○		○	
Vardenafil								●
Venlafaxine				○	○	●		●
Verapamil	○		○	○			○	●
VinBLAStine						○		●
VinCRIStine								●
Vinorelbine						○		●
Voriconazole				●	●			○
Warfarin	○			●	○			○
Yohimbine						○		
Zafirlukast				●				
Zaleplon								○
Zidovudine		○		○	○			○
Zileuton	○			○				○
Ziprasidone	○							○
Zolmitriptan	○							
Zolpidem	○			○	○	○		●
Zonisamide					○			●
Zopiclone				●				●
Zuclopenthixol						●		

[1]This opioid analgesic is bioactivated *in vivo* via CYP2D6. Inhibiting this enzyme would decrease the effects of the analgesic. The active metabolite might also affect, or be affected by, CYP enzymes.

[2]Cyclophosphamide is bioactivated *in vivo* to acrolein via CYP2B6 and 3A4. Inhibiting these enzymes would decrease the effects of cyclophosphamide.

[3]Ifosfamide is bioactivated *in vivo* to acrolein via CYP3A4. Inhibiting this enzyme would decrease the effects of ifosfamide.

[4]Mestranol is bioactivated *in vivo* to ethinyl estradiol via CYP2C8/9. See Ethinyl Estradiol for additional CYP information.

CYP Inhibitors

● = strong inhibitor
◑ = moderate inhibitor
○ = weak inhibitor

Drug	1A2	2A6	2B6	2C8/9	2C19	2D6	2E1	3A4
Acebutolol						○		
Acetaminophen								○
AcetaZOLAMIDE								○
Albendazole	○							
Alosetron	○						○	
Amiodarone	●	◑	○	◑	○	◑		◑
Amitriptyline	○			○	○	○	○	
Amlodipine	◑	○	○	○		○		○
Amphetamine						○		
Amprenavir					○			●
Anastrozole	○			○				○
Aprepitant				○	○			◑
Atazanavir	○			○				●
Atorvastatin								○
Azelastine			○	○	○	○		○
Azithromycin								○
Bepridil						○		
Betamethasone								○
Betaxolol						○		
Biperiden						○		
Bortezomib	○			○	◑	○		○
Bromazepam							○	
Bromocriptine	○							○
Buprenorphine	○	○			○	○		
BuPROPion						○		
Caffeine	●							◑
Candesartan				○				
Celecoxib						○		
Cerivastatin								○
Chloramphenicol				○				○
Chloroquine						◑		
Chlorpheniramine						○		
ChlorproMAZINE						●	○	
Chlorzoxazone							○	○
Cholecalciferol				○	○	○		
Cimetidine	◑			○	◑	◑	○	◑
Cinacalcet						○		
Ciprofloxacin	●							○
Cisapride						○		○
Citalopram	○		○		○	○		
Clarithromycin	○							●
Clemastine						○		○
Clofazimine								○
Clofibrate		○						

CYTOCHROME P450 ENZYMES: SUBSTRATES, INHIBITORS, AND INDUCERS *(Continued)*

CYP Inhibitors *(continued)*

Drug	1A2	2A6	2B6	2C8/9	2C19	2D6	2E1	3A4
ClomiPRAMINE						◑		
Clopidogrel				○				
Clotrimazole	○	○	○	○	○	○	○	◑
Clozapine	○			○	○	◑	○	○
Cocaine						●		○
Codeine						○		
Cyclophosphamide								○
CycloSPORINE				○				◑
Danazol								○
Delavirdine	○			●	●	●		●
Desipramine		◑	◑			◑	○	◑
Dexmedetomidine	○			○		●		○
Dextromethorphan						○		
Diazepam					○			○
Diclofenac	◑			○			○	●
Dihydroergotamine								○
Diltiazem				○		○		◑
Dimethyl sulfoxide				○	○			
DiphenhydrAMINE						◑		
Disulfiram	○	○	○	○		○	●	○
Docetaxel								○
Dolasetron						○		
DOXOrubicin			◑			○		○
Doxycycline								◑
Drospirenone	○			○	○			○
Duloxetine						◑		
Econazole							○	
Efavirenz				◑	◑			◑
Enoxacin	●							●
Entacapone	○	○		○	○	○	○	○
Eprosartan				○				
Ergotamine								○
Erythromycin	○							◑
Escitalopram						○		
Estradiol	○							
Estrogens, conjugated A/synthetic	○							
Estrogens, conjugated equine	○							
Ethinyl estradiol	○		○		○			○
Ethotoin					○			
Etoposide				○				○
Felbamate					○			
Felodipine				○		○		○
Fenofibrate		○		○	○			
Fentanyl								○

CYP Inhibitors *(continued)*

Drug	1A2	2A6	2B6	2C8/9	2C19	2D6	2E1	3A4
Fexofenadine						○		
Flecainide						○		
Fluconazole	○			●	●			◑
Fluoxetine	◑		○	○	◑	●		○
Fluphenazine	○			○		○	○	
Flurazepam							○	
Flurbiprofen				●				
Flutamide	○							
Fluvastatin	○			◑		○		○
Fluvoxamine	●		○	○	●	○		○
Fosamprenavir (as amprenavir)					○			●
Gefitinib					○	○		
Gemfibrozil	◑			●	●			
Glyburide								○
Grapefruit juice								◑
Halofantrine						○		
Haloperidol						◑		◑
HydrALAZINE								○
HydrOXYzine						○		
Ibuprofen				●				
Ifosfamide								○
Imatinib				○		○		●
Imipramine	○				○	◑	○	
Indinavir				○	○	○		●
Indomethacin				●	○			
Interferon alfa-2a	○							
Interferon alfa-2b	○							
Interferon gamma-1b	○						○	
Irbesartan				◑		○		○
Isoflurane			○					
Isoniazid	○	◑		◑	●	◑	◑	●
Isradipine								○
Itraconazole								●
Ketoconazole	●	◑	○	●	◑	◑		●
Ketoprofen				○				
Labetalol						○		
Lansoprazole				○	◑	○		○
Leflunomide				○				
Letrozole		●			○			
Lidocaine	●					◑		◑
Lomefloxacin	○							
Lomustine						○		○
Loratadine					◑	○		
Losartan	○			◑	○			○
Lovastatin				○		○		○
Mefenamic acid				●				
Mefloquine						○		○

CYTOCHROME P450 ENZYMES: SUBSTRATES, INHIBITORS, AND INDUCERS *(Continued)*

CYP Inhibitors *(continued)*

Drug	1A2	2A6	2B6	2C8/9	2C19	2D6	2E1	3A4
Meloxicam				○				
Mephobarbital					○			
Mestranol	○		○		○			○
Methadone						◑		○
Methimazole	○	○	○	○	○	◑	○	○
Methotrimeprazine						○		
Methoxsalen	●	●		○	○	○	○	○
Methsuximide					○			
Methylphenidate						○		
MethylPREDNISolone								○
Metoclopramide						○		
Metoprolol						○		
Metronidazole				○				◑
Metyrapone		○						
Mexiletine	●							
Miconazole	◑	●	○	●	●	●	◑	●
Midazolam				○				○
Mifepristone						○		○
Mirtazapine	○							○
Mitoxantrone								○
Moclobemide	○				○	○		
Modafinil	○	○		○	●		○	○
Montelukast				○				
Nalidixic acid	○							
Nateglinide				○				
Nefazodone	○		○			○		●
Nelfinavir	○		○	○	○	○		●
Nevirapine	○					○		○
NiCARdipine				●	◑	◑		●
Nicotine		○					○	
NIFEdipine	◑			○		○		○
Nilutamide					○			
Nisoldipine	○							○
Nitrendipine								○
Nizatidine								○
Norfloxacin	●							◑
Nortriptyline						○	○	
Ofloxacin	●							
Olanzapine	○			○	○	○		○
Omeprazole	○			◑	●	○		○
Ondansetron	○			○		○		
Orphenadrine	○	○	○	○	○	○	○	○
Oxcarbazepine					○			
Oxprenolol						○		
Oxybutynin						○		○

CYP Inhibitors *(continued)*

Drug	1A2	2A6	2B6	2C8/9	2C19	2D6	2E1	3A4
Pantoprazole				◑				
Paroxetine	○		◑	○	○	●		○
Peginterferon alfa-2a	○							
Peginterferon alfa-2b	○							
Pentamidine				○	○	○		○
Pentoxifylline	○							
Pergolide						●		○
Perphenazine	○					○		
Phencyclidine								○
Pilocarpine		○					○	○
Pimozide					○	○	○	○
Pindolol						○		
Pioglitazone				●	○	◑		
Piroxicam				●				
Pravastatin				○		○		○
Praziquantel						○		
PrednisoLONE								○
Primaquine	●					○		○
Probenecid					○			
Progesterone				○	○			○
Promethazine						○		
Propafenone	○			○		○		
Propofol	◑			○	◑	○	○	●
Propoxyphene				○		○		○
Propranolol	○					○		
Pyrimethamine				◑		◑		
Quinidine				○		●		●
Quinine				◑		●		○
Quinupristin								○
Rabeprazole					◑	○		○
Ranitidine	○					○		
Risperidone						○		○
Ritonavir				○	○	●	○	●
Rofecoxib	○							
Ropinirole	○					●		
Rosiglitazone				◑	○	○		
Saquinavir				○	○	○		◑
Selegiline	○	○		○	○	○	○	○
Sertraline	○		◑	○	◑	◑		◑
Sildenafil	○			○	○	○	○	○
Simvastatin				○		○		
Sirolimus								○
Sulconazole	○	○		○	○	○	○	○
SulfaDIAZINE				●				
Sulfamethoxazole				◑				
Sulfinpyrazone				◑				
SulfiSOXAZOLE				●				
Tacrine	○							

CYTOCHROME P450 ENZYMES: SUBSTRATES, INHIBITORS, AND INDUCERS *(Continued)*

CYP Inhibitors *(continued)*

Drug	1A2	2A6	2B6	2C8/9	2C19	2D6	2E1	3A4
Tacrolimus								○
Tamoxifen			○	○				○
Telithromycin						○		●
Telmisartan					○			
Teniposide				○				○
Tenofovir	○							
Terbinafine						●		
Testosterone								○
Tetracycline								◑
Theophylline	○							
Thiabendazole	●							
Thioridazine	○			○		◑	○	
Thiotepa			○					
Thiothixene						○		
Ticlopidine	○			○	●	◑	○	○
Timolol						○		
Tioconazole	○	○		○	○	○	○	
Tocainide	○							
TOLBUTamide				●				
Tolcapone				○				
Topiramate					○			
Torsemide					○			
Tranylcypromine	◑	●		○	◑	◑	○	○
Trazodone						◑		○
Tretinoin				○				
Triazolam				○				
Trimethoprim				◑				
Tripelennamine						◑		
Triprolidine						○		
Troleandomycin								◑
Valdecoxib				○	○			
Valproic acid				○	○	○		○
Valsartan				○				
Venlafaxine			○			○		○
Verapamil	○			○		○		◑
VinBLAStine						○		○
VinCRIStine								○
Vinorelbine						○		○
Voriconazole				○	○			◑
Warfarin				◑	○			
Yohimbine						○		
Zafirlukast	○			◑	○	○		○
Zileuton	○							
Ziprasidone						○		○

CYP Inducers

● = effectively induced
○ = not effectively induced

Drug	1A2	2A6	2B6	2C8/9	2C19	2D6	2E1	3A4
Aminoglutethimide	●				●			●
Amobarbital		●						
Aprepitant				○				○
Bexarotene								○
Bosentan				○				○
Calcitriol								○
Carbamazepine	●		●	●	●			●
Clofibrate			○				○	○
Colchicine				○			○	○
Cyclophosphamide			○	○				
Dexamethasone		○	○	○				○
Dicloxacillin								○
Efavirenz (in liver only)			○					●
Estradiol								○
Estrogens, conjugated A/synthetic								○
Estrogens, conjugated equine								○
Exemestane								○
Felbamate								○
Fosphenytoin (as phenytoin)			●	●	●			●
Griseofulvin	○			○				○
Hydrocortisone								○
Ifosfamide				○				
Insulin preparations	○							
Isoniazid (after D/C)							○	
Lansoprazole	○							
MedroxyPROGESTERone								○
Mephobarbital		○						
Metyrapone								○
Modafinil	○		○					○
Moricizine	○							○
Nafcillin								●
Nevirapine			●					●
Norethindrone					○			
Omeprazole	○							
Oxcarbazepine								●
Paclitaxel								○
Pantoprazole	○							○
Pentobarbital		●						●
Phenobarbital	●	●	●	●				●
Phenytoin			●	●	●			●
Pioglitazone								○
PredniSONE					○			○
Primaquine	○							

CYTOCHROME P450 ENZYMES: SUBSTRATES, INHIBITORS, AND INDUCERS *(Continued)*

CYP Inducers *(continued)*

Drug	1A2	2A6	2B6	2C8/9	2C19	2D6	2E1	3A4
Primidone[1]	●		●	●				●
Rifabutin								●
Rifampin	●	●	●	●	●			●
Rifapentine				●				●
Ritonavir (long-term)	○			○				○
Rofecoxib								○
Secobarbital		●		●				
Sulfinpyrazone								○
Terbinafine								○
Topiramate								○
Tretinoin							○	
Troglitazone								○
Valproic acid		○						

[1]Primidone is partially metabolized to phenobarbital. See Phenobarbital for additional CYP information.

EXTRAVASATION TREATMENT

Medication Extravasated	Cold/Warm Pack	Antidote
	VESICANTS	
Direct Cellular Toxins – Chemotherapeutic Agents		
DNA Intercalators		
Daunorubicin Doxorubicin Epirubicin Idarubicin	Cold	DMSO: Apply to area twice the size of the extravasation; repeat every 6 hours for up to 14 days; allow to air dry; do not cover with dressing
Vinca alkaloids		
Paclitaxel[1] Vinblastine Vincristine Vinorelbine	Warm	*Hyaluronidase 1. Add 1 mL NS to 150 units vial to make 150 units/mL concentration 2. Administer 0.2 mL injection subcutaneously or intradermally into the extravasation site at the leading edge **Note:** Some institutions utilize a 1:10 dilution in infants and children; prepare by mixing 0.1 mL of 150 units/mL solution with 0.9 mL NS in 1 mL syringe to make final concentration = 15 units/mL *Currently unavailable; expected availability late 2004 or early 2005
Alkylating agents		
Cisplatin	Cold	Sodium thiosulfate 1/6 molar solution: mix 4 mL of 10% sodium thiosulfate with 6 mL of sterile water; inject 3-5 mL (use only for large cisplatinum infiltrates >20 mL and when using cisplatinum concentrations >0.5 mg/mL; no data for use in cisplatinum infusions in children)
Mechlorethamine (Nitrogen mustard)		Sodium thiosulfate 1/6 molar solution: mix 4 mL of 10% sodium thiosulfate with 6 mL of sterile water; inject 0.5 mL for each mg mechlorethamine extravasated
Other vesicant chemotherapeutic agents		
Dactinomycin Mitomycin C Mitoxantrone Plicamycin	Cold	None
Ischemic Inducers		
Dobutamine Dopamine Epinephrine Norepinephrine Phenylephrine Vasopressin	None	Phentolamine (Regitine®) Mix 5 mg with 9 mL of NS Inject a small amount of this dilution into extravasated area. Blanching should reverse immediately. Monitor site. If blanching should recur, additional injections of phentolamine may be needed.

EXTRAVASATION TREATMENT *(Continued)*

Medication Extravasated	Cold/Warm Pack	Antidote
Miscellaneous Agents		
Aminophylline Calcium salts Dextrose (>10%) Mannitol (>5%) Phenytoin Contrast media Sodium bicarbonate (8.4%) Sodium chloride (>0.9%) Tetracycline	Cold	Hyaluronidase As described above
	IRRITANTS	
Arsenic trioxide	Warm	
Bleomycin	Cold	
Carboplatin ≥10 mg/mL	Cold	
Carmustine	Cold	
Cisplatin (concentration <0.5 mg/mL or <20 mL of more concentrated solution)	Cold	
Cyclophosphamide	Cold	Inject 5 mL 1/6 molar sodium thiosulfate (mix 4 mL 10% sodium thriosulfate with 6 mL sterile water)
Dacarbazine	Cold	DMSO as described above
Daunorubicin citrate (liposomal)	Cold	
Dexrazoxane	None	
Docetaxel	Warm	
Doxorubicin, liposomal	Cold	
Etoposide	Warm	Hyaluronidase as described above; use only for large infiltration
Fluorouracil	Cold	
Gemcitabine	Warm	
Gemtuzumab	None	
Ifosfamide	Cold	DMSO as described above
Irinotecan	Cold	
Oxaliplatin	None	Inject 5 mL 1/6 molar sodium thiosulfate (mix 4 mL 10% soldium thiosulfate with 6 mL sterile water)
Teniposide	Warm	Hyaluronidase as described above
Topotecan	Cold	

Note:

Extravasation: The unintentional leakage of pharmacologic and physiologic solutions into the perivascular, subcutaneous, or interstitial space.

Vesicants: Agents that cause redness, pain, and blistering when infiltrated and can progress to ulceration and tissue necrosis.

Irritants: Agents that cause redness at the injection site or along the vein and often include a mild pruritic allergic reaction related to histamine release. These reaction "flares" usually do not require intervention and subside in 30 minutes.

[1]Some references consider agent as an irritant instead of vesicant.

References

Bertelli G, "Prevention and Management of Extravasation of Cytotoxic Drugs, *Drug Saf*, 1995, 12(4):245-55.

Camp-Sorrell D, "Developing Extravasation Protocols and Monitoring Outcomes," *J Intraven Nurs*, 1998, 21(4):232-9.

Cohan RH, Ellis JH, and Garner WL, "Extravasation of Radiographic Contrast Material: Recognition, Prevention, and Treatment", *Radiology*, 1996, 200(3):593-604.

Dorr RT, "Pharmacologic Management of Vesicant Chemotherapy Extravasations," *Cancer Chemotherapy Handbook*, 2nd ed, Norwalk CT: Appleton & Lange, 1994.

Finely RS, et al, *Concepts in Oncology and Therapeutics*, 2nd ed, Bethesda MS: Am Soc Heal Sys Rx, 1998.

Fenchel K and Karthaus M, "Cytotoxic Drug Extravasation," *Antibiot Chemother*, 2000, 50:144-8.

Kassner E, "Evaluation and Treatment of Chemotherapy Extravasation Injuries," *J Pediatr Oncol Nurs*, 2000, 17(3):135-48.

NIH, Standards of Practice: Care of the Patient Receiving I.V. Cytoxic or Biologic Agents, 2001.

Mullin S, Beckwith M, and Tyler L, "Prevention and Management of Antineoplastic Extravasation Injury," *Hosp Pharm*, 2000, 35:57-74.

BURN MANAGEMENT

Modified Lund-Browder Burn Assessment Chart
Estimation of Total Body Surface Area of Burn Involvement[1]
(% by site and age)

The total body surface area of burn involvement is determined by the sum of the percentages of each site.

Site[2]	0-1 years	1-4 years	5-9 years	10-14 years	15 years	Adult
Head	9.5	8.5	6.5	5.5	4.5	3.5
Neck	0.5	0.5	0.5	0.5	0.5	0.5
Trunk	13	13	13	13	13	13
Upper arm	2	2	2	2	2	2
Forearm	1.5	1.5	1.5	1.5	1.5	1.5
Hand	1.5	1.5	1.5	1.5	1.5	1.5
Perineum	1	1	1	1	1	1
Buttock (each)	2.5	2.5	2.5	2.5	2.5	2.5
Thigh	2.75	3.25	4	4.25	4.5	4.75
Leg	2.5	2.5	2.75	3	3.25	3.5
Foot	1.75	1.75	1.75	1.75	1.75	1.75

[1]Applies only to second- and third-degree burns

[2]Percentage for each site is only for **a single extremity with** anterior **OR** posterior involvement. Percentage should be **doubled if both anterior and posterior** involvement of a single extremity.

Adapted from Coren CV, "Burn Injuries in Children," *Pediatric Annals*, 1987, 16(4):328-39.

Parkland Fluid Replacement Formula

A guideline for replacement of deficits and ongoing losses (**Note:** For infants, maintenance fluids may need to be added to this): Administer 4 mL/kg/% burn of Ringer's lactate (glucose may be added but beware of stress hyperglycemia) over the first 24 hours; half of this total is given over the first 8 hours **calculated from the time of injury**; the remaining half is given over the next 16 hours. The second 24-hour fluid requirements average 50% to 75% of first day's requirement. Concentrations and rates best determined by monitoring weight, serum electrolytes, urine output, NG losses, etc.

Colloid may be added after 18-24 hours (1 g/kg/day of albumin) to maintain serum albumin >2 g/100 mL.

Potassium is generally withheld for the first 48 hours due to the large amount of potassium that is released from damaged tissues. To manage serum electrolytes, monitor urine electrolytes twice weekly and replace calculated urine losses.

ORAL CONTRACEPTIVES

Brand Name	Type	Progestin	Estrogen	Availability
Alesse® Aviane™ Lessina™ Levlite™	Combo	Levonorgestrel 0.1 mg	Ethinyl estradiol 20 mcg	21, 28
Brevicon® Modicon® Necon® 0.5/35 Nortrel™ 0.5/35	Combo	Norethindrone 0.5 mg	Ethinyl estradiol 35 mcg	21, 28
Demulen® 1/35 Zovia™ 1/35E	Combo	Ethynodiol diacetate 1 mg	Ethinyl estradiol 35 mcg	21, 28
Demulen® 1/50 [DSC] Zovia™ 1/50E	Combo	Ethynodiol diacetate 1 mg	Ethinyl estradiol 50 mcg	21, 28
Levlen® Levora® Nordette® Portia™ Seasonale®	Combo	Levonorgestrel 0.15 mg	Ethinyl estradiol 30 mcg	21, 28
Lo/Ovral® Cryselle™ Low-Ogestrel®	Combo	Norgestrel 0.3 mg	Ethinyl estradiol 30 mcg	21, 28
Loestrin 21® 1/20	Combo	Norethindrone acetate 1 mg	Ethinyl estradiol 20 mcg	21
Loestrin 21® 1.5/30	Combo	Norethindrone acetate 1.5 mg	Ethinyl estradiol 30 mcg	21
Necon® 1/35 Nortrel™ 1/35 Norinyl® 1+35 Ortho-Novum® 1/35	Combo	Norethindrone 1 mg	Ethinyl estradiol 35 mcg	21, 28
Necon® 1/50 Norinyl® 1+50	Combo	Norethindrone 1 mg	Mestranol 50 mcg	21, 28
Ortho-Cept® Apri® Desogen®	Combo	Desogestrel 0.15 mg	Ethinyl estradiol 30 mcg	28
Ortho-Cyclen® MonoNessa™ Sprintec™	Combo	Norgestimate 0.25 mg	Ethinyl estradiol 35 mcg	21, 28
Ovcon® 35	Combo	Norethindrone 0.4 mg	Ethinyl estradiol 35 mcg	21, 28
Ovcon® 50	Combo	Norethindrone 1 mg	Ethinyl estradiol 50 mcg	21, 28
Ogestrel® 0.5/50 Ovral® [DSC]	Combo	Norgestrel 0.5 mg	Ethinyl estradiol 50 mcg	21, 28
Yasmin®	Combo	Drospirenone 3 mg	Ethinyl estradiol 30 mcg	28
Loestrin® Fe 1/20 Junel™ Fe 1/20 Microgestin™ Fe 1/20	Combo / Iron 21-28 d	Norethindrone acetate 1 mg	Ethinyl estradiol 20 mcg	28
Loestrin® Fe 1.5/30 Junel™ Fe 1.5/30 Microgestin™ Fe 1.5/30	Combo / Iron 21-28 d	Norethindrone acetate 1.5 mg	Ethinyl estradiol 30 mcg	28
Nelova™ 10/11 [DSC]	Biphasic			
	1-10 d	Norethindrone 0.5 mg	Ethinyl estradiol 35 mcg	21, 28
	11-21 d	Norethindrone 1 mg	Ethinyl estradiol 35 mcg	
	22-28 d	Inert	—	

ORAL CONTRACEPTIVES *(Continued)*

Brand Name	Type	Progestin	Estrogen	Availability
Ortho-Novum® 10/11 Necon® 10/11	Biphasic			
	1-10 d	Norethindrone 0.5 mg	Ethinyl estradiol 35 mcg	21, 28
	11-21 d	Norethindrone 1 mg	Ethinyl estradiol 35 mcg	
	22-28 d	Inert	—	
Estrostep® 21	Triphasic			
	1-5 d	Norethindrone acetate 1 mg	Ethinyl estradiol 20 mcg	21
	6-12 d	Norethindrone acetate 1 mg	Ethinyl estradiol 30 mcg	
	13-21 d	Norethindrone acetate 1 mg	Ethinyl estradiol 35 mcg	
Ortho-Novum® 7/7/7 Necon® 7/7/7	Triphasic			
	1-7 d	Norethindrone 0.5 mg	Ethinyl estradiol 35 mcg	21, 28
	8-14 d	Norethindrone 0.75 mg	Ethinyl estradiol 35 mcg	
	15-21 d	Norethindrone 1 mg	Ethinyl estradiol 35 mcg	
	22-28 d	Inert	—	
Ortho Tri-Cyclen® TriNessa™ Tri-Sprintec™	Triphasic			
	1-7 d	Norgestimate 0.18 mg	Ethinyl estradiol 35 mcg	21, 28
	8-14 d	Norgestimate 0.215 mg	Ethinyl estradiol 35 mcg	
	15-21 d	Norgestimate 0.25 mg	Ethinyl estradiol 35 mcg	
	22-28 d	Inert	—	
Ortho Tri-Cyclen® Lo	Triphasic			
	1-7 d	Norgestimate 0.18 mg	Ethinyl estradiol 25 mcg	21, 28
	8-14 d	Norgestimate 0.215 mg	Ethinyl estradiol 25 mcg	
	15-21 d	Norgestimate 0.25 mg	Ethinyl estradiol 25 mcg	
Tri-Norinyl®	Triphasic			
	1-7 d	Norethindrone 0.5 mg	Ethinyl estradiol 35 mcg	21, 28
	8-16 d	Norethindrone 1 mg	Ethinyl estradiol 35 mcg	
	17-21 d	Norethindrone 0.5 mg	Ethinyl estradiol 35 mcg	
	22- 28 d	Inert	—	
Triphasil® Tri-Levlen® Enpresse™ Trivora®	Triphasic			
	1-6 d	Levonorgestrel 0.05 mg	Ethinyl estradiol 30 mcg	21, 28
	7-11 d	Levonorgestrel 0.075 mg	Ethinyl estradiol 40 mcg	
	12-21 d	Levonorgestrel 0.125 mg	Ethinyl estradiol 30 mcg	
	22-28 d	Inert	—	

Brand Name	Type	Progestin	Estrogen	Availability
Velivet™ Cyclessa®	Triphasic 1-7 d 8-14 d 15-21 d 22-28 d	 Desogestrel 0.1 mg Desogestrel 0.125 mg Desogestrel 0.15 mg Inert	 Ethinyl estradiol 25 mcg Ethinyl estradiol 25 mcg Ethinyl estradiol 25 mcg —	28
Estrostep® Fe	Triphasic / Iron 22-28 d 1-5 d 6-12 d 13-21 d	 Norethindrone acetate 1 mg Norethindrone acetate 1 mg Norethindrone acetate 1 mg	 Ethinyl estradiol 20 mcg Ethinyl estradiol 30 mcg Ethinyl estradiol 35 mcg	28
Micronor® Camila™ Errin™ Jolivette™ Nora-BE™ Nor-QD®	Progestin only	Norethindrone 0.35 mg	—	28
Ovrette®	Progestin only	Norgestrel 0.075 mg	—	28

Combo = monophasic combination.

Monophasic Oral Contraceptives in Order of Decreasing Estrogen Content

Estrogen	Brand Name (Progestin Content)
Mestranol 50 mcg	Necon® 1/50, Norinyl® 1+50 **(Norethindrone 1 mg)**
Ethinyl estradiol 50 mcg	Demulen® 1/50 [DSC], Zovia™ 1/50E **(Ethynodiol diacetate 1 mg)**
	Ovcon®-50 **(Norethindrone 1 mg)**
	Ogestrel® 0.5/50, Ovral® [DSC] **(Norgestrel 0.5 mg)**
Ethinyl estradiol 35 mcg	Necon® 1/35, Nelova® 1/35E [DSC], Norinyl® 1+35, Nortrel® 1/35, Ortho-Novum® 1/35 **(Norethindrone 1 mg)**
	Brevicon®, Modicon®, Necon® 0.5/35, Nortrel® 0.5/35 **(Norethindrone 0.5 mg)**
	Ovcon®-35 **(Norethindrone 0.4 mg)**
	MonoNessa™, Ortho-Cyclen®, Sprintec™ **(Norgestimate 0.25 mg)**
	Demulen® 1/35, Zovia™ 1/35E **(Ethynodiol diacetate 1 mg)**
Ethinyl estradiol 30 mcg	Junel™ Fe 1.5/30, Loestrin 21® 1.5/30, Loestrin® Fe 1.5/30, Microgestin™ Fe 1.5/30 **(Norethindrone acetate 1.5 mg)**
	Cryselle™, Lo/Ovral®, Low-Ogestrel™ **(Norgestrel 0.3 mg)**
	Apri®, Desogen®, Ortho-Cept® **(Desogestrel 0.15 mg)**
	Levlen®, Levora®, Nordette®, Portia™, Seasonale® **(Levonorgestrel 0.15 mg)**
	Yasmin® **(Drospirenone 3 mg)**
Ethinyl estradiol 20 mcg	Alesse®, Aviane™, Lessina™, Levlite™ **(Levonorgestrel 0.1 mg)**
	Junel™ Fe 1/20, Loestrin 21® 1/20, Loestrin® Fe 1/20, Microgestin™ Fe 1/20 **(Norethindrone acetate 1 mg)**

ORAL CONTRACEPTIVES *(Continued)*

Hormonal Effects of Progestins

	Progestin Effect	Estrogen Effect	Antiestrogen Effect	Androgen Effect
Norethynodrel	+1	+3	0	0
Norethindrone	+1	+1 (low dose)	+1 (higher doses)	+2
Norethindrone acetate	+1	+1	+3	+2
Ethynodiol diacetate	+2	+1 (low dose)	+1 (higher doses)	+2
Norgestimate	+3	0	+3	0
Desogestrel	+3	0/+1	+3	0/+1
Norgestrel/ levonorgestrel	+3	0	+2	+3

0 = no effect; +1 = slight effect; +2 = moderate effect; +3 = pronounced effect.

Adapted from *Facts and Comparisons*, St Louis, MO: Facts and Comparisons, Inc, 1996.

Signs / Symptoms of Hormonal Imbalance With Oral Contraceptives

Estrogen Excess	Fluid retention, edema, cyclic weight gain, "bloating," hypertension, breast fullness/tenderness, nausea, migraine headache, melasma, telangiectasia, cervical mucorrhea, and polyposis
Estrogen Deficiency	Increased spotting, early or midcycle breakthrough bleeding, hypomenorrhea
Progestin Excess	Fatigue, lethargy, depression, decreased libido, increased appetite, weight gain, breast regression, monilial vaginitis, hypomenorrhea, hair loss, hirsutism, acne, oily scalp. **Note:** Hair loss, hirsutism, acne, and oily scalp are effects of the androgenic activity of progestins.
Progestin Deficiency	Amenorrhea, late breakthrough bleeding, hypermenorrhea

FLUIDS, ELECTROLYTES, AND NUTRITION

ENTERAL NUTRITIONAL PRODUCT FORMULARY, INFANTS

Milk Based Formulas[1]

(Indications: Feeding normal term infants or sick infants without special nutritional requirements)

	Human Milk	Enfamil® With Iron	Similac® With Iron
Calories /100 mL	67	68	68
Protein g/100 mL	1.0	1.45	1.40
Protein source	Mature Term human milk	Nonfat milk whey	Nonfat milk whey protein concentrate
Carbohydrate g/100 mL	6.8	7.3	7.3
Carbohydrate source	Lactose	Lactose	Lactose
Fat g/100 mL	4.0	3.6	3.65
Fat source	Human milk, fat	Palm olein, coconut, soy, and high oleic sunflower oils	High oleic safflower, soy and coconut oils
Osmolality mOsm/kg	300	300	300
Sodium mEq/L (mg/L)	7.8 (180)	8 (183)	6.8 (162)
Potassium mEq/L (mg/L)	13.5 (525)	18.7 (730)	18.2 (710)
Chloride mEq/L (mg/L)	11.9 (420)	12 (426)	12.2 (433)
Calcium mEq/L (mg/L)	14 (280)	26.4 (528)	26.4 (527)
Phosphorus mEq/L (mg/L)	9 (140)	20.5 (358)	18.8 (284)
Iron mg/L	0.3	12.2 (4.7)[2]	12.2 (4.7)[2]

[1]Information based on manufacturer's literature as of 2001 and is subject to change.

[2]Low iron formulation in parenthesis.

FLUIDS, ELECTROLYTES, AND NUTRITION *(Continued)*

Hypercaloric Milk Based Formulas – 24[1,2]
(Indications: Fluid restriction, increased caloric demands)

	Enfamil® 24	Similac® 24
Calories /100 mL	81	80.6
Protein g/100 mL	1.74	2.2
Protein source	Nonfat milk and whey	Nonfat milk
Carbohydrate g/100 mL	8.8	8.5
Carbohydrate source	Lactose	Lactose
Fat g/100 mL	4.3	4.25
Fat source	Palm olein, coconut, soy, and high oleic sunflower oils	Soy and coconut oils
Osmolality mOsm/kg	360	380
Sodium mEq/L (mg/L)	9.6 (220)	12.1 (280)
Potassium mEq/L (mg/L)	22.3 (870)	27.4 (1070)
Chloride mEq/L (mg/L)	14.4 (510)	18.6 (660)
Calcium mEq/L (mg/L)	31.4 (628)	36.4 (730)
Phosphorus mEq/L (mg/L)	27.6 (427)	36.5 (565)
Iron mg/L	14.6 (5.7)[3]	14.5

[1]Information based on manufacturer's literature as of 2001 and is subject to change; 24 calories/oz

[2]To approximate values for the content of a 30 cal/oz formula (made by dilution of a powder formulation) multiply the value desired, found in a 20 cal/oz formula, by 1.5 (20 cal/oz formula contents for Enfamil® and Similac® are listed in preceding Milk Based Formula chart). For example, the fat in a 30 cal/oz Enfamil® formula = 1.5 x 3.6 = 5.4 g/100 mL.

[3]Low iron formulation in parentheses

Soy Formulas[1]

(Indications: Lactose deficiency, milk intolerance, or galactosemia)

	Prosobee®	Isomil®
Calories /100 mL	68	67.6
Protein g/100 mL	2	1.7
Protein source	Soy protein isolate L-methionine	Soy protein isolate L-methionine
Carbohydrate g/100 mL	6.8	6.9
Carbohydrate source	Corn syrup solids	Corn syrup and sucrose
Fat g/100 mL	3.6	3.69
Fat source	Palm olein, coconut, soy, and high oleic sunflower oils	High oleic safflower, soy and coconut oils
Osmolality mOsm/kg	200	200
Sodium mEq/L (mg/L)	10.6 (240)	12.8 (297)
Potassium mEq/L (mg/L)	20.6 (810)	18.9 (730)
Chloride mEq/L (mg/L)	14.7 (540)	11.5 (419)
Calcium mEq (mg/L)	35.5 (710)	35.1 (710)
Phosphorus mEq/L (mg/L)	36 (560)	32.9 (507)
Iron mg/L	12.2	12

[1]Information based on manufacturer's literature as of 2001 and is subject to change.

FLUIDS, ELECTROLYTES, AND NUTRITION *(Continued)*

Hypercaloric Soy Formulas – 24[1,2]
(Indications: Fluid restriction, increased caloric demands)

	Prosobee® 24
Calories /100 mL	81.1
Protein g/100 mL	2.4
Protein source	Soy protein isolate
Carbohydrate g/100 mL	8.2
Carbohydrate source	Corn syrup solids
Fat g/100 mL	4.3
Fat source	Palm olein, coconut, soy, and high oleic sunflower oils
Osmolality mOsm/kg	240
Sodium mEq/L (mg/L)	12.7 (292)
Potassium mEq/L (mg/L)	25.2 (990)
Chloride mEq/L (mg/L)	19 (672)
Calcium mEq/L (mg/L)	38 (761)
Phosphorus mEq/L (mg/L)	38.9 (602)
Iron mg/L	15.2

[1]Information based on manufacturer's literature as of 2001 and is subject to change.

[2]To approximate values for the content of a 27 or 30 cal/oz formula (made by dilution of a powder based formulation), multiply the value desired, found in the 20 cal/oz formula (20 cal/oz formula contents for Prosobee® are listed in the preceding Soy Formulas chart), by the following factors: 1.35 (27 cal/oz) or 1.5 (30 cal/oz).

Casein Hydrolysate Formulas[1]

(Indication: For infants whose renal or cardiovascular functions would benefit from lowered mineral levels)

	Similac® PM 60/40
Calories /100 mL	67.6
Protein g/100 mL	1.5
Protein source	Whey and caseinate
Carbohydrate g/100 mL	6.9
Carbohydrate source	Lactose
Fat g/100 mL	3.78
Fat source	Corn, soy and coconut oils
Osmolality mOsm/kg	280
Sodium mEq/L (mg/L)	6.8 (162)
Potassium mEq/L (mg/L)	14.9 (580)
Chloride mEq/L (mg/L)	11.5 (400)
Calcium mEq/L (mg/L)	19 (380)
Phosphorus mEq/L (mg/L)	12.3 (190)
Iron mg/L	4.7
Special uses	Renal and cardiovascular disease

[1]Information based on manufacturer's literature as of 2001 and is subject to change.

FLUIDS, ELECTROLYTES, AND NUTRITION *(Continued)*

Casein Hydrolysate Formulas[1,2]

(Indication: For infants requiring low molecular weight peptides or amino acids)

	Nutramigen®	Pregestimil®	Alimentum®
Calories /100 mL	68	68	67.6
Protein g/100 mL	1.9	1.9	1.9
Protein source	Casein hydrolysate, L-cystine, L-tyrosine, and L-tryptophan	Casein hydrolysate, L-cystine, L-tyrosine, and L-tryptophan	Casein hydrolysate, L-cystine, L-tyrosine, and L-tryptophan
Carbohydrate g/100 mL	7.4	6.8	6.9
Carbohydrate source	Corn syrup solids and modified corn starch	Corn syrup solids, dextrose, and modified corn starch	Sucrose and modified tapioca starch
Fat g/100 mL	3.4	3.8	3.7
Fat source	Palm olein, soy, coconut, and high oleic sunflower oils	MCT oil, corn oil, and high oleic sunflower oil	Safflower, medium chain triglycerides, and soy oils
Osmolality mOsm/kg	320	320	370
Sodium mEq/L (mg/L)	13.8 (318)	11.5 (264)	12.8 (297)
Potassium mEq/L (mg/L)	19 (744)	18.9 (737)	20.3 (797)
Chloride mEq/L (mg/L)	16.4 (582)	16.4 (581)	15.5 (540)
Calcium mEq/L (mg/L)	31.8 (636)	31.8 (636)	35 (709)
Phosphorus mEq/L (mg/L)	27.3 (426)	28 (430)	32.7 (507)
Iron mg/L	12.2	12.8	12.2
Special uses	Sensitivity to intact proteins, galactosemia	Malabsorption, cystic fibrosis	Sensitivity to intact proteins, protein maldigest or fat malabsorption

[1]Information based on manufacturer's literature as of 2001 and is subject to change.

[2]To approximate values for the content of a 24, 27, or 30 cal/oz formula (made by dilution of a powder based formulation), multiply the value desired, found in the above 20 cal/oz formula, by the following factors: 1.2 (24 cal/oz), 1.35 (27 cal/oz), or 1.5 (30 cal/oz).

Other Infant and Pediatric Formulas[1] – Special Care

(Indication: Premature infant formulas designed for rapidly growing LBW infants)

	Preterm Human Milk	Preterm Human Milk + Similac® HMF[2] (1 pkt: 50 mL)	Special Care 20 With Fe	Special Care 24 With Fe	Neosure
Calories /100 mL	67	73	67.6	81	74.6
Protein g/100 mL	1.4	1.9	1.83	2.2	2
Protein source	Preterm human milk	Preterm human milk, nonfat milk and whey protein concentrate	Nonfat milk and whey protein concentrate	Nonfat milk and whey protein concentrate	Nonfat milk and whey protein concentrate
Carbohydrate g/100 mL	6.6	7.4	7.17	8.6	7.7
Carbohydrate source	Lactose	Corn syrup solids and lactose	Corn syrup solids and lactose	Corn syrup solids and lactose	Maltodextrin and lactose
Fat g/100 mL	3.9	4.0	3.67	4.4	4
Fat source	Preterm human milk	Preterm human milk, medium chain triglycerides	Medium chain triglycerides, soy, and coconut oils	Medium chain triglycerides, soy, and coconut oils	Medium chain triglycerides, soy, and coconut oils
Osmolality mOsm/kg	290	343	235	280	250
Sodium mEq/L (mg/L)	10.7 (248)	13.9 (321)	12.8 (290)	15.2 (350)	10.4 (246)
Potassium mEq/L (mg/L)	14.8 (570)	26.6 (1040)	22.3 (870)	26.6 (1045)	27 1060
Chloride mEq/L (mg/L)	15.4 (550)	20.4 (730)	15.5 (550)	18.6 (660)	15.7 (560)
Calcium mEq/L (mg/L)	15.4 (550)	40.9 (818)	60.8 (1220)	72.6 (1452)	39 (784)
Phosphorus mEq/L (mg/L)	8.2 (128)	29 (453)	43.7 (676)	47 (726)	29.6 (460)
Iron mg/L	1.2	2.9	12.2 (2.7)[3]	14.6 (3.2)[3]	13.4

[1]Information based on manufacturer's literature as of 2001 and is subject to change.

[2]HMF = human milk fortifier

[3]Low iron formulation in parentheses.

FLUIDS, ELECTROLYTES, AND NUTRITION *(Continued)*

ENTERAL FORMULAS – PEDIATRIC

(A selection of the commonly used enteral feedings for children 1-10 years of age)

	Pediasure®	**Peptamen Junior®**	**Vivonex® Pediatric**	**Boost®**	**Carnation Instant Breakfast®[1]**	**Ensure®**	**Kindercal®**
Calories/oz	30	30	24	30	27	31	30
Calories/mL	1.0	1.06	0.8	1.0	0.93	1.04	1.0
Carbohydrate g/100 mL	11	13.8	13	17.4	14.4	16.7	13.5
Carbohydrate source	Maltodextrin, sucrose	Maltodextrin, corn starch	Maltodextrin, modified starch	Sucrose, corn syrup solids	Maltodextrin, sucrose, lactose	Maltodextrin, sucrose	Maltodextrin, sucrose
Protein g/100 mL	3.0	3.0	2.4	4.2	4.4	3.7	3.4
Protein source	Caseinate, whey protein conc	Hydrolyzed whey protein	L-amino acids	Milk protein conc	Nonfat milk	Caseinates, soy protein isolate	Caseinates
Fat g/100 mL	5.0	3.8	2.4	1.7	1.9	2.5	4.4
Fat source	High oleic safflower, soy, and MCT oils	MCT, soy, and canola oils	MCT and soy solids	Canola, sunflower, and corn oils	Butterfat	Corn oil	Canola, high oleic sunflower, corn, and MCT oils
Osmolality mOsm/kg	335	260 unflavored 360 vanilla	360	590-620	661-747	590	310
Sodium mg/100 mL (mEq/100 mL)	38 (1.7)	46 (2)	40 (1.7)	55 (2.4)	90 (3.9)	83 (3.6)	37 (1.6)
Potassium mg/100 mL (mEq/100 mL)	131 (3.4)	132 (3.4)	120 (3.1)	169 (4.3)	250 (6.4)	154 (3.9)	131 (3.3)
Iron (mg/100 mL)	1.4	1.4	1.0	1.5	—	1.9	1.1

[1]Mixed with 2% milk as directed.

ENTERAL FORMULAS – ADOLESCENTS, ADULTS

	Isocal®	**Osmolite®**	**Osmolite HN®**	**Jevity®**
Calories/mL	1.06	1.06	1.06	1.06
Carbohydrate g/100 mL	13.5	14.8	14.4	15.0
Carbohydrate source	Maltodextrin	Maltodextrin and corn syrup solids	Maltodextrin and corn syrup solids	Maltodextrin and corn syrup solids
Protein g/100 mL	3.4	3.7	4.4	4.4
Protein source	Caseinate, soy protein isolate	Caseinate, soy protein isolate	Caseinate, soy protein isolate	Caseinates
Fat g/100 mL	4.4	3.4	3.5	3.5
Fat source	Soy oil, MCT oil	High oleic safflower, canola, and MCT oils	High oleic safflower, canola, and MCT oils	High oleic safflower, canola, and MCT oils
Osmolality mOsm/kg	270	300	300	300
Sodium mg/100 mL (mEq/100 mL)	53 (2.3)	63 (2.7)	92 (4.0)	91.6 (4.0)
Potassium mg/100 mL (mEq/100 mL)	132 (3.4)	100 (2.6)	157 (4.0)	157 (4.0)

[1]Contains 13.6 g/L soy fiber.

FLUIDS, ELECTROLYTES, AND NUTRITION *(Continued)*

ENTERAL FORMULAS WITH HIGH CALORIC DENSITY

	Ensure Plus®	Ensure Plus HN®	Comply®	TraumaCal®	Deliver®
Calories/mL	1.5	1.5	1.5	1.5	2
Carbohydrate g/100 mL	20.8	19.7	18	14.2	20
Carbohydrate source	Corn syrup solids, maltodextrin, sucrose	Maltodextrin, sucrose	Maltodextrin	Corn syrup solids, sucrose	Corn syrup
Protein g/100 mL	5.4	6.2	6.0	8.2	7.5
Protein source	Caseinate, soy protein isolate	Caseinate, soy protein isolate	Caseinates	Caseinates	Caseinates
Fat g/100 mL	4.8	4.9	6.1	6.8	10.2
Fat source	Canola, high oleic safflower and corn oils	Corn oil	Canola, high oleic sunflower, MCT and corn oils	Soy oil, MCT oil	Soy oil, MCT oil
Osmolality mOsm/kg	690	650	460	580	640
Sodium mg/100 mL (mEq/100 mL)	100 (4.3)	117 (5.1)	120 (5.2)	118 (5.1)	80 (3.5)
Potassium mg/100 mL (mEq/100 mL)	183 (4.7)	179 (4.6)	185 (4.7)	140 (3.6)	168 (4.3)

ENTERAL FORMULAS WITH MODIFIED PROTEIN – "ELEMENTAL"

Adolescents and Adults

	Criticare HN®	**Peptamen®**	**Tolerex®**	**Vivonex Plus®**
Calories/mL	1.06	1.0	1.0	1.0
Carbohydrate g/100 mL	22	12.7	23	19.0
Carbohydrate source	Maltodextrin, modified corn starch	Maltodextrin, corn starch	Maltodextrin	Maltodextrin, modified starch
Protein g/100 mL	3.8	4.0	2.1	4.5
Protein source	Hydrolyzed casein, L-amino acids	Hydrolyzed whey	L-amino acids	L-amino acids
Fat g/100 mL	0.53	3.9	0.15	0.67
Fat source	Safflower oil	Sunflower and MCT oils	Safflower oil	Soy oil
Osmolality mOsm/kg	650	270 unflavored 380 vanilla	550 unflavored 617-678 flavored	650
Sodium mg/100 mL (mEq/100 mL)	63 (2.7)	50 (2.2)	47 (2.0)	61 (2.7)
Potassium mg/100 mL (mEq/100 mL)	132 (3.4)	125 (3.2)	117 (3.0)	106 (2.7)

FLUIDS, ELECTROLYTES, AND NUTRITION *(Continued)*

Nutritional Modules[1]

	Polycose® Liquid	Polycose® Powder	Promod® Powder[2]
Indication	Carbohydrate additive for use as a caloric supplement which is readily mixable in most foods, enteral formulas or beverages without appreciably altering their taste	Carbohydrate additive for use as a caloric supplement which is readily mixable in most foods, enteral formulas or beverages without appreciably altering their taste	Protein supplement which mixes readily in enteral formulas, most foods, or beverages without appreciably altering their taste
Calories	2/mL	3.8/g[3]	4.2/g
Protein (g)	—	—	0.76/g
Protein source	—	—	Whey protein concentrate
Carbohydrate (g)	0.5/mL	0.94/g	<0.1/g
Carbohydrate source	Glucose polymers	Glucose polymers	Lactose
Fat (g)	—	—	<0.09/g
Fat source	—	—	Soy lecithin
Osmolality mOsm/kg	900	900 in solution	—
Sodium mEq/L (mg/L)	<0.03/mL (<0.7/mL)	<0.05/g (<1.1/g)	<0.099/g (<2.3/g)
Potassium mEq/L (mg/L)	<0.002/mL (<0.06/mL)	<0.003/g (<0.1/g)	<0.25/g (<9.85/g)
Chloride mEq/L (mg/L)	<0.04/mL (<1.4/mL)	<0.06/g (<2.23/g)	—
Calcium mEq/L (mg/L)	<0.01/mL (<0.2/mL)	<0.02/g (<0.3/g)	<0.33/g (<6.67/g)
Phosphorus mEq/L (mg/L)	(<0.03/mL)	(<0.05/g)	(<5/g)
Iron mg/L	—	—	—

[1]These products are not complete formulations and should not be used as a sole source of nutrition.

[2]1 scoop = 6.6 g, 1 tsp = 1.3 g, 1 tbsp = 4 g.

[3]1 tsp (2 g) = 8 calories, 1 tbsp (6 g) = 23 calories, 1/4 cup (24 g) = 95 calories.

Nutritional Modules[1]

	Vegetable Oil[2]	Microlipid®	MCT Oil®[3]	Whole Milk
Indications	Inexpensive fat source for calories and essential fatty acids	50% fat emulsion for use as a source of calories or essential fatty acids; it mixes easily and stays in emulsion	Fat supplement for use for patients who cannot efficiently digest and absorb long-chain fats	
Calories	8/mL	4.5/mL	7.67/mL	157/8 oz
Protein (g)	—	—	—	8/8 oz
Protein source	—	—	—	82% casein, 18% whey
Carbohydrate (g)	—	—	—	11/8 oz
Carbohydrate source	—	—	—	Lactose
Fat (g)	0.93/mL	0.5/mL[4]	0.93/mL	8.9/8 oz
Fat source	Corn, soybean, sunflower or safflower oils[5]	Safflower oil, polyglycerol esters, soy lecithin	Lipid fraction of coconut oil (consists primarily of C_8 and C_{10} saturated fatty acids)	Butter fat
Osmolality mOsm/kg	—	60	—	288
Sodium mEq/L (mg/L)	—	—	—	5.3/8 oz (122/8 oz)
Potassium mEq/L (mg/L)	—	—	—	9/8 oz (351/8 oz)
Chloride mEq/L (mg/L)	—	—	—	7/8 oz (247/8 oz)
Calcium mEq/L (mg/L)	—	—	—	14.4/8 oz (288/8 oz)
Phosphorus mEq/L (mg/L)	—	—	—	14.6/8 oz (227/8 oz)
Iron mg/L	—	—	—	0.12/8 oz

[1]These products are not complete formulations and should not be used as a sole source of nutrition.

[2]1 tbsp = 14 g.

[3]Does not contain essential fatty acids.

[4]1 tbsp = 5.9 g linoleic.

[5]% of linoleic from fat: soybean oil 51%, corn oil 58%, sunflower oil 65%, safflower oil 77%.

FLUID AND ELECTROLYTE REQUIREMENTS IN CHILDREN

Maintenance Fluids (Two methods)

Surface area method (most commonly used in children >10 kg): 1500-2000 mL/m^2/day

Body weight method

<10 kg	100 mL/kg/day
11-20 kg	1000 mL + 50 mL/kg (for each kg >10)
>20 kg	1500 mL + 20 mL/kg (for each kg >20)

Maintenance Electrolytes (See specific electrolyte in Alphabetical Listing of Drugs for more detailed information)

Sodium: 3-4 mEq/kg/day **or** 30-50 mEq/m^2/day
Potassium: 2-3 mEq/kg/day **or** 20-40 mEq/m^2/day

Dehydration Fluid Therapy

Goals of therapy:

- Restore circulatory volume to prevent shock (10% to 15% dehydration)
- Restore combined intracellular and extracellular deficits of water and electrolytes within 24 hours
- Maintain adequate water and electrolytes
- Resolve homeostatic distortions (eg, acidosis)
- Replace ongoing losses

Analysis of the Severity of Dehydration by Physical Signs

Clinical Sign	Mild[1]	Moderate[1]	Severe[1]
Pre-illness body weight	5% loss	10% loss	15% loss
Skin turgor	↓	Tenting	Tenting
Mucous membranes	Dry	Very dry	Parched
Skin color	Pale	Grey	Mottled
Urine output	↓	↓↓	Azotemic
Blood pressure	Normal	Normal, ↓	↓↓
Heart rate	Normal, ↑	↑	↑↑
Fontanelle (<7 mo)	Flat	Soft	Sunken
CNS	Consolable	Irritable	Lethargic/coma

[1]Postpubertal children and adults experience the same symptoms with mild, moderate, and severe dehydration associated with 3%, 6%, and 9% losses in body weight respectively.

Restoration of Circulatory Volume (10% to 15% dehydration estimate)

Fluid boluses of 20 mL/kg using crystalloid (eg, normal saline) or 10 mL/kg colloid (eg, 5% albumin) administered as rapidly as possible; repeat until improved circulation (eg, warm skin, decreased heart rate (towards normal), improved capillary refill time, urine output restored).

Classification of Dehydration (based upon the serum sodium concentration)

Isotonic	130-150 mEq/L
Hypotonic	<130 mEq/L
Hypertonic	>150 mEq/L

Estimated Water & Electrolyte Deficits in Dehydration
(moderate to severe)

Type of Dehydration	Water (mL/kg)	Na+ (mEq/kg)	K+ (mEq/kg)	Cl^- and HCO_3^- (mEq/kg)
Isotonic	100-150	8-10	8-10	16-20
Hypotonic	50-100	10-14	10-14	20-28
Hypertonic	120-180	2-5	2-5	4-10

Current Pediatric Diagnosis & Treatment, 10th ed, 1991.

Water deficit may also be calculated (in isotonic dehydration):

$$\text{Water deficit (mL)} = \frac{\text{\% dehydration} \times \text{wt (kg)} \times 1000 \text{ g/kg}}{100}$$

Assessment of Water Loss in Relation to Serum Na^+ Concentrations Degree of Dehydration as % Body Weight

Serum Na^+	Mild	Moderate	Severe
Isotonic	5%	10%	15%
Hypotonic ($Na^+ < 130$)	4%	6%	8%
Hypertonic ($Na^+ > 150$)	7%	12%	17%

Example of Fluid Replacement
(assume 10 kg infant with 10% isotonic dehydration)

	Water	Sodium (mEq)	Potassium (mEq)
Maintenance	1000 mL	40	20
Deficit[1]	1000 mL	80	80
Total	2000 mL	120	100

[1]Reduce this total by any fluid boluses given initially.

First 8 hours:

Replace 1/3 maintenance water = 330 mL
Replace 1/2 deficit water = 500 mL
Total 830 mL/8 h = 103 mL/h

Replace 1/2 of Na^+ & K^+ = 60 mEq sodium/803 mL; 50 mEq potassium/803 mL (It is suggested that the maximum potassium initially used is 40 mEq/L and is **not** started until urine output has been established.)

The actual order would appear as: $D_5$1/2NS at 103 mL/hour for 8 hours; add 40 mEq/L KCl after patient voids.

Second 16 hours:

Replace 2/3 maintenance water = 670 mL
Replace 1/2 deficit water = 500 mL
Total 1260 mL/16 h = 79 mL/h

Replace remainder of sodium and potassium.

The actual order would appear as: $D_5$1/3NS with KCl 40 mEq/L at 79 mL/hour for 16 hours. (Use of 1/4NS may be more desirable for convenience.)

FLUID AND ELECTROLYTE REQUIREMENTS IN CHILDREN *(Continued)*

Analysis of Ongoing Losses

Electrolyte Composition of Biological Fluids (mEq/L)

Fluid Type	Sodium	Potassium	Chloride	Total HCO_3^-
Stomach	20-120	5-25	90-160	0-5
Duodenal drainage	20-140	3-30	30-120	10-50
Biliary tract	120-160	3-12	70-130	30-50
Small intestine Initial drainage	100-140	4-40	60-100	30-100
Small intestine Established drainage	4-20	4-10	10-100	40-120
Pancreatic	110-160	4-15	30-80	70-130
Diarrheal stool	10-25	10-30	30-120	10-50

Current Pediatric Diagnosis & Treatment, 9th ed, Appleton & Lange, 1987.

Because of the wide range of normal values, specific analyses are suggested in individual cases.

Alterations of Maintenance Fluid Requirements

Fever	Increase maintenance fluids by 5 mL/kg/day for each degree of temperature above 38°C
Hyperventilation	Increase maintenance fluids by 10-60 mL/100 kcal BEE (basal energy expenditure)
Sweating	Increase maintenance fluids by 10-25 mL/100 kcal BEE (basal energy expenditure)
Hyperthyroidism	Variable increase in maintenance fluids: 25%-50%
Renal disease	Monitor and analyze output; adjust therapy accordingly
Renal failure	Maintenance fluids are equal to insensible losses (300 mL/m^3) + urine replacement (mL for mL)
Diarrhea	Increase maintenance fluids on a mL/mL loss basis

Oral Rehydration

Due to the high worldwide incidence of dehydration from infantile diarrhea, effective, inexpensive oral rehydration solutions have been developed. In the U.S., a typical effective solution for rehydration contains 50-60 mEq/L sodium, 20-30 mEq/L potassium, 30 mEq/L bicarbonate or its equivalent, and sufficient chloride to provide electroneutrality. Two percent to 3% glucose facilitates electrolyte absorption and short-term calories. The following table describes the electrolyte/sugar content of commonly used oral rehydration solutions.

Composition of Frequently Used Oral Electrolyte Replacement Solutions

Solutions	% CHO	Na^+ (mEq/L)	K^+ (mEq/L)	Cl^- (mEq/L)	HCO^- (mEq/L)
Normal saline		154		154	
Ringer's lactate		130	4	109	28
Dextrose 5% in 0.25% NaCl	5% glucose	38		38	
WHO solution	2% glucose or 4% sucrose	90	20	80	30 citrate
WHO solution, modified	2% glucose	55	25	30	50
Rehydralyte®	2.5% glucose	75	20	65	30 citrate
Ricelyte®	3% carbohydrate	50	25	45	34 citrate
Resol®	2% glucose	50	20	50	34 citrate
Rice water	2.5% carbohydrate	90	20	30	80
Pedialyte® (Ross)	2.5% glucose	45	20	35	30 citrate
Infalyte® (Penwalt)	3% glucose	50	25	45	34
Gatorade®	2.6% glucose, 2% fructose	23.5	<1	17	
Apple juice	3.2% glucose, 1.3% sucrose, 7.5% fructose	<1	25		
Orange juice 1:3 (dilution with water)	1% glucose, 1.2% fructose	<1	50		50 citrate
Grape juice	1.6% glucose, 2.1% fructose	0.2-0.7	8-11		8
One package cherry gelatin dissolved in 4 cups water		24	Needs added K^+		
Coca-Cola®		1.6	<1		13.4 citrate
Pepsi-Coal®		6.5	0.8		
Beef broth		120	10		
Chicken broth		250	8		

Adapted from Aranda-Michel, J and Giannella RA, "Acute Diarrhea" A Practical Review," *Am J of Med,* 1999, 106:670-6.

PARENTERAL NUTRITION (PN)

The following information is intended as a brief overview of the use of PN in infants and children.

Goal: The therapeutic goal of PN in infants and children is both to maintain nutrition status and to achieve balanced somatic growth.

General Indications for Use

PN is the provision of required nutrients by the intravenous route to replenish, optimize, or maintain nutritional status.

Specific Indications

PN of **all** required nutrients (total parenteral nutrition) is indicated in patients for whom it is expected that it would be impossible or dangerous to enterally administer nutrition. PN in combination with enteral nutrition is indicated in patients who are expected to be unable to meet their nutritional needs by the enteral route alone within 5 days. Peripheral PN is indicated only for partial nutritional supplementation or as bridge therapy for patients awaiting central venous access.

1. Patients with an inability to absorb nutrients via the gastrointestinal tract which may include the following: severe diarrhea, short bowel syndrome, developmental anomalies of the GI tract, inflammatory bowel disease, cystic fibrosis, or anatomic or functional loss of GI integrity.
2. Severe malnutrition.
3. Severe catabolic states such as: burns, trauma, or sepsis.
4. Patients undergoing high dose chemotherapy, radiation, and bone marrow transplantation.
5. Patients whose clinical condition may necessitate complete bowel rest (eg, necrotizing enterocolitis, pancreatitis, GI fistulas, or recent GI surgery).
6. Intensive care low-birth-weight infants.
7. Neonatal asphyxia.
8. Meconium ileus.
9. Respiratory distress syndrome (RDS).

Nutritional Assessment

As many as 33% of hospitalized pediatric patients are malnourished and require nutritional therapy. The type of nutritional support indicated depends on the underlying disease, the degree of gastrointestinal function, and the severity of malnutrition. Acutely malnourished patients have an increased risk for serious infection, postoperative complications, and death. Indicators of acute protein-calorie malnutrition include low weight for height, low serum albumin, lymphopenia, decreased body fat folds, and decreased arm muscle area. Nutritional screening may be done by the dietitian. Those patients who are at nutritional risk should receive a complete nutritional assessment.

Nutritional Requirements

Approximate requirements for energy and protein at various ages for normal subjects are listed in the first table at the end of this section. Patients who are severely malnourished or markedly catabolic may require higher levels to achieve catch-up growth or meet increased requirements. Patients who are well-nourished and/or inactive may require less.

During parenteral nutrition, 10% to 16% of calories should be in the form of amino acids to achieve optimal benefit (approximately 2-3 g/kg/day in infants and 1.5-2.5 g/kg/day ideal body weight in older patients). Exceptions include patients with renal or hepatic failure (where less protein is indicated), or in the treatment of severe trauma, head injury, or sepsis (where more protein may be indicated).

PN ORDERING

Fluid Intake

The patient should be given a total volume of fluid reasonable for his/her age and cardiovascular status. It is generally safe to start with the fluid maintenance level of 1500 mL/m^2/day in children (see Fluid and Electrolyte Requirements in Children). The fluid requirements in preterm infants are extremely variable due to much greater insensible water losses from radiant warmers and bili-lights. While the standard fluid maintenance of 100 mL/kg/day may be sufficient for term infants, intakes of up to 150 mL/kg/day may be necessary in the very low birth weight infants. Be sure to consider significant fluid intake from medications or other I.V. fluids and enteral diets in planning the fluids available for PN.

Dextrose

For central PN, dextrose is usually begun with a 10% to 12.5% solution or a solution providing dextrose at no more than 5 mg/kg/minute (in neonates and premature infants). The concentration is advanced, if tolerated, by 2.5% to 5% per day (2-2.5 mg/kg/minute increments in neonates and premature infants) to the desired caloric density, usually 20% to 25% dextrose. Fluid restricted patients often need 30% to 35% dextrose to meet their energy needs. For peripheral PN, 5% to 12.5% dextrose is utilized.

Dextrose calculations:

% Dextrose = dextrose (g)/100 mL

Dextrose calorie value = 3.4 kcal/g

$$\text{Dextrose infusion rate (mg/kg/minute)} = \frac{\text{rate (mL/h)} \times \text{\% dextrose} \times 0.166}{\text{weight (kg)}}$$

$$\text{\% Dextrose desired}^1 = \frac{\text{desired rate (mg/kg/min)} \times \text{weight (kg)}}{0.166 \times \text{rate (mL/h)}}$$

[1]Do not use dextrose concentrations <5% due to hypotonicity.

Amino Acids

Amino acids may be described as either a "standard" mixture of essential and nonessential amino acids or "specialized" mixtures. Specialized mixtures are intended for use in patients whose physiologic or metabolic needs may not be met with the "standard" amino acid compositions. Examples of specialized solutions include:

TrophAmine®, Aminosyn® PF	Indicated for use in premature infants and young children due to addition of taurine, L-glutamic acid, L-aspartic acid, increased amounts of histidine, and reduction in amounts of methionine, alanine, phenylalanine, and glycine. Supplementation with a cysteine additive has been recommended.
HepatAmine®	Indicated for treatment in patients with hepatic encephalopathy due to cirrhosis or hepatitis or in patients with liver disease who are intolerant of standard amino acid solutions. Contains higher percentage of branched-chain amino acids and a lower percentage of aromatic amino acids than standard mixtures.

PARENTERAL NUTRITION (PN) *(Continued)*

(continued)

NephrAmine®, Aminosyn® RF	Indicated for use in patients with compromised renal function who are intolerant of standard amino acid solutions. Contains a mixture of essential amino acids and histidine.

Amino acid calculations:

% amino acid	=	amino acid (g)/100mL
Grams of protein	=	grams of nitrogen x 6.25
% amino acid desired	=	(g amino acid/kg) x weight (kg) x 100 / total PN fluid volume (mL)

Fat Emulsion (FE)

There are three roles for intravenous fat in parenteral nutrition:

1. to provide nonprotein calories
2. to provide essential fatty acids and a "balanced" calorie source
3. to provide calories in catabolic patients with limited ability to excrete CO_2

The FE dosage is increased as tolerated daily (see General Guidelines for Initiation and Advancement for PN following). The maximum fat intake is 4 g/kg/day and no more than 60% of the total daily caloric intake. It is administered as a continuous infusion over 24 hours or at a rate no greater than 0.15-0.2 g/kg/hour via a Y-connector with the dextrose-amino acid I.V. line. In patients receiving cyclic PN, the FE should be administered over the duration of the PN infusion. The triglyceride concentration should be checked before the first infusion and daily as the dose is increased. Subsequently, it should be monitored at least weekly. Triglyceride concentrations should be maintained at <200 mg/dL in neonates, <350 mg/dL in renal patients, and <250 mg/dL in other patients. FE should be used cautiously in neonates with hyperbilirubinemia due to displacement of bilirubin from albumin by the free fatty acids. An increase in free bilirubin may increase the risk of kernicterus. Significant displacement occurs when the free fatty acid to serum albumin molar ratio (FFA/SA) >6. For example, infants with a total bilirubin >8-10 mg/dL (assuming an albumin concentration of 2.5-3 g/dL) should not receive more parenteral FE than required to meet the essential fatty acid requirement of 0.5-1 g/kg/day.

Note: Avoid use of 10% FE in preterm infants because a greater accumulation of plasma lipids occurs due to the greater phospholipid load of the 10% concentration.

Fat emulsion calculations:

20% FE = 20 g fat/100 mL = 2 kcal/mL

$$\text{Desired 20\% FE (mL)} = \frac{\text{(\% total kcal as fat) x (total kcal)}}{\text{2 kcal/mL}}$$

or as an alternative

Desired 20% FE (mL) = FE (g/kg) x weight (kg) x 5 mL/g

General Guidelines for Initiation and Advancement of PN[1]

Age	Initiation and Advancement[2]	Dextrose	Protein (g/kg/d)	Fat (g/kg/d)
Premature infant	Initial	4-6 mg/kg/min	0.5-1.5	0.5
	Daily increase	1-2.5 mg/kg/min	0.5-1	0.5
	Maximum	18 mg/kg/min	2.5-3	3
Term infant - 1 y	Initial	7-9 mg/kg/min	1-1.5	0.5-1
	Daily increase	1-2.5 mg/kg/min	1	0.5-1
	Maximum	21 mg/kg/min	2.5-3	4
Children 1-10 y	Initial dextrose concentration	10%-12.5%	1-1.5	1
	Daily increase	5% increments	1	1
	Maximum	15 mg/kg/min	2-2.5	3
>10 y	Initial dextrose concentration	10%-15%	1-1.5	1
	Daily increase	5% increments	1	1
	Maximum	8.5 mg/kg/min	1.5-2	3

[1]Rate of advancement may be limited by metabolic tolerance (eg, hyperglycemia, azotemia, hypertriglyceridemia)

[2]Timely intervention in premature infants is essential with initiation of dextrose as soon as possible after birth, amino acids within the first 12 hours, and fat emulsion within 24-48 hours of life.

MINERALS, TRACE ELEMENTS, AND VITAMINS

Guideline for Daily Electrolyte Requirements

	Neonates (mEq/kg)	Infants/Children (mEq/kg)	Adolescents
Sodium	2-5[1]	2-6	1-2 mEq/kg
Potassium	2-4	2-4	1-2 mEq/kg
Calcium gluconate[2]	3-4[3]	1-2.5	10-20 mEq/d
Magnesium	0.3-0.5	0.3-0.5	10-30 mEq/d
Phosphate[2]	1-2 mmol/kg[3]	0.5-1 mmol/kg	10-40 mmol/d

[1]Premature infants lose sodium in urine due to the immature resorptive function of kidney and diuretic use. Hyponatremia may lead to poor tissue growth and adverse developmental outcomes. Sodium content in PN may be adjusted to a maximum of 154 mEq/L (NS) to achieve normal sodium serum levels.

[2]Calcium-phosphate stability in parenteral nutrition solutions is dependent upon the pH of the solution, temperature, and relative concentration of each ion. The pH of the solution is primarily dependent upon the amino acid concentration. The higher the percentage amino acids the lower the pH, the more soluble the calcium and phosphate. Individual commercially available amino acid solutions vary significantly with respect to pH lowering potential and consequent calcium phosphate compatibility. See the pharmacist for specific calcium phosphate stability information.

[3]A 1.7:1 calcium to phosphate ratio in PN allows for the highest absolute retention of both minerals and simulates the in utero accretion of calcium and phosphate.

Vitamins

A pediatric parenteral multivitamin product is indicated for children <11 years of age. Children >11 years of age may receive adult multivitamin formulations.

Dosage:

Pediatric MVI:

Neonates: 2 mL/kg/d; maximum 5 mL/d

Infants and children ≤11 y: 5 mL

Children >11 y and adults: Use adult formulation 10 mL/d

PARENTERAL NUTRITION (PN) *(Continued)*

Trace Mineral Daily Requirements[1]

	Infants	**Children (≥3 mo to ≤5 y)**	**Older Children and Adolescents**
Chromium[2]	0.2 mcg/kg	0.14-0.2 mcg/kg (max: 5 mcg)	10-15 mcg
Copper[3]	20 mcg/kg	20 mcg/kg (max: 300 mcg)	0.3-0.5 mg
Iodide[4]	1 mcg/kg	1 mcg/kg	1 mcg/kg
Manganese[3]	1 mcg/kg	2-10 mcg/kg (max: 50 mcg)	60-150 mcg
Selenium[2,5]	2-3 mcg/kg	2-3 mcg/kg (max: 30 mcg)	20-60 mcg
Zinc	400 mcg/kg (preterm) 300 mcg/kg (term <3 mo)	100 mcg/kg (max: 5 mg)	2.5-5 mg

[1]Recommended intakes of trace elements cannot be achieved through the use of a single pediatric trace element product. Only through the use of individualized trace element products can recommended intakes be achieved.

[2]Omit in patients with renal dysfunction.

[3]Omit in patients with impaired biliary excretion or cholestatic liver disease.

[4]Percutaneous absorption from protein-bound iodine may be adequate.

[5]Indicated for use in long-term parenteral nutrition patients.

These are recommended daily trace mineral requirements. Additional supplementation may be indicated in clinical conditions resulting in excessive losses. For example, additional zinc may be needed in situations of excessive gastrointestinal losses.

Developing the PN Goal Regimen

The purpose of this example is to illustrate the thought process in determining what dextrose and amino acid solution and fat emulsion intake would provide the desired daily fluid calorie and protein goals.

1. Calculate the fluid, protein, and caloric goals. Example:

   Weight = 10 kg
   Fluids = 100 mL/kg/day = 1000 mL
   Calories = 100 kcal/kg/day = 1000 kcal
   Protein = 2.5 g/kg/day = 25 g

2. If fat emulsion (FE) comprises 40% to 60% of the total daily calories, using the above example: 40% of 1000 kcal = 400 kcal.

   400 kcal ÷ 2 kcal/mL (20% FE) = 200 mL

3. To determine the goal dextrose concentration calculate the total daily calories remaining. Example:

   1000 kcal (total daily calories)
   - 400 kcal (daily calories from fats)
   600 kcal (total daily calories remaining)

4. Determine the concentration of dextrose to achieve the total daily calories remaining. Example:

$$600 \text{ kcal} \div 3.4 \text{ kcal/g} \times [100 \div 800 \text{ mL}^{1}] = 22\%$$

[1]Total daily fluids desired minus that from fats.

5. Calculate percent amino acid solution to achieve goal protein intake. Example:

$$[25 \text{ g (total protein)} \div 800 \text{ mL (total fluid)}] \times 100 = 3.1\%$$

This patient's goal regimen would be: dextrose 22%, amino acid 3.1%, 800 mL/day plus fat emulsion 20% 200 mL/day.

Suggested PN Monitoring Guidelines

	Suggested Frequency	
Parameter	**Initial/Hospitalized**	**Follow-up/Outpatient**
Growth		
Weight	Daily	Daily to q visit
Height/length	Weekly	Weekly to q visit
Body composition (triceps skinfold, bone age)	Initially	Monthly to annually
Metabolic (Serum[1])		
Electrolytes	Twice weekly	Weekly to q visit
BUN/creatinine	Weekly	Weekly to q visit
Acid-base status	Until stable	As indicated
Albumin/prealbumin	Weekly	Weekly to q visit
Glucose	Daily to weekly	Weekly to q visit
Triglyceride	Initially daily	Weekly to q visit
Liver function tests	Weekly	Weekly to q visit
Complete blood count/differential	Weekly	Weekly to q visit
Platelets, PT/PTT	Weekly	As indicated
Iron indices	As indicated	Biannually to annually
Trace elements	As indicated	Annually
Carnitine	As indicated	As indicated
Folate/vitamin B_{12}	As indicated	As indicated
Ammonia	As indicated	As indicated
Bilirubin, direct	Weekly	As indicated
Metabolic (Urine)		
Glucose	Twice daily	Daily to weekly
Ketone	Twice daily	Daily to weekly
Specific gravity	As indicated	As indicated
Urea nitrogen	As indicated	As indicated
Clinical Calculations		
Fluid balance	Daily	As indicated
Projected vs actual intake	Daily	Weekly to q visit
Calorie/protein intake	Daily	As indicated

Frequency depends on clinical condition.

[1]For metabolically unstable patients, need to check more frequently.

Adapted from "Guidelines for the Use of Parenteral and Enteral Nutrition in Adult and Pediatric Patients. ASPEN Board of Directors and The Clinical Guidelines Task Force," *JPEN J Parenter Enteral Nutr*, 2002, 26(1 Suppl):1-138SA.

PARENTERAL NUTRITION (PN) *(Continued)*

Nutritional Guidelines for Pediatric Patients

Age	kcal/kg/d	Protein g/kg/d
Preterm neonate	120-140	3-4
Term infant - 1 y	90-120	2-3
1-7 y	75-90	1-1.2
12 y	60-75	1-1.2
12-18 y	30-60	0.8-0.9
>18 y	25-30	0.8

PN kcal/mL[1]

Dextrose Concentration						
5%	10%	15%	20%	25%	30%	35%
0.17	0.34	0.51	0.68	0.85	1.02	1.19

Dextrose provides 3.4 kcal/g.

Fat emulsion 10% provides 1.1 kcal/mL.

Fat emulsion 20% provides 2 kcal/mL.

[1]Calories derived from amino acids are not included.

Reference

"Guidelines for the Use of Parenteral and Enteral Nutrition in Adult and Pediatric Patients. ASPEN Board of Directors and The Clinical Guidelines Task Force," *JPEN J Parenter Enteral Nutr*, 2002, 26(1 Suppl):1-138SA.

Y-Site Compatibility of Medications With TPN and Lipid[1]

(Administered in D_5W or NS via Y-connector into PN line)

Medication	PN	Lipid	Comments
Acetazolamide	I	—	Visual precipitate forms
Acyclovir	I	—	Visual precipitate forms
Albumin	C	I	May crack emulsion
Aldesleukin	C	C	
Allopurinol	—	—	
Alprostadil	—	—	
Amikacin	C	I	May cause oiling out of fat emulsion
Aminophylline	C	C	Incompatible with insulin
Amphotericin B	I	I	Visual precipitate forms
Ampicillin	I	I	Visual precipitate forms
Ampicillin/sulbactam	C	C	
Amrinone	—	—	
Atracurium	C	—	
Atropine	—	—	
Aztreonam	C	C	
Bicarbonate	I	I	Incompatible with many electrolytes; precipitate forms
Bumetanide	C	—	

Y-Site Compatibility of Medications With TPN and Lipid[1] *(continued)*

Medication	PN	Lipid	Comments
Buprenorphine	C	—	
Butorphanol	C	—	
Caffeine citrate	—	—	
Carboplatin	C	—	
Cefamandole	C	C	
Cefazolin	C	C	
Cefepime	—	—	
Cefonicid	—	—	
Cefoperazone	C	C	
Cefotaxime	C	C	
Cefotetan	C	C	
Cefoxitin	C	C	
Ceftazidime	C	C	
Ceftizoxime	C	C	
Ceftriaxone	C	C	
Cefuroxime	C	C	
Cephalothin	C	C	
Cephapirin	C	C	
Cephradine	I	—	Heavy precipitate of Ca/Phos due to increased pH
Chloramphenicol	C	C	
Chlorothiazide	I	—	Precipitate forms
Chlorpromazine	C	C	
Cimetidine	C	C	
Ciprofloxacin	C	C	
Cisatracurium	—	—	
Cisplatin	C	C	
Clindamycin	C	C	
Cyanocobalamin	C	C	
Cyclophosphamide	C	C	
Cyclosporine	C[2]	C	
Cytarabine	C[2]	C	
Dexamethasone (sodium phosphate)	C	C	
Digoxin	C	C	
Diphenhydramine	C	C	
Dobutamine	C	C	
Dopamine	C	C[2]	
Doxacurium	—	—	
Doxapram	—	—	
Doxorubicin	I	I	
Doxycycline	C	I	Free oil formation
Droperidol	C	I	

PARENTERAL NUTRITION (PN) *(Continued)*

Y-Site Compatibility of Medications With TPN and Lipid[1] *(continued)*

Medication	PN	Lipid	Comments
Enalaprilat	C	C	
Epinephrine	C	—	
Epoetin alfa	C	—	
Erythromycin lactobionate	C	C	
Etoposide	—	—	
Famotidine	C	C	
Fentanyl	C	C	
Filgrastim	I	C	Incompatible with salt solutions
Fluconazole	C	C	
Fluorouracil	C[2]	C[2]	
Folic acid	C	C	
Foscarnet	C	—	
Fosphenytoin	—	—	
Furosemide	C	C	
Ganciclovir	I	I	Precipitate forms
Gentamicin	C	C	
Granisetron	C	C	
Haloperidol (lactate)	C	I	Free oil formation
Heparin	C	I	Free oil formation with 100 units/mL heparin
Hydralazine	—	—	
Hydrocortisone sodium phosphate	C	C	
Hydrocortisone sodium succinate	C	C	
Hydromorphone	C	I[2]	Free oil formation
Hydroxyzine	C	C	
Idarubicin	C	—	
Ifosfamide	C	C	
IL-2	C	—	
Imipenem/cilastatin	C	C	
Indomethacin	I	—	
Insulin, regular	C	C	
Iron dextran	C[2]	I	Causes oiling out of fat emulsion
Isoproterenol	C	C	
Kanamycin	C	C	
Leucovorin	C	C	
Levofloxacin	—	—	
Levorphanol	C	I	Free oil formation
Lidocaine	C	C	
Linezolid	C	—	

Y-Site Compatibility of Medications With TPN and Lipid[1] *(continued)*

Medication	PN	Lipid	Comments
Lorazepam (0.1 mg/mL)	C	I	
Mannitol (15%)	C	C	
Meperidine	C	C	
Meropenem	C	C	
Mesna	C	C	
Methotrexate	C[2]	C	Hazy subvisual precipitate
Methyldopa	C	I[2]	May crack emulsion
Methylprednisolone sodium succinate	C	C	
Metoclopramide	C[2]	C	
Metronidazole	C	C	
Midazolam	I	I	Precipitate forms
Milrinone	C	—	
Minocycline	I	I	
Mitoxantrone	C[2]	C	
Morphine	C	C[2]	
Nafcillin	C	C	
Nalbuphine	C	I	Free oil formation
Netilmicin	C	C	
Nitroglycerin	C	C	
Norepinephrine	C	C	
Octreotide	I	C	Formation of glycosyl octreotide conjugate may reduce efficacy
Ofloxacin	C	C	
Ondansetron	C	I	Free oil formation
Oxacillin	C	C	
Paclitaxel	C	C	
Penicillin G Na/K	C	C	
Pentobarbital	C	I	Free oil formation
Phenobarbital	C	I	Free oil formation
Phenytoin	I	I	Immediate precipitate
Phytonadione	C	C	
Piperacillin	C	C	
Piperacillin/tazobactam	C	C	
Promethazine	C	C	
Propofol	C	—	
Ranitidine	C	C	
Sargramostim	C	—	
Sodium bicarbonate	I	C	Incompatible with many electrolytes; precipitate forms
Sodium nitroprusside	C	C	
Tacrolimus	C	C	
Thiamine	C	C	

PARENTERAL NUTRITION (PN) *(Continued)*

Y-Site Compatibility of Medications With TPN and Lipid[1] *(continued)*

Medication	PN	Lipid	Comments
Ticarcillin	C	C	
Ticarcillin/clavulanate	C	C	
Thiotepa	C	—	
Trimethoprim/ sulfamethoxazole	C	C	
Tobramycin	C	C	
Urokinase	C	—	
Vancomycin	C	C	
Vecuronium	C	—	
Verapamil	—	—	
Vitamin K	C	C	
Zidovudine	C	C	

C = compatible, may simultaneously infuse drug and TPN/lipid.

I = incompatible; drug should be given through a **separate** I.V. line or turn off the TPN/liquid during drug administration. Flush I.V. line with normal saline **before** and **after** drug administration.

— = information on compatibility not available. Give drug through a **separate** I.V. line or turn off TPN infusion during drug administration. Flush line with normal saline **before** and **after** drug administration.

[1]Compatibility does not reflect 3-in-one total nutrient admixture (including fat emulsion) solutions.

[2]Variable stability depending upon TPN composition (see Trissel, 2005).

Reference

Trissel LA, "Handbook on Injectable Drugs," 13th ed, Bethesda, MD: American Society of Health-System Pharmacists, Inc, 2005.

Pharmacologic considerations of mixing medications with PN solutions include:

- Adsorption — bag, bottle, tubing, filter
- Blood levels
- Site of injection/administration
- Flush
- Amino acid-dextrose concentrations
- pH factors
- Temperature
- Additives in solution
- Heparin dose

GROWTH CHARTS

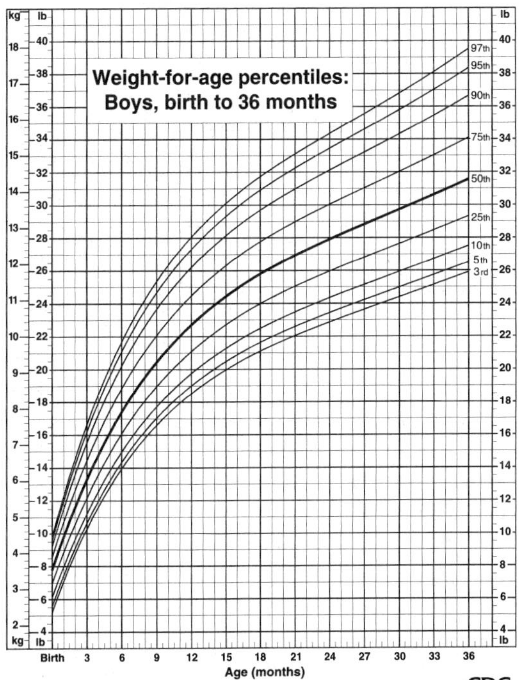

SOURCE: Developed by the National Center for Health Statistics in collaboration with the National Center for Chronic Disease Prevention and Health Promotion (2000). Available at http://www.cdc.gov/growthcharts

GROWTH CHARTS *(Continued)*

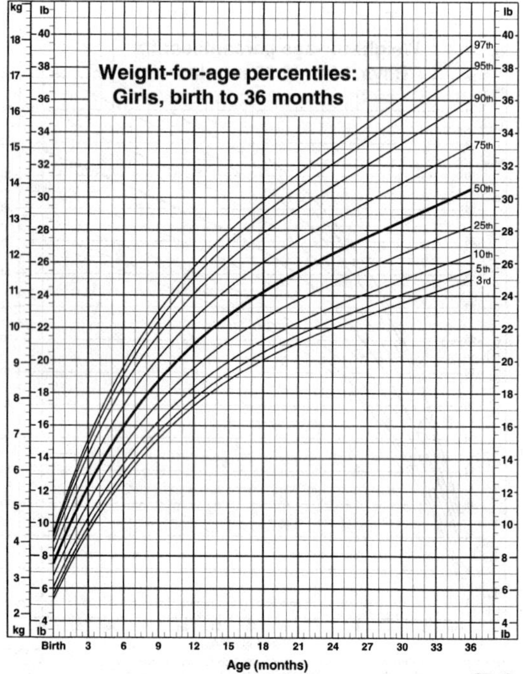

SOURCE: Developed by the National Center for Health Statistics in collaboration with the National Center for Chronic Disease Prevention and Health Promotion (2000). Available at http://www.cdc.gov/growthcharts

CDC Growth Charts: United States

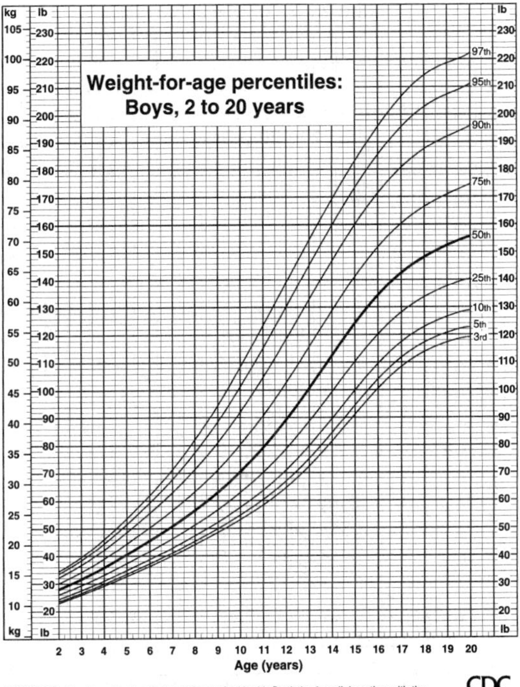

Weight-for-age percentiles: Boys, 2 to 20 years

Age (years)

SOURCE: Developed by the National Center for Health Statistics in collaboration with the National Center for Chronic Disease Prevention and Health Promotion (2000). Available at http://www.cdc.gov/growthcharts

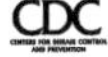

GROWTH CHARTS *(Continued)*

CDC Growth Charts: United States

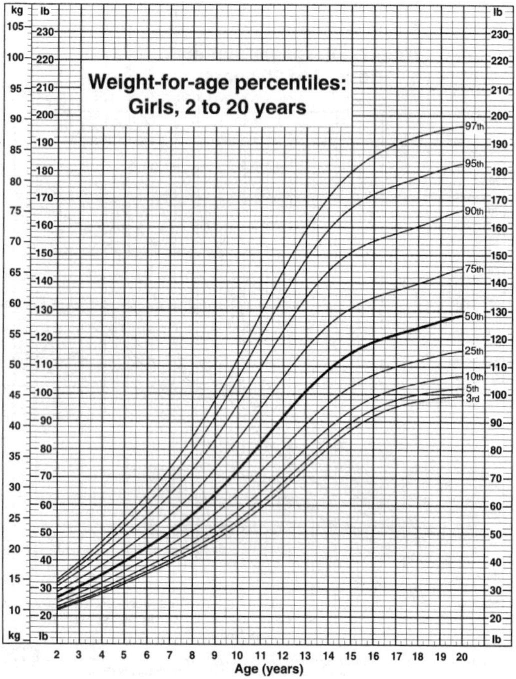

Weight-for-age percentiles: Girls, 2 to 20 years

kg | lb

97th, 95th, 90th, 75th, 50th, 25th, 10th, 5th, 3rd

Age (years): 2 3 4 5 6 7 8 9 10 11 12 13 14 15 16 17 18 19 20

SOURCE: Developed by the National Center for Health Statistics in collaboration with the National Center for Chronic Disease Prevention and Health Promotion (2000). Available at http://www.cdc.gov/growthcharts

CDC Growth Charts: United States

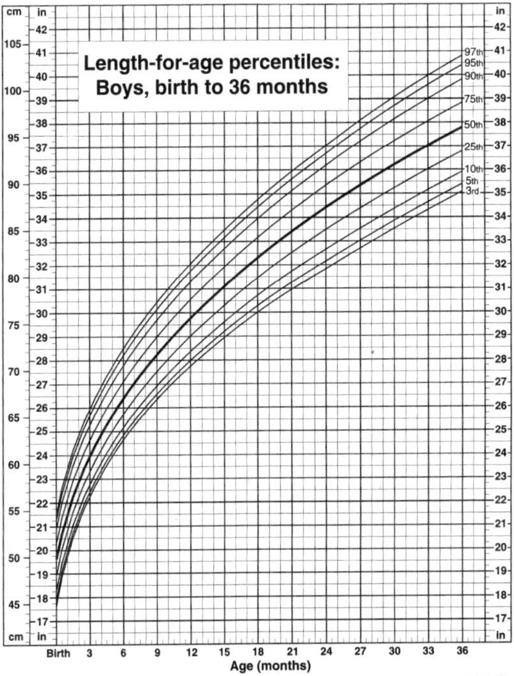

SOURCE: Developed by the National Center for Health Statistics in collaboration with the National Center for Chronic Disease Prevention and Health Promotion (2000). Available at http://www.cdc.gov/growthcharts

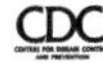

GROWTH CHARTS *(Continued)*

CDC Growth Charts: United States

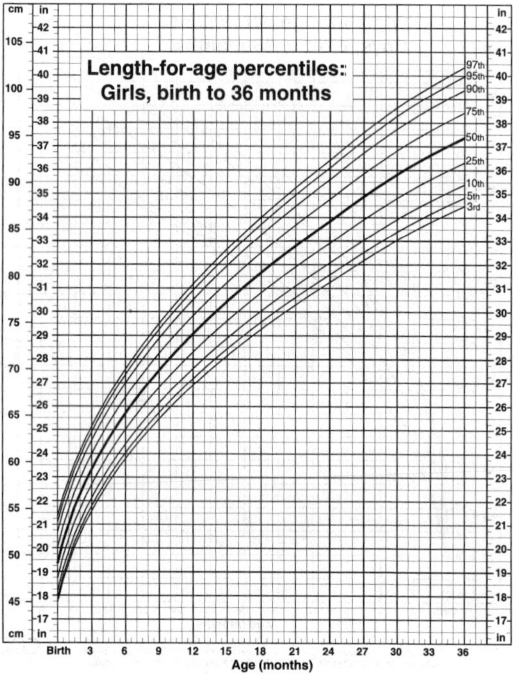

Length-for-age percentiles: Girls, birth to 36 months

cm: 45 50 55 60 65 70 75 80 85 90 95 100 105

in: 17 18 19 20 21 22 23 24 25 26 27 28 29 30 31 32 33 34 35 36 37 38 39 40 41 42

97th 95th 90th 75th 50th 25th 10th 5th 3rd

Birth 3 6 9 12 15 18 21 24 27 30 33 36

Age (months)

SOURCE: Developed by the National Center for Health Statistics in collaboration with the National Center for Chronic Disease Prevention and Health Promotion (2000). Available at http://www.cdc.gov/growthcharts

CDC Growth Charts: United States

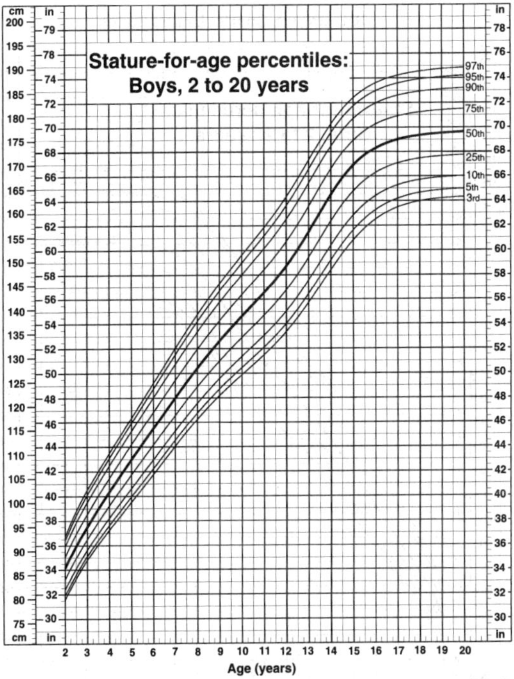

Stature-for-age percentiles: Boys, 2 to 20 years

cm: 75, 80, 85, 90, 95, 100, 105, 110, 115, 120, 125, 130, 135, 140, 145, 150, 155, 160, 165, 170, 175, 180, 185, 190, 195, 200

in: 30, 32, 34, 36, 38, 40, 42, 44, 46, 48, 50, 52, 54, 56, 58, 60, 62, 64, 66, 68, 70, 72, 74, 76, 78, 79

Percentiles: 97th, 95th, 90th, 75th, 50th, 25th, 10th, 5th, 3rd

Age (years): 2, 3, 4, 5, 6, 7, 8, 9, 10, 11, 12, 13, 14, 15, 16, 17, 18, 19, 20

SOURCE: Developed by the National Center for Health Statistics in collaboration with the National Center for Chronic Disease Prevention and Health Promotion (2000). Available at http://www.cdc.gov/growthcharts

GROWTH CHARTS *(Continued)*

CDC Growth Charts: United States

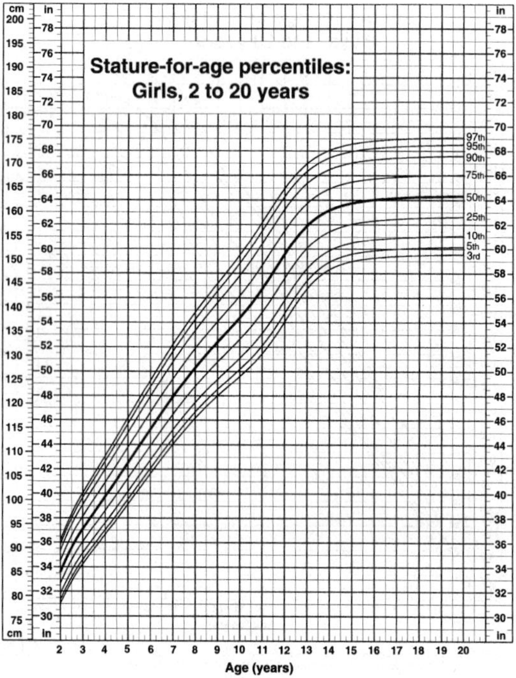

Stature-for-age percentiles: Girls, 2 to 20 years

cm: 75, 80, 85, 90, 95, 100, 105, 110, 115, 120, 125, 130, 135, 140, 145, 150, 155, 160, 165, 170, 175, 180, 185, 190, 195, 200

in: 30, 32, 34, 36, 38, 40, 42, 44, 46, 48, 50, 52, 54, 56, 58, 60, 62, 64, 66, 68, 70, 72, 74, 76, 78

97th, 95th, 90th, 75th, 50th, 25th, 10th, 5th, 3rd

2 3 4 5 6 7 8 9 10 11 12 13 14 15 16 17 18 19 20

Age (years)

SOURCE: Developed by the National Center for Health Statistics in collaboration with the National Center for Chronic Disease Prevention and Health Promotion (2000). Available at http://www.cdc.gov/growthcharts

CDC Growth Charts: United States

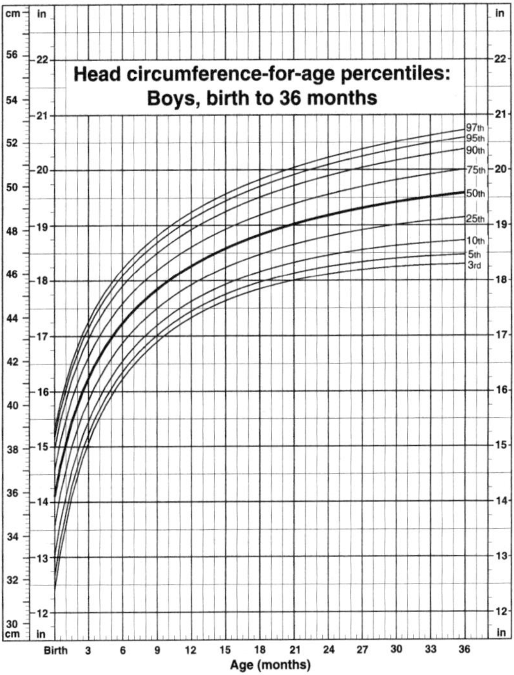

Head circumference-for-age percentiles: Boys, birth to 36 months

cm: 30 32 34 36 38 40 42 44 46 48 50 52 54 56

in: 12 13 14 15 16 17 18 19 20 21 22

97th
95th
90th
75th
50th
25th
10th
5th
3rd

Birth 3 6 9 12 15 18 21 24 27 30 33 36

Age (months)

SOURCE: Developed by the National Center for Health Statistics in collaboration with the National Center for Chronic Disease Prevention and Health Promotion (2000).
Available at http://www.cdc.gov/growthcharts

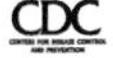

GROWTH CHARTS *(Continued)*

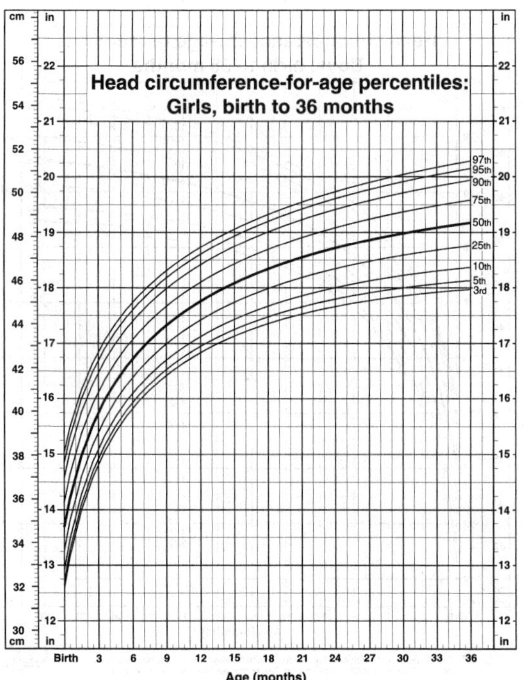

SOURCE: Developed by the National Center for Health Statistics in collaboration with the National Center for Chronic Disease Prevention and Health Promotion (2000). Available at http://www.cdc.gov/growthcharts

IDEAL BODY WEIGHT CALCULATION

Adults (18 years and older)

IBW (male) = 50 + (2.3 x height in inches over 5 feet)
IBW (female) = 45.5 + (2.3 x height in inches over 5 feet)

IBW is in kg.

Children

a. 1-18 years (Traub and Johnson, 1980)

$$\text{IBW} = \frac{(\text{height}^2 \times 1.65)}{1000}$$

IBW is in kg.
Height is in cm.

b. 5 feet and taller (Traub and Johnson, 1980)

IBW (male) = 39 + (2.27 x height in inches over 5 feet)
IBW (female) = 42.2 + (2.27 x height in inches over 5 feet)

IBW is in kg.

c. 1-17 years (Traub and Kichen, 1983)

$$\text{IBW} = 2.396e^{0.01883\ (\text{height})}$$

IBW is in kg.
Height is in cm.

References

Traub SL and Johnson CE, "Comparison of Methods of Estimating Creatinine Clearance in Children," *Am J Hosp Pharm*, 1980, 37(2):195-201.

Traub SL and Kichen L, "Estimating Ideal Body Mass in Children," *Am J Hosp Pharm*, 1983, 40(1):107-10.

BODY SURFACE AREA OF ADULTS AND CHILDREN

Calculating Body Surface Area in Children

In a child of average size, find weight and corresponding surface area on the boxed scale to the left; or, use the nomogram to the right. Lay a straightedge on the correct height and weight points for the child, then read the intersecting point on the surface area scale.

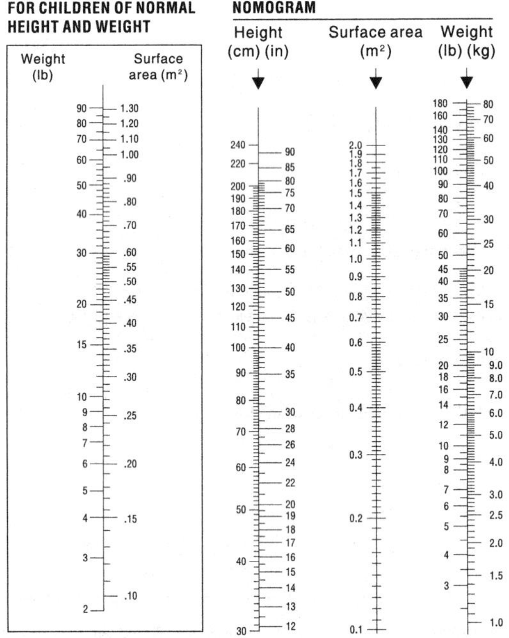

BODY SURFACE AREA FORMULA
(Adult and Pediatric)

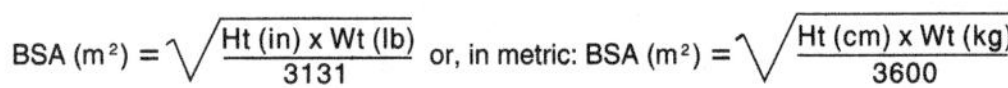

$$BSA\ (m^2) = \sqrt{\frac{Ht\ (in) \times Wt\ (lb)}{3131}}\ \text{or, in metric: } BSA\ (m^2) = \sqrt{\frac{Ht\ (cm) \times Wt\ (kg)}{3600}}$$

References

Lam TK and Leung DT, "More on Simplified Calculation of Body Surface Area," *N Engl J Med*, 1988, 318(17):1130 (Letter).

Mosteller RD, "Simplified Calculation of Body Surface Area", *N Engl J Med*, 1987, 317(17):1098 (Letter).

AVERAGE WEIGHTS AND SURFACE AREAS

Average Weight and Surface Area of Preterm Infants, Term Infants, and Children

Age	Average Weight (kg)[1]	Approximate Surface Area (m^2)
Weeks Gestation		
26	0.9-1	0.1
30	1.3-1.5	0.12
32	1.6-2	0.15
38	2.9-3	0.2
40 (term infant at birth)	3.1-4	0.25
Months		
3	5	0.29
6	7	0.38
9	8	0.42
Year		
1	10	0.49
2	12	0.55
3	15	0.64
4	17	0.74
5	18	0.76
6	20	0.82
7	23	0.90
8	25	0.95
9	28	1.06
10	33	1.18
11	35	1.23
12	40	1.34
Adults	70	1.73

[1]Weights from age 3 months and over are rounded off to the nearest kilogram.

PHYSICAL DEVELOPMENT

Weight gain first 6 weeks

20 g/day

Birth weight

regained by day 14

doubles by age 4 mo

triples by age 12 mo

quadruples by age 2 y

Teeth

1st tooth 6-18 mo

teeth = age (mo) – 6
(until 30 mo)

Head circumference

35 cm at birth

44 cm by 6 mo

47 cm by 1 y

1 cm/mo for 1st y

3 cm/mo 2nd y

Length

increases 50% by age 1 y

doubles by age 4 y

triples by age 13 y

Tanner Stages of Sexual Development

Stage	Characteristics	Age at Onset (mean ± SD)
Genital stages: Male		
1	Prepubertal	
2	Scrotum and testes enlarge; skin of scrotum reddens and rugations appear	11.4 ± 1.1 y
3	Penis lengthens; testes enlarge further	12.9 ± 1 y
4	Penis growth continues in length and width; glans develops adult form	13.8 ± 1 y
5	Development completed; adult appearance	14.9 ± 1.1 y
Breast development: Female		
1	Prepubertal	
2	Breast buds appear; areolae enlarge	11.2 ± 1.1 y
3	Elevation of breast contour; areolae enlarge	12.2 ± 1.1 y
4	Areolae and papilla form a secondary mound on breast	13.1 ± 1.2 y
5	Adult form	15.3 ± 1.7 y
Menarche		
Pubic hair: Both sexes		13.5 ± 1 y
1	Prepubertal, no coarse hair	
2	Longer, silky hair appears at base of penis or along labia	F: 11.7 ± 1.2 y M: 12 ± 1 y
3	Hair coarse, kinky, spreads over pubic bone	F: 12.4 ± 1.1 y M: 13.9 ± 1 y
4	Hair of adult quality but not spread to junction of medial thigh with perineum	F: 13 ± 1 y M: 14.4 ± 1.1 y
5	Spread to medial thigh	F: 14.4 ± 1.1 y M: 15.2 ± 1.1 y
6	"Male escutcheon"	Variable if occurs
Maximum growth rate		
Male at 14.1±0.9 y		
Female at 12.1±0.9 y		

EMETOGENIC POTENTIAL OF SINGLE CHEMOTHERAPEUTIC AGENTS

Class I — Low (<10%)

Asparaginase/Pegaspargase
Bleomycin
Busulfan
Chlorambucil (oral)
Cladribine
Corticosteroids
Cyclophosphamide (oral)
Fludarabine
Hydroxyurea
Melphalan (oral)
Mercaptopurine
Methotrexate <50 mg/m^2
Thioguanine (oral)
Vinblastine
Vincristine

Class II — Moderately Low (10% to 30%)

Cytarabine <500 mg/m^2
Doxorubicin ≤20 mg/m^2
Etoposide
Fluorouracil <1000 mg/m^2
Gemcitabine
Interferon-beta
Lomustine
Methotrexate ≥50-250 mg/m^2
Mitomycin <8 mg/m^2
Paclitaxel
Raltitrexed
Thiotepa

Class III — Moderate (30% to 60%)

Amsacrine
Azacitidine
Cyclophosphamide <750 mg/m^2
Cytarabine 500-1000 mg/m^2
Daunorubicin
Docetaxel
Doxorubicin >20 mg to <60 mg/m^2
Epirubicin
Fluorouracil ≥1000 mg/m^2
Idarubicin
Ifosfamide
Irinotecan
Methotrexate >250 mg/m^2 to ≤1000 mg/m^2
Mitomycin ≥8 mg/m^2
Mitoxantrone
Teniposide
Topotecan
Tretinoin
Vinorelbine

Class IV — Moderately High (60% to 90%)

Actinomycin D
Aldesleukin
Carboplatin 200-400 mg/m^2
Carmustine <250 mg
Cisplatin <50 mg/m^2
Cyclophosphamide 750-1500 mg/m^2
Cytarabine >1000 mg/m^2
Dacarbazine <500 mg/m^2
Doxorubicin ≥60 mg/m^2
Melphalan 20-80 mg/m^2
Methotrexate >1000 mg/m^2
Procarbazine (oral)

Class V — High (>90%)

Busulfan (as part of BMT regimen)
Carboplatin >500 mg/m^2
Carmustine ≥250 mg/m^2
Cisplatin ≥50 mg/m^2
Cyclophosphamide ≥1500 mg/m^2
Dacarbazine ≥500 mg/m^2
Mechlorethamine
Melphalan >80 mg/m^2
Pentostatin

COMPATIBILITY OF CHEMOTHERAPY AND RELATED SUPPORTIVE CARE MEDICATIONS

Compatible: The drugs are physically compatible when mixed in the same container or infused through the same I.V. line simultaneously.

Y-site compatible: The drugs are physically compatible when infused through the same I.V. line simultaneously.

Incompatible: The drugs are physically incompatible when mixed in the same container, or infused through the same I.V. line simultaneously.

Variable compatibility: The compatibility of the drugs varies according to the concentration and/or diluent of the drugs. Please refer to the table at the end of this section for more information on variable compatibility.

Abbreviations

AA	Amino acid solution
BNS	Bacteriostatic normal saline
BWI	Bacteriostatic water for injection
D_5W	5% dextrose in water
D_5/NS	5% dextrose in 0.9% sodium chloride
$D_5/^1/_4NS$	5% dextrose in 0.225% sodium chloride
$D_5/^1/_2NS$	5% dextrose in 0.45% sodium chloride
D_5LR	5% dextrose in lactated Ringer's injection
$D_{10}W$	10% dextrose in water
$D_{10}W$/0.01% albumin	10% dextrose in water with 0.01% albumin
$D_{10}W$/0.05% albumin	10% dextrose in water with 0.05% albumin
$D_{10}W$/0.1% albumin	10% dextrose in water with 0.1% albumin
D_{10}/NS	10% dextrose in water in 0.9% sodium chloride
LR	Lactated Ringer's injection
NS	0.9% sodium chloride (normal saline)
SWI	Sterile water for injection
TPN	Total parenteral nutrition solution

Reported Compatibilities and Incompatibilities of Parenteral Dosage Forms

Aldesleukin

Compatible:

- D_5W
- SWI

Y-Site Compatible:

- Amikacin
- Amphotericin
- Calcium gluconate
- Cotrimoxazole
- Diphenhydramine
- Dopamine
- Fat emulsion
- Fluconazole
- Foscarnet
- Gentamicin
- Heparin
- Magnesium sulfate
- Metoclopramide
- Morphine
- Ondansetron
- Piperacillin
- Potassium chloride
- Ranitidine
- Thiethylperazine
- Ticarcillin
- Tobramycin

Incompatible:

- Ganciclovir
- Heparin
- Pentamidine
- Prochlorperazine
- Promethazine

Amifostine

Compatible:

- NS

Y-Site Compatible:

- Amikacin
- Aminophylline
- Ampicillin
- Ampicillin/sulbactam
- Aztreonam
- Bleomycin
- Bumetanide
- Buprenorphine
- Butorphanol
- Calcium gluconate
- Carboplatin
- Carmustine
- Cefamandole
- Cefepime
- Cefotaxime
- Cefotetan
- Cefoxitin
- Ceftazidime
- Ceftizoxime
- Ceftriaxone
- Cefuroxime
- Cimetidine
- Ciprofloxacin
- Clindamycin
- Cotrimoxazole
- Cyclophosphamide
- Cytarabine
- Dacarbazine
- Dactinomycin
- Daunomycin
- Dexamethasone
- Diphenhydramine
- Dobutamine
- Dopamine
- Doxorubicin
- Doxycycline
- Droperidol
- Enalaprilat
- Etoposide
- Famotidine
- Floxuridine
- Fluconazole
- Fludarabine
- Fluorouracil
- Furosemide
- Gallium nitrate
- Gemcitabine
- Gentamicin
- Granisetron
- Haloperidol
- Heparin
- Hydrocortisone sodium phosphate
- Hydrocortisone sodium succinate
- Hydromorphone
- Idarubicin
- Ifosfamide
- Imipenem/cilastatin
- Leucovorin
- Lorazepam
- Magnesium sulfate
- Mannitol
- Mechlorethamine
- Meperidine
- Mesna
- Methotrexate
- Methylprednisolone
- Metoclopramide
- Metronidazole
- Mezlocillin
- Mitomycin
- Mitoxantrone
- Morphine
- Nalbuphine
- Netilmicin
- Ondansetron
- Piperacillin
- Plicamycin
- Potassium chloride
- Promethazine
- Ranitidine
- Sodium bicarbonate
- Streptozocin
- Teniposide
- Thiotepa
- Ticarcillin
- Ticarcillin/clavulanate
- Tobramycin
- Trimetrexate
- Vancomycin
- Vinblastine
- Vincristine

Incompatible:

- Acyclovir
- Amphotericin
- Chlorpromazine
- Cisplatin
- Ganciclovir
- Hydroxyzine
- Minocycline
- Prochlorperazine

COMPATIBILITY OF CHEMOTHERAPY AND RELATED SUPPORTIVE CARE MEDICATIONS *(Continued)*

Asparaginase

Compatible:

D_5W
NS
SWI

Y-Site Compatible:

Methotrexate
Sodium bicarbonate

Bleomycin

Compatible:

BNS
BWI
SWI
Amikacin
Amsacrine
Ceftazidime
Cephapirin
Cimetidine
Dacarbazine
Dexamethasone
Diphenhydramine
Droperidol
Fluorouracil
Furosemide
Gentamicin
Heparin
Hydrocortisone sodium phosphate
Leucovorin
Metoclopramide
Phenytoin
Streptomycin
Tobramycin
Vinblastine
Vincristine

Y-Site Compatible:

Allopurinol
Amifostine
Aztreonam
Cefepime
Cisplatin
Cyclophosphamide
Doxorubicin
Doxorubicin, liposomal
Filgrastim
Fludarabine
Gemcitabine
Methotrexate
Mitomycin
Ondansetron
Paclitaxel
Piperacillin
Sargramostim
Teniposide
Thiotepa
Vinorelbine

Incompatible:

Aminophylline
Ascorbic acid
Cefazolin
Cephalothin
Diazepam
Doxapram
Hydrocortisone sodium succinate
Nafcillin
Penicillin G
Terbutaline

Variable Compatibility:

D_5W
NS

Busulfan

Compatible:

D_5W
NS

Carboplatin

Compatible:

D_5W
SWI
Etoposide
Floxuridine
Ifosfamide

Y-Site Compatible:

Allopurinol
Amifostine
Aztreonam
Cefazolin
Doxorubicin, liposomal
Filgrastim
Fludarabine
Gemcitabine
Granisetron
Ondansetron
Piperacillin
Piperacillin/tazobactam
Propofol
Sargramostim
Teniposide
Thiotepa
TPN
Vinorelbine

Incompatible:

Fluorouracil
Mesna
Sodium bicarbonate

Variable Compatibility:

D_5/NS
$D_5/{}^1/_4$NS
$D_5/{}^1/_2$NS
NS

Carmustine

Compatible:

- D_5W
- NS
- SWI
- Dacarbazine

Y-Site Compatible:

- Amifostine
- Aztreonam
- Cefepime
- Filgrastim
- Fludarabine
- Gemcitabine
- Ondansetron
- Piperacillin
- Piperacillin/tazobactam
- Sargramostim
- Teniposide
- Thiotepa
- Vinorelbine

Incompatible:

- Allopurinol
- Sodium bicarbonate

Cisplatin

Compatible:

- D_5/NS
- $D_5/\frac{1}{4}NS$
- $D_5/\frac{1}{2}NS$
- NS
- Cefazolin
- Cephalothin
- Cyclophosphamide
- Floxuridine
- Hydroxyzine
- Hydroxyurea
- Ifosfamide
- Leucovorin
- Mannitol
- Mechlorethamine
- Ondansetron

Y-Site Compatible:

- Allopurinol
- Aztreonam
- Bleomycin
- Bumetanide
- Chlorpromazine
- Cimetidine
- Dexamethasone
- Diphenhydramine
- Doxapram
- Doxorubicin
- Doxorubicin, liposomal
- Droperidol
- Famotidine
- Filgrastim
- Fludarabine
- Fluorouracil
- Furosemide
- Ganciclovir
- Gemcitabine
- Granisetron
- Heparin
- Hydromorphone
- Lorazepam
- Methotrexate
- Methylprednisolone
- Metoclopramide
- Mitomycin
- Morphine
- Paclitaxel
- Potassium chloride
- Prochlorperazine
- Promethazine
- Propofol
- Ranitidine
- Sargramostim
- Teniposide
- Thiotepa
- Vinorelbine

Incompatible:

- Amifostine
- Amsacrine
- Cefepime
- Gallium nitrate
- Mesna
- Oxacillin
- Piperacillin
- Piperacillin/tazobactam
- Sodium bicarbonate

Variable Compatibility:

- D_5W
- SWI
- Etoposide

Cladribine

Compatible:

- NS

Cyclophosphamide

Compatible:

- D_5W
- D_5/NS
- D_5/LR
- NS
- LR
- SWI
- AA 4.25%/$D_{25}W$
- Cisplatin
- Dacarbazine
- Etoposide
- Fluorouracil
- Hydroxyzine
- Mesna
- Methotrexate
- Mitoxantrone
- Ondansetron

Y-Site Compatible:

- Allopurinol
- Amifostine
- Amikacin
- Ampicillin
- Azlocillin
- Aztreonam
- Bleomycin
- Cefamandole
- Cefazolin
- Cefepime
- Cefoperazone
- Cefotaxime
- Cefoxitin
- Ceftriaxone
- Cephalothin
- Cephapirin
- Chloramphenicol
- Chlorpromazine
- Cimetidine
- Clindamycin
- Cotrimoxazole
- Dexamethasone
- Diphenhydramine
- Doxapram
- Doxorubicin
- Doxorubicin, liposomal
- Doxycycline

COMPATIBILITY OF CHEMOTHERAPY AND RELATED SUPPORTIVE CARE MEDICATIONS *(Continued)*

Droperidol
Erythromycin
Famotidine
Filgrastim
Fludarabine
Furosemide
Gallium nitrate
Ganciclovir
Gemcitabine
Gentamicin
Granisetron
Heparin
Hydromorphone
Idarubicin
Kanamycin
Leucovorin
Lorazepam
Methylprednisolone
Metoclopramide
Metronidazole
Mezlocillin
Minocycline
Mitomycin
Morphine
Moxalactam
Nafcillin
Oxacillin
Paclitaxel
Penicillin G
Piperacillin
Piperacillin/tazobactam
Prochlorperazine
Promethazine
Propofol
Ranitidine
Sargramostim
Sodium bicarbonate
Teniposide
Thiotepa
Ticarcillin
Ticarcillin/clavulanate
Tobramycin
TPN
Vancomycin
Vinblastine
Vincristine
Vinorelbine

Cytarabine

Compatible:

BNS
BWI
D_5W
D_5/NS
$D_5/{}^1/_4$NS
$D_5/{}^1/_2$NS
D_5/LR
D_{10}/NS
NS
LR
AA 4.25%/$D_{25}W$
Corticotropin
Dacarbazine
Daunomycin
Etoposide
Hydroxyzine
Hydroxyurea
Lincomycin
Mitoxantrone
Ondansetron
Potassium chloride
Prednisolone
Sodium bicarbonate
Vincristine

Y-Site Compatible:

Amifostine
Amsacrine
Aztreonam
Cefepime
Chlorpromazine
Cimetidine
Dexamethasone
Diphenhydramine
Doxorubicin, liposomal
Droperidol
Famotidine
Filgrastim
Fludarabine
Furosemide
Gemcitabine
Granisetron
Heparin
Idarubicin
Lorazepam
Metoclopramide
Morphine
Paclitaxel
Piperacillin
Piperacillin/tazobactam
Prochlorperazine
Promethazine
Propofol
Ranitidine
Sargramostim
Teniposide
Thiotepa
TPN
Vinorelbine

Incompatible:

Allopurinol
Ceftazidime
Fluorouracil
Gallium nitrate
Ganciclovir
Insulin
Nafcillin
Oxacillin
Penicillin G

Variable Compatibility:

Cephalothin
Gentamicin
Hydrocortisone sodium phosphate
Methylprednisolone

Dacarbazine

Compatible:

NS
SWI
Bleomycin
Carmustine
Cimetidine
Cyclophosphamide
Cytarabine
Dactinomycin
Doxorubicin
Fluorouracil
Mercaptopurine
Methotrexate
Ondansetron
Vinblastine

Y-Site Compatible:

Amifostine
Aztreonam
Doxorubicin, liposomal
Filgrastim
Fludarabine
Granisetron
Hydrocortisone sodium phosphate
Lidocaine
Paclitaxel
Sargramostim
Teniposide
Thiotepa
Vinorelbine

Incompatible:

D_5W
Allopurinol
Cefepime
Hydrocortisone sodium succinate
Piperacillin
Piperacillin/tazobactam

Variable Compatibility:

Heparin

Dactinomycin

Compatible:

D_5W
NS
SWI
Dacarbazine

Y-Site Compatible:

Allopurinol
Amifostine
Aztreonam
Cefepime
Fludarabine
Gemcitabine
Ondansetron
Sargramostim
Teniposide
Thiotepa
Vinorelbine

Incompatible:

BNS
BWI
Filgrastim

Daunomycin

Compatible:

D_5W
NS
LR
SWI
Cytarabine
Etoposide
Hydrocortisone sodium succinate

Y-Site Compatible:

Amifostine
Filgrastim
Gemcitabine
Methotrexate
Ondansetron
Sodium bicarbonate
Teniposide
Thiotepa
Vinorelbine

Incompatible:

Allopurinol
Aztreonam
Cefepime
Dexamethasone
Fludarabine
Piperacillin
Piperacillin/tazobactam

Dexrazoxane

Compatible:

D_5W

Y-Site Compatible:

Gemcitabine

COMPATIBILITY OF CHEMOTHERAPY AND RELATED SUPPORTIVE CARE MEDICATIONS *(Continued)*

Diphenhydramine

Compatible:

Amikacin
Aminophylline
Ascorbic acid
Atropine
Bleomycin
Butorphanol
Cephapirin
Chlorpromazine
Cimetidine
Colistimethate
Dimenhydrinate
Droperidol
Erythromycin
Fentanyl
Fluphenazine
Glycopyrrolate
Hydrocortisone sodium succinate
Hydromorphone
Hydroxyzine
Lidocaine
Meperidine
Methicillin
Methyldopate
Metoclopramide
Midazolam
Morphine
Nalbuphine
Nafcillin
Netilmicin
Penicillin G (sodium and potassium)
Pentazocine
Perphenazine
Prochlorperazine
Promazine
Promethazine
Ranitidine
Scopolamine
Sufentanil
Thiothixene
Polymyxin B
Vitamin B complex with C

Y-Site Compatible:

Acyclovir
Aldesleukin
Amifostine
Amsacrine
Aztreonam
Ciprofloxacin
Cisplatin
Cyclophosphamide
Cytarabine
Doxorubicin
Filgrastim
Fluconazole
Fludarabine
Gallium nitrate
Gemcitabine
Granisetron
Heparin
Idarubicin
Melphalan
Meperidine
Methotrexate
Ondansetron
Paclitaxel
Piperacillin/tazobactam
Potassium chloride
Sargramostim
Tacrolimus
Teniposide
Thiotepa
Vinorelbine

Incompatible:

Allopurinol
Amobarbital
Amphotericin
Cefepime
Cephalothin
Dexamethasone
Foscarnet
Haloperidol
Pentobarbital
Secobarbital
Thiopental

Variable Compatibility:

Diatrizoate
Iodipamide

Docetaxel

Compatible:

D_5W
NS

Y-Site Compatible:

Gemcitabine

Incompatible:

Doxorubicin, liposomal

Doxorubicin

Compatible:

D_5W
NS
LR
Dacarbazine
Ondansetron
Vincristine

Y-Site Compatible:

Amifostine
Aztreonam
Bleomycin
Chlorpromazine
Cimetidine
Cisplatin
Cyclophosphamide
Dexamethasone
Diphenhydramine
Famotidine
Filgrastim
Fludarabine
Gemcitabine
Granisetron
Hydromorphone
Leucovorin
Lorazepam
Methotrexate
Methylprednisolone
Metoclopramide
Mitomycin
Morphine
Paclitaxel
Prochlorperazine
Promethazine
Propofol
Ranitidine
Sargramostim
Sodium bicarbonate
Teniposide
Thiotepa
Vinorelbine

Incompatible:

Allopurinol
Aminophylline
Cefepime
Cephalothin
Diazepam
Furosemide
Gallium nitrate
Ganciclovir
Heparin
Hydrocortisone sodium succinate
Piperacillin/tazobactam
TPN
Paclitaxel
Tobramycin

Variable Compatibility:

Fluorouracil
Vinblastine

Doxorubicin, Liposomal

Compatible:

D_5W

Y-Site Compatible:

Allopurinol
Aldesleukin
Aminophylline
Ampicillin
Aztreonam
Bleomycin
Calcium chloride
Calcium gluconate
Cefazolin
Cefepime
Cefoperazone
Cefoxitin
Ceftizoxime
Ceftriaxone
Chlorpromazine
Cimetidine
Ciprofloxacin
Cisplatin
Clindamycin
Cotrimoxazole
Cyclophosphamide
Cytarabine
Dacarbazine
Dexamethasone
Diphenhydramine
Dobutamine
Dopamine
Droperidol
Enalaprilat
Etoposide
Famotidine
Fluconazole
Fluorouracil
Furosemide
Ganciclovir
Gentamicin
Granisetron
Haloperidol
Heparin
Hydrocortisone sodium succinate
Hydromorphone
Ifosfamide
Leucovorin
Lorazepam
Magnesium sulfate
Mesna
Methotrexate
Methylprednisolone
Metronidazole
Mezlocillin
Netilmicin
Ondansetron
Piperacillin
Potassium chloride
Prochlorperazine
Ranitidine
Ticarcillin
Ticarcillin/clavulanate
Tobramycin
Vancomycin
Vinblastine
Vincristine
Vinorelbine

Incompatible:

Amphotericin
Buprenorphine
Ceftazidime
Docetaxel
Gallium nitrate
Hydroxyzine
Mannitol
Meperidine
Metoclopramide
Miconazole
Mitoxantrone
Morphine
Ofloxacin
Piperacillin/tazobactam
Promethazine
Sodium bicarbonate

Droperidol

Compatible:

Atropine
Bleomycin
Butorphanol
Chlorpromazine
Cimetidine
Cisplatin
Cyclophosphamide
Dimenhydrinate
Diphenhydramine
Doxorubicin
Fentanyl
Glycopyrrolate
Hydroxyzine
Meperidine
Metoclopramide
Midazolam
Mitomycin
Morphine
Nalbuphine
Pentazocine
Perphenazine
Prochlorperazine
Promazine
Promethazine
Scopolamine
Vinblastine
Vincristine

Y-Site Compatible:

Amifostine
Aztreonam
Filgrastim
Fluconazole
Fludarabine
Gemcitabine
Hydrocortisone sodium succinate
Idarubicin
Melphalan
Ondansetron
Paclitaxel
Potassium chloride
Sargramostim
Teniposide
Thiotepa
Vinorelbine
Vitamin B complex with C

COMPATIBILITY OF CHEMOTHERAPY AND RELATED SUPPORTIVE CARE MEDICATIONS *(Continued)*

Incompatible:

Allopurinol
Cefepime
Fluorouracil
Foscarnet
Furosemide
Heparin
Leucovorin
Methotrexate
Nafcillin
Pentobarbital
Piperacillin/tazobactam

Erythropoietin

Compatible:

BNS
D_{10}/0.05% albumin
D_{10}/0.1% albumin

Incompatible:

$D_{10}W$
D_{10}/0.01% albumin
NS
SWI

Etoposide

Compatible:

D_5W
NS
LR
Carboplatin
Cyclophosphamide
Cytarabine
Daunomycin
Floxuridine
Fluorouracil
Hydroxyzine
Ifosfamide
Ondansetron

Y-Site Compatible:

Allopurinol
Amifostine
Aztreonam
Doxorubicin, liposomal
Fludarabine
Gemcitabine
Granisetron
Haloperidol
Methotrexate
Paclitaxel
Piperacillin
Piperacillin/tazobactam
Sargramostim
Sodium bicarbonate
Teniposide
Vinorelbine

Incompatible:

Cefoperazone
Ceftazidime
Cefepime
Filgrastim
Gallium nitrate
Idarubicin

Variable Compatibility:

Cisplatin
Mannitol
Potassium chloride

Filgrastim

Compatible:

D_5W
SWI

Y-Site Compatible:

Acyclovir
Allopurinol
Amikacin
Aminophylline
Ampicillin
Ampicillin/sulbactam
Aztreonam
Bleomycin
Bumetanide
Buprenorphine
Butorphanol
Calcium gluconate
Carboplatin
Carmustine
Cefazolin
Cefotetan
Ceftazidime
Chlorpromazine
Cimetidine
Cisplatin
Cotrimoxazole
Cyclophosphamide
Cytarabine
Dacarbazine
Daunomycin
Dexamethasone
Diphenhydramine
Doxorubicin
Doxycycline
Droperidol
Enalaprilat
Fat emulsion
Floxuridine
Fluconazole
Fludarabine
Gallium nitrate
Ganciclovir
Gentamicin
Haloperidol
Hydrocortisone sodium phosphate
Hydrocortisone sodium succinate
Hydromorphone
Hydroxyzine
Idarubicin
Ifosfamide
Imipenem/cilastatin
Leucovorin
Lorazepam
Mechlorethamine
Meperidine
Mesna
Methotrexate
Metoclopramide
Miconazole
Minocycline
Mitoxantrone
Morphine
Nalbuphine
Netilmicin
Ondansetron
Plicamycin
Potassium chloride
Promethazine
Ranitidine
Sodium bicarbonate
Streptozocin
Ticarcillin
Ticarcillin/clavulanate
Tobramycin
Vancomycin
Vinblastine
Vincristine
Vinorelbine

Incompatible:

NS
Amphotericin
Amsacrine
Cefepime
Cefonicid
Cefoperazone
Cefotaxime
Cefoxitin
Ceftizoxime
Ceftriaxone
Cefuroxime
Dactinomycin
Etoposide
Fluorouracil
Furosemide
Heparin
Mannitol
Methylprednisolone
Metronidazole
Mezlocillin
Mitomycin
Piperacillin
Prochlorperazine
Thiotepa

Floxuridine

Compatible:

D_5W
NS
SWI
Carboplatin
Cisplatin
Etoposide
Fluorouracil
Heparin
Leucovorin

Y-Site Compatible:

Amifostine
Aztreonam
Filgrastim
Fludarabine
Gemcitabine
Ondansetron
Paclitaxel
Piperacillin/tazobactam
Sargramostim
Teniposide
Thiotepa
Vinorelbine

Incompatible:

Allopurinol
Cefepime

Fludarabine

Compatible:

D_5W
NS
SWI

Y-Site Compatible:

Allopurinol
Amifostine
Amikacin
Aminophylline
Ampicillin
Ampicillin/sulbactam
Amsacrine
Aztreonam
Bleomycin
Butorphanol
Carboplatin
Carmustine
Cefazolin
Cefepime
Cefoperazone
Cefotaxime
Cefotetan
Ceftazidime
Ceftizoxime
Ceftriaxone
Cefuroxime
Cimetidine
Cisplatin
Cotrimoxazole
Cyclophosphamide
Cytarabine
Dacarbazine
Dactinomycin
Dexamethasone
Diphenhydramine
Doxorubicin
Doxycycline
Droperidol
Etoposide
Famotidine
Filgrastim
Floxuridine
Fluconazole
Fluorouracil
Furosemide
Gemcitabine
Gentamicin
Haloperidol
Heparin
Hydrocortisone sodium phosphate
Hydrocortisone sodium succinate
Hydromorphone
Ifosfamide
Imipenem/cilastatin
Lorazepam
Magnesium sulfate
Mannitol
Mechlorethamine
Meperidine
Mesna
Methotrexate
Methylprednisolone
Metoclopramide
Mezlocillin
Minocycline
Mitoxantrone
Morphine
Multivitamins
Nalbuphine
Netilmicin
Ondansetron
Pentostatin
Piperacillin
Piperacillin/tazobactam
Potassium chloride
Promethazine
Ranitidine
Sodium bicarbonate
Teniposide
Tetracycline
Ticarcillin
Ticarcillin/clavulanate
Tobramycin
Vancomycin
Vinblastine
Vincristine
Vinorelbine

Incompatible:

Acyclovir
Amphotericin
Chlorpromazine
Daunomycin
Ganciclovir
Hydroxyzine
Miconazole
Prochlorperazine

Fluorouracil

Compatible:

D_5W
D_5/LR
NS
Bleomycin
Cephalothin
Cyclophosphamide
Dacarbazine
Etoposide
Floxuridine
Ifosfamide
Magnesium sulfate
Methotrexate
Mitoxantrone
Prednisolone
Vincristine

COMPATIBILITY OF CHEMOTHERAPY AND RELATED SUPPORTIVE CARE MEDICATIONS *(Continued)*

Y-Site Compatible:

Allopurinol
Amifostine
Aztreonam
Cefepime
Cisplatin
Doxorubicin, liposomal
Fludarabine
Furosemide
Gemcitabine
Granisetron
Heparin
Hydrocortisone sodium succinate
Mannitol
Metochlopramide
Mitomycin
Paclitaxel
Piperacillin
Piperacillin/tazobactam
Potassium chloride
Propofol
Sargramostim
Teniposide
Thiotepa
Vinblastine
Vitamin B complex

Incompatible:

Carboplatin
Cytarabine
Diazepam
Droperidol
Epirubicin
Filgrastim
Gallium nitrate
Ondansetron
TPN
Vinorelbine

Variable Compatibility:

Doxorubicin
Leucovorin

Gemcitabine

Compatible:

NS

Y-Site Compatible:

Amifostine
Amikacin
Aminophylline
Ampicillin
Ampicillin/sulbactam
Aztreonam
Bleomycin
Bumetanide
Buprenorphine
Butorphanol
Calcium gluconate
Carboplatin
Carmustine
Cefazolin
Cefonicid
Cefotetan
Cefoxitin
Ceftazidime
Ceftizoxime
Ceftriaxone
Cefuroxime
Chlorpromazine
Cimetidine
Ciprofloxacin
Cisplatin
Clindamycin
Cyclophosphamide
Cytarabine
Dactinomycin
Daunomycin
Dexamethasone
Dexrazoxane
Diphenhydramine
Dobutamine
Docetaxel
Dopamine
Doxorubicin
Doxycycline
Droperidol
Enalaprilat
Etoposide
Etoposide phosphate
Famotidine
Floxuridine
Fludarabine
Fluorouracil
Fluconazole
Gallium nitrate
Gentamicin
Granisetron
Haloperidol
Heparin
Hydrocortisone sodium phosphate
Hydrocortisone sodium succinate
Hydromorphone
Hydroxyzine
Idarubicin
Ifosfamide
Leucovorin
Lorazepam
Mannitol
Meperidine
Mesna
Metoclopramide
Metronidazole
Miconazole
Minocycline
Mitoxantrone
Morphine
Nalbuphine
Netilmicin
Ofloxacin
Ondansetron
Paclitaxel
Plicamycin
Potassium chloride
Promethazine
Ranitidine
Sodium bicarbonate
Streptozocin
Teniposide
Thiotepa
Ticarcillin
Ticarcillin/clavulanate
Tobramycin
Topotecan
Trimethoprim
Vancomycin
Vinblastine
Vincristine
Vinorelbine
Zidovudine

Incompatible:

Acyclovir
Amphotericin
Cefoperazone
Cefotaxime
Furosemide
Ganciclovir
Imipenem/cilastatin
Irinotecan
Methotrexate
Methylprednisolone
Mezlocillin
Mitomycin
Piperacillin
Piperacillin/tazobactam
Prochlorperazine

Haloperidol

Compatible:

Hydromorphone
Sufentanil

Y-Site Compatible:

Amifostine
Amsacrine
Aztreonam
Cimetidine
Dobutamine
Dopamine
Famotidine
Filgrastim
Fludarabine
Gemcitabine
Lidocaine
Lorazepam
Melphalan
Midazolam
Nitroglycerin
Norepinephrine bitartrate
Ondansetron
Paclitaxel
Phenylephrine
Tacrolimus
Teniposide
Theophylline
Thiotepa
TPN
Vinorelbine

Incompatible:

Allopurinol
Cefepime
Diphenhydramine
Fluconazole
Foscarnet
Gallium nitrate
Heparin
Hydroxyzine
Ketorolac
Piperacillin/tazobactam
Sargramostim

Variable Compatibility:

Benztropine
Cyclizine
Diamorphine
Sodium nitroprusside

Heparin

Compatible:

Aminophylline
Amphotericin
Ascorbic acid
Bleomycin
Calcium gluconate
Cefepime
Cephapirin
Chloramphenicol
Cibenzoline
Clindamycin
Cloxacillin
Colistimethate
Dimenhydrinate
Dopamine
Enalaprilat
Erythromycin
Esmolol
Floxacillin
Fluconazole
Flumazenil
Furosemide
Isoproterenol
Lidocaine
Lincomycin
Methyldopate
Methylprednisolone
Metronidazole
Nafcillin
Norepinephrine
Octreotide
Potassium chloride
Prednisolone
Promazine
Ranitidine
Sodium bicarbonate
Verapamil
Vitamin B complex with C

Y-Site Compatible:

Acyclovir
Aldesleukin
Allopurinol
Amifostine
Ampicillin
Ampicillin/sulbactam
Atracurium
Atropine
Aztreonam
Betamethasone sodium phosphate
Cefazolin
Cefotetan
Ceftazidime
Ceftriaxone
Cephalothin
Chlordiazepoxide
Chlorpromazine
Cimetidine
Cisplatin
Cyanocobalamin
Cyclophosphamide
Cytarabine
Digoxin
Diphenhydramine
Edrophonium
Epinephrine
Erythromycin
Esmolol
Estrogens, conjugated
Ethacrynate
Famotidine
Fentanyl
Fludarabine
Fluorouracil
Foscarnet
Gallium nitrate
Gemcitabine
Hydralazine
Hydrocortisone sodium succinate
Insulin
Kanamycin
Leucovorin
Lorazepam
Magnesium sulfate
Melphalan
Menadiol sodium diphos-phate
Methicillin
Methotrexate
Methoxamine
Methyldopate
Metoclopramide
Metronidazole
Midazolam
Minocycline
Mitomycin
Morphine
Neostigmine
Nitroglycerin
Ondansetron
Oxacillin
Oxytocin
Paclitaxel
Pancuronium
Penicillin G potassium
Pentazocine
Phytonadione
Piperacillin
Piperacillin/tazobactam
Procainamide
Prochlorperazine
Propranolol
Pyridostigmine
Sargramostim
Scopolamine
Sodium nitroprusside
Streptokinase
Succinylcholine
Tacrolimus
Teniposide
Theophylline
Thiotepa
Ticarcillin
Ticarcillin/clavulanate
TPN
Trimethobenzamide
Trimethaphan
Vercuronium
Vinblastine
Vincristine
Vinorelbine
ZIdovudine

COMPATIBILITY OF CHEMOTHERAPY AND RELATED SUPPORTIVE CARE MEDICATIONS *(Continued)*

Incompatible:

Alteplase
Amikacin
Amiodarone
Amsacrine
Ciprofloxacin
Codeine phosphate
Daunomycin
Diazepam
Dobutamine
Doxorubicin
Doxycycline
Ergotamine
Filgrastim
Gentamicin
Haloperidol
Hyaluronidase
Idarubicin
Labetatol
Levorphanol
Methadone
Methotrimeprazine
Phenytoin
Polymyxin B
Streptomycin
Tobramycin
Triflupromazine

Variable Compatibility:

Cephalothin
Dacarbazine
Diltiazem
Droperidol
Hydrocortisone sodium succinate
Methylprednisolone
Penicillin G sodium
Promethazine
Quinidine gluconate
Vancomycin

Hydroxyzine

Compatible:

Atropine
Benzquinamide
Bupivacaine
Butorphanol
Chlorpromazine
Cimetidine
Cisplatin
Codeine
Cyclophosphamide
Cytarabine
Diphenhydramine
Doxapram
Droperidol
Etoposide
Fentanyl
Fluphenazine
Glycopyrrolate
Hydromorphone
Lidocaine
Meperidine
Methotrimeprazine
Metoclopramide
Midazolam
Morphine
Nalbuphine
Oxymorphone
Pentazocine
Mesna
Methotrexate
Nafcillin
Perphenazine
Procaine
Prochlorperazine
Promazine
Promethazine
Scopolamine
Sufentanil
Thiothixene

Y-Site Compatible:

Aztreonam
Ciprofloxacin
Filgrastim
Foscarnet
Gemcitabine
Melphalan
Ondansetron
Sufentanil
Teniposide
Thiotepa
Vinorelbine

Incompatible:

Allopurinol
Amifostine
Aminophylline
Amobarbital
Cefepime
Chloramphenicol
Diphenhydramine
Fluconazole
Fludarabine
Haloperidol
Ketorolac
Paclitaxel
Penicillin G (sodium and potassium)
Pentobarbital
Phenobarbital
Piperacillin/tazobactam
Ranitidine
Sargramostim

Idarubicin

Compatible:

D_5W
D_5/NS
NS
LR

Y-Site Compatible:

Amifostine
Amikacin
Aztreonam
Ciprofloxacin
Cyclophosphamide
Cytarabine
Diphenhydramine
Droperidol
Erythromycin
Filgrastim
Gemcitabine
Imipenem/cilastatin
Magnesium sulfate
Mannitol
Metoclopramide
Potassium chloride
Ranitidine
Sargramostim
Thiotepa
Vinorelbine

Incompatible:

Acyclovir
Allopurinol
Ampicillin/sulbactam
Cefazolin
Cefepime
Ceftazidime
Dexamethasone
Etoposide
Furosemide
Gentamicin
Heparin
Hydrocortisone sodium succinate
Lorazepam
Meperidine
Methotrexate
Mezlocillin
Piperacillin/tazobactam
Sodium bicarbonate
Teniposide
Vancomycin
Vincristine

Ifosfamide

Compatible:

D_5W
D_5/NS
D_5/$^1/_4$NS
D_5/LR
NS
LR
SWI
Carboplatin
Cisplatin
Etoposide
Fluorouracil

Y-Site Compatible:

Allopurinol
Amifostine
Aztreonam
Doxorubicin, liposomal
Filgrastim
Fludarabine
Gallium nitrate
Gemcitabine
Granisetron
Ondansetron
Paclitaxel
Piperacillin
Piperacillin/tazobactam
Propofol
Sargramostim
Sodium bicarbonate
Teniposide
Thiotepa
TPN
Vinorelbine

Incompatible:

Cefepime
Methotrexate

Variable Compatibility:

Epirubicin
Mesna

Irinotecan

Compatible:

D_5W

Incompatible:

Gemcitabine

Leucovorin

Compatible:

BWI
D_5W
D_{10}/NS
NS
LR
SWI
Bleomycin
Cisplatin
Floxuridine

Y-Site Compatible:

Amifostine
Aztreonam
Cefepime
Cyclophosphamide
Doxorubicin
Doxorubicin, liposomal
Filgrastim
Fluconazole
Furosemide
Gemcitabine
Heparin
Methotrexate
Metoclopramide
Mitomycin
Piperacillin
Piperacillin/tazobactam
Sodium bicarbonate
Tacrolimus
Teniposide
Thiotepa
TPN
Vinblastine
Vincristine

Incompatible:

Droperidol
Foscarnet
Trimetrexate

Variable Compatibility:

Fluorouracil

Lorazepam

Compatible:

Cimetidine
Hydromorphone

Y-Site Compatible:

Acyclovir
Albumin
Amifostine
Amikacin
Amoxicillin
Amoxicillin/clavulanate
Amsacrine
Atracurium
Bumetanide
Cefepime
Cefotaxime
Ciprofloxacin
Cisplatin
Cotrimoxazole
Cyclophosphamide
Cytarabine
Dexamethasone
Diltiazem
Doxorubicin
Erythromycin
Etomidate
Fentanyl
Filgrastim
Fluconazole
Fludarabine
Furosemide
Gemcitabine
Gentamicin
Granisetron
Haloperidol
Heparin
Hydrocortisone sodium succinate
Kantaserin
Melphalan
Methotrexate
Metronidazole
Morphine
Paclitaxel

COMPATIBILITY OF CHEMOTHERAPY AND RELATED SUPPORTIVE CARE MEDICATIONS *(Continued)*

Pancuronium
Piperacillin
Piperacillin/tazobactam
Potassium chloride
Ranitidine
Tacrolimus
Teniposide
Thiotepa
Vancomycin
Vercuronium
Vinorelbine
Zidovudine

Incompatible:

Aldesleukin
Aztreonam
Buprenorphine
Floxacillin
Gallium nitrate
Idarubicin
Imipenem/cilastatin
Ondansetron
Sargramostim
Sufentanil
Thiopental

Variable Compatibility:

Foscarnet

Mechlorethamine

Compatible:

NS
SWI

Y-Site Compatible:

Amifostine
Aztreonam
Filgrastim
Fludarabine
Granisetron
Ondansetron
Sargramostim
Teniposide
Vinorelbine

Incompatible:

D_5W
Allopurinol
Cefepime
Methohexital

Melphalan

Compatible:

NS

Y-Site Compatible:

Acyclovir
Amikacin
Aminophylline
Ampicillin
Aztreonam
Bleomycin
Bumetanide
Buprenorphine
Butorphanol
Calcium gluconate
Carboplatin
Carmustine
Cefazolin
Cefepime
Cefoperazone
Cefotaxime
Cefotetan
Ceftazidime
Ceftriaxone
Cefuroxime
Cimetidine
Cisplatin
Cotrimoxazole
Cyclophosphamide
Cytarabine
Dacarbazine
Dactinomycin
Daunomycin
Diazepam
Doxorubicin
Doxycycline
Droperidol
Enalaprilat
Etoposide
Famotidine
Filgrastim
Floxuridine
Fluconazole
Fludarabine
Fluorouracil
Furosemide
Gallium nitrate
Ganciclovir
Gentamicin
Haloperidol
Heparin
Hydrocortisone sodium phosphate
Hydrocortisone sodium succinate
Hydromorphone
Hydroxyzine
Idarubicin
Ifosfamide
Imipenem/cilastatin
Lorazepam
Mannitol
Mechlorethamine
Meperidine
Mesna
Methotrexate
Methylprednisolone
Metoclopramide
Metronidazole
Miconazole
Minocycline
Mitomycin
Mitoxantrone
Morphine
Nalbuphine
Netilmicin
Ondansetron
Pentostatin
Piperacillin
Plicamycin
Potassium chloride
Prochlorperazine
Promethazine
Ranitidine
Sodium bicarbonate
Streptozocin
Teniposide
Thiotepa
Ticarcillin
Ticarcillin/clavulanate
Tobramycin
Vancomycin
Vinblastine
Vincristine
Vinorelbine

Incompatible:

D_5W
LR
SWI
Amphotericin
Chlorpromazine

Mesna

Compatible:

- BWI
- D_5W
- NS
- LR
- Cyclophosphamide
- Hydroxyzine
- Ifosfamide

Y-Site Compatible:

- Allopurinol
- Amifostine
- Aztreonam
- Cefepime
- Doxorubicin, liposomal
- Filgrastim
- Fludarabine
- Gallium nitrate
- Gemcitabine
- Granisetron
- Methotrexate
- Ondansetron
- Paclitaxel
- Piperacillin/tazobactam
- Sargramostim
- Sodium acetate
- Teniposide
- Thiotepa
- TPN
- Vinorelbine

Incompatible:

- Carboplatin
- Cisplatin
- Chlorpromazine

Methadone

Incompatible:

- Aminophylline
- Ammonium chloride
- Amobarbital
- Chlorothiazide
- Phenytoin
- Heparin
- Methicillin
- Nitrofurantoin
- Pentobarbital
- Sodium bicarbonate
- Thiopental

Methotrexate

Compatible:

- D_5W
- NS
- LR
- SWI
- Amino acid 4.25%/$D_{25}W$
- Cephalothin
- Cyclophosphamide
- Cytarabine
- Dacarbazine
- Fluorouracil
- Hydroxyzine
- Imipenem/cilastatin
- Mercaptopurine
- Ondansetron
- Sodium bicarbonate
- Vincristine

Y-Site Compatible:

- Allopurinol
- Amifostine
- Asparaginase
- Aztreonam
- Bleomycin
- Cefepime
- Ceftriaxone
- Cimetidine
- Cisplatin
- Daunomycin
- Dexchlorpheniramine
- Diphenhydramine
- Doxapram
- Doxorubicin
- Doxorubicin, liposomal
- Etoposide
- Famotidine
- Filgrastim
- Fludarabine
- Furosemide
- Gallium nitrate
- Ganciclovir
- Granisetron
- Heparin
- Hydromorphone
- Leucovorin
- Lorazepam
- Mesna
- Methylprednisolone
- Mitomycin
- Morphine
- Oxacillin
- Paclitaxel
- Piperacillin/tazobactam
- Prochlorperazine
- Ranitidine
- Sargramostim
- Teniposide
- Thiotepa
- Vinblastine
- Vindesine
- Vinorelbine

Incompatible:

- Dexamethasone
- Gemcitabine
- Idarubicin
- Ifosfamide
- Midazolam
- Nalbuphine
- Prednisolone
- Promethazine
- Propofol
- TPN

Variable Compatibility:

- Droperidol
- Metoclopramide
- Vancomycin

Metoclopramide

Compatible:

- D_5W
- NS
- Clindamycin
- Mannitol
- Multivitamins
- Potassium acetate
- Potassium chloride
- Potassium phosphate
- Verapamil
- TPN

Y-Site Compatible:

- Acyclovir
- Aldesleukin
- Amifostine
- Aztreonam
- Bleomycin
- Ciprofloxacin
- Cisplatin
- Cyclophosphamide
- Cytarabine
- Diltiazem
- Doxorubicin
- Droperidol
- Famotidine
- Filgrastim
- Fluconazole

COMPATIBILITY OF CHEMOTHERAPY AND RELATED SUPPORTIVE CARE MEDICATIONS *(Continued)*

- Fludarabine
- Fluorouracil
- Foscarnet
- Gallium nitrate
- Gemcitabine
- Heparin
- Idarubicin
- Leucovorin
- Melphalan
- Meperidine
- Methotrexate
- Mitomycin
- Morphine
- Ondansetron
- Paclitaxel
- Piperacillin/tazobactam
- Sargramostim
- Sufentanil
- Tacrolimus
- Teniposide
- Thiotepa
- Vinblastine
- Vincristine
- Vinorelbine
- Zidovudine

Incompatible:

- Allopurinol
- Ampicillin
- Calcium gluconate
- Cefepime
- Cephalothin
- Chloramphenicol
- Dexamethasone
- Erythromycin
- Floxacillin
- Furosemide
- Penicillin G potassium
- Sodium bicarbonate

Metronidazole

Compatible:

- Amikacin
- Aminophylline
- Cefazolin
- Cefotaxime
- Cefotetan
- Cefoxitin
- Ceftazidime
- Ceftizoxime
- Ceftriaxone
- Cefuroxime
- Cephalothin
- Chloramphenicol
- Ciprofloxacin
- Clindamycin
- Disopyramide
- Floxacillin
- Fluconazole
- Gentamicin
- Heparin
- Hydrocortisone
- Moxalactam
- Multielectrolyte concentrate
- Multivitamins
- Netilmicin
- Penicillin G potassium
- Tobramycin

Y-Site Compatible:

- Acyclovir
- Allopurinol
- Amifostine
- Cefepime
- Cyclophosphamide
- Diltiazem
- Enalaprilat
- Esmolol
- Fluconazole
- Foscarnet
- Gemcitabine
- Heparin
- Hydromorphone
- Labetatol
- Lorazepam
- Magnesium sulfate
- Melphalan
- Meperidine
- Midazolam
- Morphine
- Perphenazine
- Piperacillin/tazobactam
- Sargramostim
- Tacrolimus
- Teniposide
- Theophylline
- Thiotepa
- TPN
- Vinorelbine

Incompatible:

- Aztreonam
- Dopamine
- Filgrastim

Variable Compatibility:

- Ampicillin
- Cefamandole

Mitomycin

Compatible:

- NS
- LR
- Dexamethasone
- Hydrocortisone sodium succinate

Y-Site Compatible:

- Allopurinol
- Amifostine
- Bleomycin
- Cisplatin
- Cyclophosphamide
- Doxorubicin
- Droperidol
- Fluorouracil
- Furosemide
- Leucovorin
- Methotrexate
- Metoclopramide
- Ondansetron
- Teniposide
- Thiotepa
- Vinblastine
- Vincristine

Incompatible:

- Aztreonam
- Cefepime
- Filgrastim
- Gemcitabine
- Piperacillin/tazobactam
- Sargramostim
- Vinorelbine

Variable Compatibility:

- D_5W
- SWI
- Heparin

Mitoxantrone

Compatible:

- D_5W
- D_5/NS
- NS
- Cyclophosphamide
- Cytarabine
- Fluorouracil
- Potassium chloride

Y-Site Compatible:

- Allopurinol
- Amifostine
- Filgrastim
- Fludarabine
- Gemcitabine
- Ondansetron
- Sargramostim
- Teniposide
- Thiotepa
- Vinorelbine

Incompatible:

- Aztreonam
- Cefepime
- Doxorubicin, liposomal
- Heparin
- Paclitaxel
- Piperacillin
- Piperacillin/tazobactam
- Propofol

Variable Compatibility:

- Hydrocortisone sodium phosphate
- Hydrocortisone sodium succinate
- TPN

Ondansetron

Compatible:

- D_5W
- NS
- LR
- Cisplatin
- Cyclophosphamide
- Cytarabine
- Dacarbazine
- Dexamethasone
- Doxorubicin
- Etoposide
- Fluconazole
- Hydrocortisone sodium succinate
- Mannitol
- Meperidine
- Methotrexate
- Morphine
- Ranitidine

Y-Site Compatible:

- Aldesleukin
- Amifostine
- Amikacin
- Aztreonam
- Bleomycin
- Carboplatin
- Carmustine
- Cefazolin
- Cefotaxime
- Cefoxitin
- Ceftazidime
- Ceftizoxime
- Cefuroxime
- Chlorpromazine
- Cimetidine
- Dactinomycin
- Daunomycin
- Diphenhydramine
- Doxorubicin, liposomal
- Doxycycline
- Droperidol
- Famotidine
- Filgrastim
- Floxuridine
- Fludarabine
- Gallium nitrate
- Gemcitabine
- Gentamicin
- Haloperidol
- Heparin
- Hydrocortisone sodium phosphate
- Hydromorphone
- Hydroxyzine
- Ifosfamide
- Imipenem/cilastatin
- Magnesium sulfate
- Mechlorethamine
- Mesna
- Metoclopramide
- Miconazole
- Mitomycin
- Mitoxantrone
- Paclitaxel
- Pentostatin
- Piperacillin/tazobactam
- Potassium chloride
- Prochlorperazine
- Promethazine
- Sodium acetate
- Streptozocin
- Teniposide
- Thiotepa
- Ticarcillin
- Ticarcillin/clavulanate
- TPN
- Vancomycin
- Vinblastine
- Vincristine
- Vinorelbine

Incompatible:

- Acyclovir
- Allopurinol
- Aminophylline
- Amphotericin
- Ampicillin
- Ampicillin/sulbactam
- Amsacrine
- Cefepime
- Cefoperazone
- Furosemide
- Ganciclovir
- Lorazepam
- Methylprednisolone
- Mezlocillin
- Piperacillin
- Sargramostim
- Sodium bicarbonate

Variable Compatibility:

- Fluorouracil

COMPATIBILITY OF CHEMOTHERAPY AND RELATED SUPPORTIVE CARE MEDICATIONS *(Continued)*

Paclitaxel

Compatible:

NS

Y-Site Compatible:

Acyclovir
Amikacin
Aminophylline
Ampicillin/sulbactam
Bleomycin
Butorphanol
Calcium chloride
Carboplatin
Cefepime
Cefotetan
Ceftazidime
Cefuroxime
Cimetidine
Cyclophosphamide
Cytarabine
Dacarbazine
Dexamethasone
Diphenhydramine
Doxorubicin
Droperidol
Etoposide
Famotidine
Floxuridine
Fluconazole
Fluorouracil
Furosemide
Ganciclovir
Gemcitabine
Gentamicin
Granisetron
Haloperidol
Heparin
Hydrocortisone sodium phosphate
Hydrocortisone sodium succinate
Hydromorphone
Ifosfamide
Lorazepam
Magnesium sulfate
Mannitol
Meperidine
Mesna
Methotrexate
Metoclopramide
Morphine
Nalbuphine
Ondansetron
Pentostatin
Potassium chloride
Prochlorperazine
Propofol
Ranitidine
Sodium bicarbonate
Thiotepa
TPN
Vancomycin
Vinblastine
Vincristine

Incompatible:

Amphotericin
Chlorpromazine
Doxorubicin, liposomal
Hydroxyzine
Methylprednisolone
Mitoxantrone

Variable Compatibility:

D_5W
Cisplatin

Pentostatin

Compatible:

NS
LR

Y-Site Compatible:

Fludarabine
Ondansetron
Paclitaxel
Sargramostim

Variable Compatibility:

D_5W

Phytonadione

Compatible:

Amikacin
Calcium gluceptate
Cefapirin
Chloramphenicol
Cimetidine
Netilmicin
Doxapram
Sodium bicarbonate
TPN

Y-Site Compatible:

Ampicillin
Epinephrine
Famotidine
Heparin
Hydrocortisone sodium succinate
Potassium chloride
Tolazoline
Vitamin B complex with C

Incompatible:

Dobutamine
Ranitidine

Plicamycin

Compatible:

D_5W
NS
SWI
Piperacillin

Y-Site Compatible:

Allopurinol
Amifostine
Aztreonam
Filgrastim
Gemcitabine
Piperacillin/tazobactam
Teniposide
Vinorelbine

Incompatible:

Cefonicid

Prochlorperazine

Compatible:

Amikacin
Ascorbic acid
Dexamethasone
Dimenhydrinate
Erythromycin
Ethacrinate
Lidocaine
Nafcillin
Sodium bicarbonate
Vitamin B complex with C

Y-Site Compatible:

Amsacrine
Cisplatin
Cyclophosphamide
Cytarabine
Doxorubicin
Fluconazole
Heparin
Hydrocortisone sodium succinate
Melphalan
Methotrexate
Ondansetron
Paclitaxel
Potassium chloride
Sargramostim
Sufentanil
Teniposide
Thiotepa
Vinorelbine

Incompatible:

Aldesleukin
Allopurinol
Amifostine
Aminophylline
Amphotericin
Ampicillin
Aztreonam
Calcium gluceptate
Cefepime
Cephalothin
Chloramphenicol
Floxacillin
Fludarabine
Foscarnet
Filgrastim
Furosemide
Gallium nitrate
Gemcitabine
Methohexital
Penicillin G sodium
Piperacillin/tazobactam
Phenobarbital
Thiopental

Variable Compatibility:

Calcium gluconate
Penicillin G potassium

Promethazine

Compatible:

Amikacin
Ascorbic acid
Chloroquine
Netilmicin
Vitamin B complex with C

Y-Site Compatible:

Amifostine
Amsacrine
Aztreonam
Ciprofloxacin
Cisplatin
Cyclophosphamide
Cytarabine
Doxorubicin
Filgrastim
Fluconazole
Fludarabine
Gemcitabine
Melphalan
Ondansetron
Sargramostim
Teniposide
Thiotepa
Vinorelbine

Incompatible:

Aldesleukin
Allopurinol
Aminophylline
Cefepime
Cefoperazone
Cefotetan
Ceftizoxime
Chloramphenicol
Chlorothiazide
Floxacillin
Foscarnet
Furosemide
Heparin
Hydrocortisone sodium succinate
Methicillin
Methohexital
Methotrexate
Penicillin G (sodium and potassium)
Pentobarbital
Piperacillin/tazobactam
Thiopental

Variable Compatibility:

Potassium chloride

COMPATIBILITY OF CHEMOTHERAPY AND RELATED SUPPORTIVE CARE MEDICATIONS *(Continued)*

Sargramostim

Compatible:

BWI
D_5W
NS
SWI

Y-Site Compatible:

Allopurinol
Amikacin
Aminophylline
Aztreonam
Bleomycin
Butorphanol
Calcium gluconate
Carboplatin
Carmustine
Cefazolin
Cefepime
Cefotetan
Cefoxitin
Ceftizoxime
Ceftriaxone
Cefuroxime
Cimetidine
Cisplatin
Cotrimoxazole
Cyclophosphamide
Cyclosporine
Cytarabine
Dacarbazine
Dactinomycin
Dexamethasone
Diphenhydramine
Dobutamine
Doxorubicin
Doxycycline
Droperidol
Etoposide
Famotidine
Fentanyl
Floxuridine
Fluconazole
Fluorouracil
Furosemide
Gentamicin
Heparin
Human immune globulin
Idarubicin
Ifosfamide
Magnesium sulfate
Mannitol
Mechlorethamine
Meperidine
Mesna
Methotrexate
Metoclopramide
Metronidazole
Mezlocillin
Miconazole
Minocycline
Mitoxantrone
Netilmicin
Pentostatin
Piperacillin/tazobactam
Potassium chloride
Prochlorperazine
Promethazine
Ranitidine
Teniposide
Ticarcillin
Ticarcillin/clavulanate
Vinblastine
Vincristine

Incompatible:

Acyclovir
Ampicillin
Ampicillin/sulbactam
Cefonicid
Cefoperazone
Chlorpromazine
Ganciclovir
Haloperidol
Hydrocortisone sodium phosphate
Hydrocortisone sodium succinate
Hydromorphone
Hydroxyzine
Imipenem/cilastatin
Methylprednisolone
Mitomycin
Morphine
Nalbuphine
Ondansetron
Piperacillin
Sodium bicarbonate
Tobramycin

Variable Compatibility:

Amphotericin
Amsacrine
Ceftazidime
Vancomycin

Streptozocin

Compatible:

D_5W
NS
SWI

Y-Site Compatible:

Filgrastim
Gemcitabine
Granisetron
Ondansetron
Teniposide
Thiotepa
Vinorelbine

Incompatible:

Allopurinol
Aztreonam
Cefepime
Piperacillin
Piperacillin/tazobactam

Teniposide

Compatible:

D_5W
NS
LR

Y-Site Compatible:

Acyclovir
Allopurinol
Amifostine
Amikacin
Aminophylline
Amphotericin
Ampicillin
Ampicillin/sulbactam
Aztreonam
Bleomycin
Bumetanide
Buprenorphine
Butorphanol
Calcium gluconate
Carboplatin
Carmustine
Cefazolin
Cefonicid
Cefoperazone
Cefotaxime
Cefotetan
Cefoxitin
Ceftazidime
Ceftizoxime

Ceftriaxone
Cefuroxime
Chlorpromazine
Cimetidine
Cisplatin
Corticotropin
Cotrimoxazole
Cyclophosphamide
Cytarabine
Dacarbazine
Dactinomycin
Daunomycin
Dexamethasone
Diphenhydramine
Doxorubicin
Doxycycline
Droperidol
Enalaprilat
Etoposide
Famotidine
Floxuridine
Fluconazole
Fludarabine
Fluorouracil
Furosemide
Gallium nitrate
Ganciclovir
Gemcitabine
Gentamicin
Haloperidol
Heparin
Hydrocortisone sodium phosphate
Hydrocortisone sodium succinate
Hydromorphone
Hydroxyzine
Ifosfamide
Imipenem/cilastatin
Leucovorin
Lorazepam
Mannitol
Mechlorethamine
Meperidine
Mesna
Methotrexate
Methylprednisolone
Metoclopramide
Metronidazole
Mezlocillin
Miconazole
Midazolam
Mitomycin
Mitoxantrone
Morphine
Nalbuphine
Netilmicin
Ondansetron
Piperacillin
Plicamycin
Potassium chloride
Prochlorperazine
Promethazine
Ranitidine
Sargramostim
Sodium bicarbonate
Streptozocin
Thiotepa
Ticarcillin
Ticarcillin/clavulanate
Tobramycin
Vancomycin
Vinblastine
Vincristine
Vinorelbine

Incompatible:
Idarubicin

Thiethylperazine

Compatible:
NS
Butorphanol
Hydromorphone
Midazolam
Ranitidine

Y-Site Compatible:
Aldesleukin

Incompatible:
Ketorolac
Perphenazine

Variable Compatibility:
Nalbuphine

Thiotepa

Compatible:
NS
SWI

Y-Site Compatible:
Acyclovir
Allopurinol
Amifostine
Amikacin
Aminophylline
Amphotericin
Ampicillin
Ampicillin/sulbactam
Aztreonam
Bleomycin
Bumetanide
Buprenorphine
Butorphanol
Calcium gluconate
Carboplatin
Carmustine
Cefazolin
Cefepime
Cefonicid
Cefoperazone
Cefotaxime
Cefotetan
Cefoxitin
Ceftazidime
Ceftizoxime
Ceftriaxone
Cefuroxime
Chlorpromazine
Cimetidine
Ciprofloxacin
Cotrimoxazole
Cyclophosphamide
Cytarabine
Dacarbazine
Dactinomycin
Daunomycin
Dexamethasone
Diphenhydramine
Dobutamine
Dopamine
Doxorubicin
Doxycycline
Droperidol
Enalaprilat
Etoposide
Famotidine
Floxuridine
Fluconazole
Fludarabine
Fluorouracil
Furosemide
Gallium nitrate
Ganciclovir
Gemcitabine
Gentamicin
Granisetron
Haloperidol
Heparin
Hydrocortisone sodium phosphate
Hydrocortisone sodium succinate
Hydromorphone
Hydroxyzine
Idarubicin
Ifosfamide
Imipenem/cilastatin
Leucovorin
Lorazepam
Magnesium sulfate
Mannitol
Meperidine
Mesna
Methotrexate
Methylprednisolone
Metoclopramide
Metronidazole
Mezlocillin
Miconazole
Mitomycin
Mitoxantrone

COMPATIBILITY OF CHEMOTHERAPY AND RELATED SUPPORTIVE CARE MEDICATIONS *(Continued)*

Morphine
Nalbuphine
Netilmicin
Ofloxacin
Ondansetron
Paclitaxel
Piperacillin
Piperacillin/tazobactam
Plicamycin
Potassium chloride
Prochlorperazine
Promethazine
Ranitidine
Sodium bicarbonate
Streptozocin
Teniposide
Ticarcillin
Ticarcillin/clavulanate
Tobramycin
TPN
Vancomycin
Vinblastine
Vincristine

Incompatible:

Cisplatin
Filgrastim
Minocycline

Topotecan

Compatible:

D_5W
NS
LR

Y-Site Compatible:

Gemcitabine

Trimetrexate

Compatible:

D_5W

Y-Site Compatible:

Amifostine

Incompatible:

BNS
D_5/NS
$D_5/^1/_4NS$
$D_5/^1/_2NS$
D_5/LR
D_{10}/NS
NS
LR
Calcium chloride
Chloride ion
Leucovorin
Potassium chloride

Vinblastine

Compatible:

BNS
D_5W
NS
LR
Bleomycin
Dacarbazine

Y-Site Compatible:

Allopurinol
Amifostine
Aztreonam
Cisplatin
Cyclophosphamide
Doxorubicin, liposomal
Droperidol
Filgrastim
Fludarabine
Fluorouracil
Gemcitabine
Leucovorin
Methotrexate
Metoclopramide
Mitomycin
Ondansetron
Paclitaxel
Piperacillin
Piperacillin/tazobactam
Sargramostim
Teniposide
Vincristine
Vinorelbine

Incompatible:

Cefazolin
Furosemide

Variable Compatibility:

Doxorubicin
Heparin

Vincristine

Compatible:

D_5W
NS
LR
Bleomycin
Cytarabine
Doxorubicin
Fluorouracil
Methotrexate

Y-Site Compatible:

Allopurinol
Amifostine
Aztreonam
Cisplatin
Cyclophosphamide
Doxapram
Doxorubicin, liposomal
Droperidol
Filgrastim

Fludarabine
Gemcitabine
Granisetron
Heparin
Leucovorin
Metoclopramide
Mitomycin
Ondansetron
Paclitaxel
Piperacillin/tazobactam
Sargramostim
Teniposide
Vinblastine
Vinorelbine

Incompatible:

Cefepime
Furosemide
Idarubicin
Sodium bicarbonate

Vinorelbine

Compatible:

D_5W
$D_5/^1/_2NS$
NS
LR

Y-Site Compatible:

Amikacin
Aztreonam
Bleomycin
Bumetanide
Buprenorphine
Butorphanol
Calcium gluconate
Carboplatin
Carmustine
Cefotaxime
Ceftazidime
Ceftizoxime
Chlorpromazine
Cimetidine
Cisplatin
Cyclophosphamide
Cytarabine
Dacarbazine
Dactinomycin
Daunomycin
Dexamethasone
Diphenhydramine
Doxorubicin
Doxorubicin, liposomal
Doxycycline
Droperidol
Enalaprilat
Etoposide
Famotidine
Filgrastim
Fluconazole
Fludarabine
Fluorouracil
Gallium nitrate
Gemcitabine
Gentamicin
Haloperidol
Heparin
Hydrocortisone sodium phosphate
Hydrocortisone sodium succinate
Hydromorphone
Hydroxyzine
Idarubicin
Ifosfamide
Imipenem/cilastatin
Lorazepam
Mannitol
Mechlorethamine
Meperidine
Mesna
Methotrexate
Metoclopramide
Metronidazole
Minocycline
Mitoxantrone
Morphine
Nalbuphine
Netilmicin
Ondansetron
Plicamycin
Streptozocin
Teniposide
Ticarcillin
Ticarcillin/clavulanate
Tobramycin
Vinblastine
Vincristine
Vindesine

Incompatible:

Acyclovir
Allopurinol
Aminophylline
Amphotericin
Ampicillin
Cefazolin
Cefoperazone
Cefotetan
Ceftriaxone
Cefuroxime
Cotrimoxazole
Fluorouracil
Furosemide
Ganciclovir
Methylprednisolone
Mitomycin
Sodium bicarbonate
Thiotepa

COMPATIBILITY OF CHEMOTHERAPY AND RELATED SUPPORTIVE CARE MEDICATIONS *(Continued)*

Drug	Variable Compatibility
Carboplatin	Solutions in saline are less stable than in dextrose.
Carmustine	Solutions should be dispensed in glass and protected from light. Solutions are stable for <8 hours under most circumstances.
Cisplatin	Must have a chloride concentration of at least 0.2% in the final solution. The commercial product has a NS concentration. Etoposide + mannitol + potassium chloride in normal saline precipitates within 24 hours; when in $D_5/^1/_2$NS, it is stable for 24 hours.
Dacarbazine	Heparin 100 units/mL with dacarbazine 25 mg/mL is **incompatible**. Heparin 100 units/mL with dacarbazine 10 mg/mL is **compatible.**
Filgrastim	Gentamicin is reported to be physically **compatible** for Y-site injection, but with a decrease in biologic activity. Imipenem/cilastatin with filgrastim 40 mcg/mL is reported to be physically **compatible** for Y-site injection, but with a decrease in biologic activity.
Fluorouracil	Doxorubicin 2 mg/mL with fluorouracil 50 mg/mL is **compatible** for 13 minutes. Doxorubicin 0.5-1 mg/mL with fluorouracil 50 mg/mL is **incompatible**. Fluorouracil with doxorubicin is **Y-site compatible.** Variable compatibility with leucovorin.
Mesna	**Compatible** with ifosfamide. **Incompatible** with ifosfamide and epinephrine.
Leucovorin	Variable compatibility with fluorouracil.
Mitomycin	Mitomycin 50 mg/L in NS has a color change and 10% loss of drug concentration in 12 hours. Mitomycin 1 g/L in SWI precipitates in 24 hours under refrigeration. Other temperatures and concentrations are reported to be stable. Mitomycin in D_5W is **incompatible** in 20 mg/L; **compatible** in 40 mg/L. Mitomycin 500 mg/L with heparin 33,300 units/L in NS is **compatible**. PVC containers of mitomycin 167 mg/L with heparin 33,300 units/L in NS is **compatible**. Glass containers of mitomycin 167 mg/L with heparin 33,300 units/L in NS are **incompatible**.
Pentostatin	Pentostatin 20 mg/mL in D_5W at room temperature: a 2% loss of drug in 24 hours; 8% to 10% loss in 48 hours; and a 10% loss in 54 hours. Under refrigeration, there is no loss in 96 hours. There is a 10% loss in 23 hours at room temperature of pentostatin 2 mg/mL in D_5W
Sargramostim	Amphotericin B 0.6 mg/mL in D_5W with sargramostim 10 mcg/mL in NS forms immediate precipitate. Amphotericin B 0.6 mg/mL in D_5W with sargramostim 10 mcg/mL in D_5W is **Y-site compatible**. Amsacrine with sargramostim in NS forms immediate precipitate. Amsacrine with sargramostim in D_5W is **Y-site compatible**. Ceftazidime 40 mg/mL in NS with sargramostim 10 mcg/mL in NS is **incompatible**, with particle formation within 4 hours. Ceftazidime 40 mg/mL with sargramostim 6 or 15 mcg/mL is **compatible** for 2 hours (Y-site **compatible**). Vancomycin 20 mg/mL and sargramostim 6 mcg/mL is **incompatible**. Vancomycin 10 mg/mL and sargramostim 10 mcg/mL is **Y-site compatible**. Vancomycin 20 mg/mL and sargramostim 15 mcg/mL is **Y-site compatible**.
Vancomycin	Vancomycin 5 mg/mL with methotrexate 30 mg/mL is **compatible** for 2 hours, precipitates within 4 hours. Other concentrations tested were **compatible** for 1 hour. Vancomycin with methotrexate is **Y-site compatible**.

Drug	Variable Compatibility
Vinblastine	In various volumes, doxorubicin 2 mg/mL with vinblastine 1 mg/mL yields erratic assay results. Vinblastine with doxorubicin is **Y-site compatible**. Heparin 200 units/mL with vinblastine 1 mg/mL is **incompatible** in a syringe for 13 minutes. Heparin 500 units/mL with vinblastine 0.5 mg/mL is **compatible** in a syringe for 13 minutes.

Suggested Readings

Hall PD, Yui D, Lyons S, et al, "Compatibility of Filgrastim With Selected Antimicrobial Drugs During Simulated Y-Site Administration," *Am J Health-System Pharm*, 1997, 54:184-9.

McGuire TR, Narducci WA, and Fox JL, "Compatibility and Stability of Ondansetron Hydrochloride, Dexamethasone and Lorazepam in Injectable Solutions," *Am J Health-System Pharm*, 1993, 50:1410-4.

Najari Z and Rucho WJ, "Compatibility of Commonly Used Bone Marrow Drugs During Y-Site Delivery," *Am J Health-System Pharm*, 1997, 54:181-4.

Trissel LA, Chandler SW, and Folstad JT, "Visual Compatibility of Amsacrine With Selected Drugs During Simulated Y-Site Injection," *Am J Hospital Pharm*, 1990, 47:2525-8.

Trissel LA, Bready BB, Kwan JW, et al, "Visual Compatibility of Sargramostim With Selected Antineoplastic Agents, Anti-infectives, or Other Drugs During Simulated Y-Site Injection," *Am J Hospital Pharm*, 1992, 49:402-6.

Trissel LA and Martinez JF, "Physical Compatibility of Melphalan With Selected Drugs During Simulated Y-Site Administration," *Am J Hospital Pharm*, 1993, 50:2359-63.

Trissel LA and Martinez JF, Visual, "Turbidimetric and Particle-Content Assessment of Compatibility of Vinorelbine Tartrate With Selected Drugs During Simulated Y-Site Injection," *Am J Hospital Pharm*, 1994, 51:495-9.

Trissel LA and Martinez JF, "Physical Compatibility of Allopurinol Sodium With Selected Drugs During Simulated Y-Site Administration," *Am J Hospital Pharm*, 1994, 51:1792-9.

Trissel LA and Martinez JF, "Compatibility of Filgrastim With Selected Drugs During Simulated Y-Site Administration," *Am J Hospital Pharm*, 1994, 51:1907-13.

Trissel LA and Martinez JF, "Screening Teniposide For Y-Site Compatibility," *Hospital Pharm*, 1994, 29:1010, 1012-4, 1017.

Trissel LA, *Handbook on Injectable Drugs*, 9th Ed. Bethesda, MD: *Am Society Health-Systems Pharmacists*, 1996.

Trissel LA, *Supplement to Handbook on Injectable Drugs*, 9th Ed. Bethesda, MD: *Am Society of Health-Systems Pharmacists*, 1997.

Trissel LA, Gilbert DL, and Martinez JF, "Compatibility of Granisetron Hydrochloride With Selected Drugs During Simulated Y-Site Administration," *Am J Health-System Pharm*, 1997, 54:56-60.

Trissel LA, Gilbert DL, and Martinez JF, "Compatibility of Propofol With Selected Drugs During Simulated Y-Site Administration," *Am J Health-System Pharm*, 1997, 54:1287-92.

Trissel LA, Gilbert DL, Martinez JF, et al, "Compatibility of Parenteral Nutrient Solutions With Selected Drugs During Simulated Y-Site Administration," *Am J Health-System Pharm*, 1997, 54:1295-300.

Trissel LA, Gilbert DL, and Martinez JF, "Compatibility of Doxorubicin Hydrochloride Liposome With Selected Other Drugs During Simulated Y-Site Administration," *Am J Health-System Pharm*, 1997; 54:2708-13.

Trissel LA, Martinez JF, and Gilbert DL, "Compatibility of Gemcitabine Hydrochloride With 107 Selected Drugs During Simulated Y-Site Administration," *J Am Pharmaceutical Association*, 1999, 39 (4):514-18.

Zhang Y, Xu QA, Trissel LA, et al, "Compatibility and Stability of Paclitaxel Combined With Cisplatin and With Carboplatin in Infusion Solutions," *Ann Pharmacother*, 1997, 31 (12):1465-70.

HEMATOLOGIC ADVERSE EFFECTS OF DRUGS

Drug	Red Cell Aplasia	Thrombocy-topenia	Neutrope-nia	Pancytope-nia	Hemolysis
Acetazolamide		+	+	+	
Allopurinol			+		
Amiodarone	+				
Amphotericin B				+	
Amrinone		++			
Asparaginase		+++	+++	+++	++
Barbiturates		+		+	
Benzocaine					++
Captopril			++		+
Carbamazepine		++	+		
Cephalosporins			+		++
Chloramphenicol		+	++	+++	
Chlordiazepoxide			+	+	
Chloroquine		+			
Chlorothiazides		++			
Chlorpropamide	+	++	+	++	+
Chlortetracycline				+	
Chlorthalidone			+		
Cimetidine		+	++	+	
Codeine		+			
Colchicine				+	
Cyclophosphamide		+++	+++	+++	+
Dapsone					+++
Desipramine		++			
Digitalis		+			
Digitoxin		++			
Erythromycin		+			
Estrogen		+		+	
Ethacrynic acid			+		
Fluorouracil		+++	+++	+++	+
Furosemide		+	+		
Gold salts	+	+++	+++	+++	
Heparin		++		+	
Ibuprofen			+		+
Imipramine			++		
Indomethacin		+	++	+	
Isoniazid		+		+	
Isosorbide dinitrate					+
Levodopa					++
Meperidine		+			
Meprobamate		+	+	+	
Methimazole			++		
Methyldopa		++			+++
Methotrexate		+++	+++	+++	++
Methylene blue					+
Metronidazole			+		
Nalidixic acid					+

Drug	Red Cell Aplasia	Thrombocy-topenia	Neutrope-nia	Pancytope-nia	Hemolysis
Naproxen				+	
Nitrofurantoin			++		+
Nitroglycerine		+			
Penicillamine		++	+		
Penicillins		+	++	+	+++
Phenazopyridine					+++
Phenothiazines		+	++	+++	+
Phenylbutazone		+	++	+++	+
Phenytoin		++	++	++	+
Potassium iodide		+			
Prednisone		+			
Primaquine					+++
Procainamide			+		
Procarbazine		+	++	++	+
Propylthiouracil		+	++	+	+
Quinidine		+++	+		
Quinine		+++	+		
Reserpine		+			
Rifampicin		++	+		+++
Spironolactone			+		
Streptomycin		+		+	
Sulfamethoxazole with trimethoprim			+		
Sulfonamides	+	++	++	++	++
Sulindac	+	+	+	+	
Tetracyclines		+			+
Thioridazine			++		
Tolbutamide		++	+	++	
Triamterene					+
Valproate	+				
Vancomycin			+		

+ = rare or single reports.

++ = occasional reports.

+++ = substantial number of reports.

Adapted from D'Arcy PF and Griffin JP, eds, *Iatrogenic Diseases*, New York, NY: Oxford University Press, 1986, 128-30.

TUMOR LYSIS SYNDROME, MANAGEMENT

Tumor lysis syndrome (TLS) may be seen with any tumor that is undergoing rapid cell turnover as a result of high growth fraction or high cell death due to therapy. It occurs most often in Burkitt's lymphoma and T-cell ALL, both of which have large tumor burdens and high sensitivity to chemotherapy. Acute lysis of tumor cells results in the rapid release of potassium, phosphates, and nucleic acids into the circulation. Hypocalcemia, hyperuricemia, and renal failure may result. Secondary acute precipitation of calcium and urates in the kidney, tumor infiltration of the kidney, obstructive uropathy, and dehydration may increase the primary metabolic disturbances. The following chart reviews the management of TLS.

Therapy	Infants & Children	Adolescents & Adults
Hydration (patients typically present with dehydration; I.V. fluids should be started immediately)	3000-6000 mL/m²/day D_5W 1/4 NS (+ sodium bicarbonate) Maintain urine output at ≥1 mL/kg/hour Maintain urine specific gravity at ≤1.010 Strict monitoring of I & O	3000-6000 mL/m²/day D_5W 1/4 NS (+ sodium bicarbonate) Maintain urine output at 100-150 mL/hour Maintain urine specific gravity at ≤1.010 Strict monitoring of I & O
Alkalinization	50-100 mEq/L sodium bicarbonate in I.V. fluid Maintain urine pH at 7.0-7.5 Reduce bicarbonate if serum bicarbonate >30 mEq/L or urine pH >7.5	50-100 mEq/L sodium bicarbonate in I.V. fluid Maintain urine pH at 7.0-7.5 Reduce bicarbonate if serum bicarbonate >30 mEq/L or urine pH >7.5
Uric acid reduction	Allopurinol: I.V., oral: 200-400 mg/m²/day in 1-3 divided doses (maximum: 600 mg/day) Urate oxidase: I.V. (investigational, see protocol): 0.2 mg/kg/dose once or twice daily	Allopurinol: I.V.: 200-400 mg/m²/day in 1-3 divided doses (maximum: 600 mg/day) Oral: 600-800 mg/day in 1-2 doses
Diuretics (avoid if hypovolemic)	Furosemide: I.V.: 1 mg/kg/dose as needed Mannitol: I.V.: 0.25-0.5 g/kg/dose as needed	Furosemide: I.V.: 20-40 mg/dose as needed Mannitol: I.V.: 0.25-0.5 g/kg/dose as needed
Phosphate reduction	Aluminum hydroxide: Oral: 50 mg/kg/dose every 8 hours	Aluminum hydroxide: Oral: 30-40 mL/dose every 6-8 hours
Dialysis indications (peritoneal dialysis is much less efficient for reducing uric acid than other modalities, and is contraindicated in patients with abdominal tumors.)	Potassium level >6 mEq/L Uric acid level >10 mg/dL Creatinine >10 times normal Uremia Phosphorus >10 mg/dL or rapidly rising Symptomatic hypocalcemia Severe, unmanageable hypertension Volume overload	

Kelly KM and Lange B, "Oncologic Emergencies," *Pediatr Clin North Am*, 1997, 44(4):809-30.

ANTITHROMBOTIC THERAPY IN CHILDREN

Recommendations From the Seventh American College of Chest Physicians (ACCP) Conference on Antithrombotic and Thrombolytic Therapy

Used with permission from Monagle P, Chan A, Massicotte P, et al, "Antithrombotic Therapy in Children: The Seventh ACCP Conference on Antithrombotic and Thrombolytic Therapy," *Chest*, 2004, 126(3 Suppl):645S-687S.

Abbreviations: ADP = adenosine diphosphate; AIS = arterial ischemic stroke; aPTT = activated partial thromboplastin time; AT = antithrombin; BT = Blalock-Taussig; CC = cardiac catheterization; CHD = congenital heart disease; CI = confidence interval; CSVT = cerebral sinovenous thrombosis; CVL = central venous line; DVT = deep venous thrombosis; FFP = fresh-frozen plasma; FXa = factor Xa; GP = glycoprotein; HIT = heparin-induced thrombocytopenia; ICH = intracranial hemorrhage; INR = international normalized ratio; IVC = inferior vena cava; LMWH = low-molecular-weight heparin; MRV = magnetic resonance venography; PC = protein C; PE = pulmonary embolism; PICU = pediatric ICU; PS = protein S; PTS = post-thrombotic syndrome; RCT = randomized controlled trial; RR = relative risk; RVT = renal vein thrombosis; SK = streptokinase; SVT = sinovenous thrombosis; TE = thromboembolic event; tPA = tissue plasminogen activator; TPN = total parenteral nutrition; UAC = umbilical arterial catheter; UFH = unfractionated heparin; UK = urokinase; UVC = umbilical vein catheter; VKA = vitamin K antagonist; VTE = venous thromboembolism

1.1 Venous Thromboembolism

Neonates with VTE

1.1.1. ACCP suggests treatment with either UFH or LMWH, or radiographic monitoring and anticoagulation therapy if extension occurs (Grade 2C).

1.1.2. ACCP suggests that if clinicians elect treatment with anticoagulation therapy, they administer UFH or LMWH, and subsequently administer LMWH for 10 days to 3 months (Grade 2C).

1.1.3. ACCP suggests that clinicians adjust the dose of UFH to prolong the aPTT corresponding to an anti-FXa level of 0.35-0.7 units/mL (Grade 2C).

1.1.4. ACCP suggests that clinicians adjust the dose of LMWH to achieve an anti-FXa level of 0.5-1.0 unit/mL (Grade 2C).

1.1.5. ACCP suggests that if the thrombus extends following the discontinuation of heparin therapy, clinicians administer VKAs or extended LMWH therapy (Grade 2C).

1.1.6. ACCP suggests that clinicians **not** use thrombolytic therapy for the treatment of VTEs in neonates unless there is major vessel occlusion that is causing the critical compromise of organs or limbs (Grade 2C). If thrombolytic therapy is used, ACCP suggests supplementation with plasminogen (ie, FFP) immediately prior to thrombolysis (Grade 2C).

1.1.7. ACCP suggests that, in general, clinicians should remove either CVLs or UVCs that are *in situ*. However, if either CVLs or UVCs are still in place at the completion of the above therapy, ACCP suggests prophylactic dosing with LMWH to prevent recurrent VTEs until such time as the CVL or UVC is removed (both Grade 2C).

ANTITHROMBOTIC THERAPY IN CHILDREN *(Continued)*

1.2. Systemic Venous Thromboembolic Disease in Children

First TE for children (>2 months of age)

1.2.1. ACCP recommends treatment with I.V. heparin sufficient to prolong the aPTT to a range that corresponds to an anti-FXa level of 0.35-0.7 units/mL or with LMWH sufficient to achieve an anti-FXa level of 0.5-1.0 unit/mL 4 h after an injection (Grade 1C+).

1.2.2. ACCP recommends initial treatment with heparin or LMWH for 5-10 days (Grade 1C+). For patients in whom subsequent VKAs will be used, ACCP recommends beginning oral therapy as early as day 1 and discontinuing heparin/ LMWH therapy on day 6 if the INR is in the therapeutic range on two consecutive days (Grade 1C+). For massive PEs or extensive DVT, ACCP recommends a longer period of heparin or LMWH therapy (Grade 1C+).

1.2.3. ACCP suggests continuing anticoagulant therapy for idiopathic TEs for at least 6 months using VKAs to achieve a target INR of 2.5 (INR range, 2.0-3.0) or, alternatively, LMWH to maintain an anti-FXa level of 0.5-1.0 unit/mL (Grade 2C). *Underlying values and preferences:* The suggestion to administer anticoagulation therapy to children with idiopathic DVT for at least 6 months rather than on a lifelong basis places a relatively high value on the avoidance of the known risk of bleeding secondary to anticoagulant therapy in young active adults, and less importance on the unknown risk of recurrence in the absence of an ongoing clinical precipitating factor.

1.2.4. ACCP suggests that for secondary TEs anticoagulant therapy be continued for at least 3 months using VKAs to achieve a target INR of 2.5 (INR range, 2.0-3.0) or, alternatively, using LMWH to maintain an anti-FXa level of 0.5-1.0 unit/mL (Grade 2C).

1.2.5. ACCP suggests that, in the presence of ongoing risk factors such as active nephrotic syndrome, ongoing asparaginase therapy, or administration of a lupus anticoagulant, anticoagulant therapy in either therapeutic or prophylactic doses continue until the risk factor has resolved (Grade 2C).

1.2.6. ACCP suggests that clinicians **not** use thrombolytic therapy routinely for the treatment of venous TE in children (Grade 2C). Treatment needs to be individualized, and based on the size and location of the thrombus, and the degree of organ compromise. If thrombolytic therapy is used, in the presence of physiologic or pathologic deficiencies of plasminogen, ACCP suggests supplementation with plasminogen (ie, FFP) (Grade 2C).

Recurrent idiopathic TEs in children

1.2.7. ACCP recommends indefinite therapy with either therapeutic or prophylactic doses of VKAs (Grade 1C+). ACCP suggests LMWH therapy as an alternative if VKA therapy is too difficult (Grade 2C).

Recurrent secondary TEs in children

1.2.8. ACCP suggests that, following the initial 3 months of therapy, anticoagulation therapy be continued for at least a further 3 months or until removal of any precipitating factors (Grade 2C).

CVL-related thrombosis

There are two aspects to the management of CVL-related thrombosis. First, management of the CVL itself and, second, anticoagulation therapy.

1.2.9. ACCP suggests that if the CVL is no longer required, or is nonfunctioning, it be removed (Grade 2C). ACCP suggests at least 3-5 days of anticoagulation therapy prior to its removal. If CVL access is required and the CVL involved is still functioning, ACCP suggests that the CVL remain *in situ* (Grade 2C). Anticoagulation therapy should be administered as described in recommendations 1.2.1-1.2.6.

1.2.10. For children with a first CVL-related DVT after the initial 3 months of therapy, ACCP suggests that prophylactic doses of VKAs (INR range, 1.5-1.8) or LMWH (anti-FXa level range, 0.1- 0.3) be administered until the CVL is removed (Grade 2C).

1.2.11. For children with recurrent CVL-related TEs after the initial 3 months of therapy, ACCP suggests prophylactic doses of VKAs (INR range, 1.5-1.8) or LMWH (anti-FXa level range, 0.1-0.3) be continued until the removal of the CVL. If the recurrence occurs while children are receiving prophylactic therapy, ACCP suggests continuing therapeutic doses until the CVL is removed or for a minimum of 3 months (Grade 2C).

1.3 Renal Vein Thrombosis

1.3.1. For unilateral RVT in the absence of uremia, and in the absence of extension into the IVC, ACCP suggests supportive care with careful monitoring of the RVT for extension (Grade 2C). Alternatively, ACCP suggests anticoagulation therapy with UFH or LMWH (Grade 2C).

1.3.2. For unilateral RVT that does extend into the IVC, ACCP suggests anticoagulation therapy with UFH or LMWH for 6 weeks to 3 months (Grade 2C). *Remark:* The therapeutic range is the same as that for the treatment of venous thrombosis.

1.3.3. For bilateral RVT with various degrees of renal failure, ACCP suggests therapy with UFH (and not LMWH) and thrombolytic therapy (Grade 2C).

1.4 Central Venous Line Prophylaxis

1.4.1. For children With CVLs, ACCP recommends **against** routine primary prophylaxis (Grade 1B).

1.4.2. For children receiving long-term home TPN, ACCP suggests antithrombotic prophylaxis. ACCP suggests continuous therapy with VKAs (target INR, 2-2.5) or, alternatively, for the first 3 months after each CVL is inserted (all Grade 2C). *Remark:* The optimal drug and dose are unknown.

1.5 Primary Prophylaxis for BT Shunts in Neonates

1.5.1. For neonates having BT shunts, ACCP suggests therapy with intraoperative heparin followed by either aspirin (5 mg/kg/d) or no further anticoagulant therapy (Grade 2C).

1.6 Primary Prophylaxis for Stage 1 Norwood Procedures in Neonates

1.6.1. For patients who have undergone the Norwood procedure, ACCP suggests heparin therapy immediately after the procedure (Grade 2C).

1.8 Primary Prophylaxis for Fontan Surgery in Children

1.8.1. For children after Fontan surgery, ACCP suggests therapy with aspirin (5 mg/kg/d) or therapeutic heparin followed by VKAs to achieve a target INR of 2.5 (INR range, 2-3) (Grade 2C). *Remark:* The optimal duration of therapy is unknown. Whether patients with fenestrations require more intensive therapy until fenestration closure is unknown.

1.9 Primary Prophylaxis for Endovascular Stents in Children

1.9.1. For children having endovascular stents inserted, ACCP suggests the administration of heparin perioperatively (Grade 2C).

ANTITHROMBOTIC THERAPY IN CHILDREN *(Continued)*

1.10 Primary Prophylaxis for Dilated Cardiomyopathy in Neonates and Children

1.10.1. For children with cardiomyopathy, ACCP suggests that they receive therapy with VKAs to achieve a target INR of 2.5 (INR range, 2-3) commencing no later than at the time of their activation on a cardiac transplant waiting list (Grade 2C). *Underlying values and preferences:* ACCP's suggestion for the administration of VKAs places a high value on avoiding thrombotic complications, and a relatively low value on avoiding the inconvenience, discomfort, and limitations of anticoagulant monitoring in children who have a potentially curative therapy (for their cardiomyopathy) available to them.

1.11 Primary Prophylaxis for Biological Prosthetic Heart Valves in Children

1.11.1. For children with biological prosthetic heart valves, ACCP recommends treatment according to the adult guidelines (Grade 1C+).

1.12 Primary Prophylaxis for Mechanical Prosthetic Heart Valves in Children

1.12.1. For children with mechanical prosthetic heart valves, ACCP recommends the administration of VKAs following adult guidelines (Grade 1C+).

1.12.2. In children in whom additional antithrombotic therapy is required due to lack of response to therapy with VKAs or a contraindication to therapy with full-dose VKAs, ACCP suggests adding therapy with aspirin (6-20 mg/kg/d) (Grade 2C).

1.14 Thromboprophylaxis for Cardiac Catheterization in Neonates and Children

1.14.1. For neonates and children requiring CC via an artery, ACCP recommends I.V. heparin prophylaxis (Grade 1A).

1.14.2. ACCP suggests the use of heparin doses of 100-150 units/kg as a bolus. Further doses may be required in prolonged procedures (both Grade 2B).

1.14.3. For prophylaxis for CC, ACCP recommends **against** aspirin therapy (Grade 1B).

1.15 Femoral Artery Thrombosis Following Cardiac Catheterization

1.15.1. For children or neonates with a femoral artery thrombosis, ACCP recommends therapeutic doses of I.V. heparin (Grade 1C). ACCP suggests treatment for at least 5-7 days (Grade 2C). *Remark:* The optimal duration of therapy is unknown.

1.15.2. For children or neonates with limb-threatening or organ-threatening (via proximal extension) femoral artery thrombosis who fail to respond to initial heparin therapy, and who have no known contraindications, ACCP recommends the administration of thrombolytic therapy (Grade 1C).

1.15.3. For children with femoral artery thrombosis in selected cases, ACCP suggests surgical intervention, in particular when there is a contraindication to thrombolytic therapy, or when organ or limb death is imminent (Grade 2C).

1.16 Peripheral Artery Thrombosis

1.16.1. For neonates and children with peripheral arterial catheters *in situ*, ACCP recommends the administration of low-dose heparin through the catheter, preferably by continuous infusion, to prolong the catheter patency (Grade 1A).

1.16.2. For children with a peripheral arterial catheter-related TE, ACCP suggests the immediate removal of the catheter (Grade 2C). ACCP suggests subsequent anticoagulation therapy with or without thrombolysis, depending on the clinical situation (Grade 2C).

1.18 Aortic Thrombosis Secondary to UACs in Neonates

1.18.1. For neonates with UACs, ACCP suggests therapy with low-dose heparin infusion (1-5 units/h) (Grade 2A).

1.18.2. ACCP suggests that aortic thrombosis secondary to UACs be managed by the same principles as those for femoral artery thrombosis secondary to cardiac catheters. If there is evidence of renal failure, then urgent restoration of renal blood flow is required, and ACCP suggests thrombolysis or thrombectomy (all Grade 2C).

1.19 Spontaneous Aortic Thrombosis in Neonates

1.19.1. For children experiencing spontaneous aortic thrombosis with evidence of renal ischemia, ACCP suggests urgent, aggressive use of thrombolytic or surgical therapy, supported by anticoagulation therapy with heparin or LMWH (Grade 2C).

1.20 Kawasaki Disease in Children

1.20.1. ACCP recommends aspirin therapy in high doses (ie, 80-100 mg/kg/d during the acute phase, for up to 14 days) as an anti-inflammatory agent, then in lower doses (ie, 3- 5 mg/kg/d for ≥7 weeks) as an antiplatelet agent (Grade 1C+).

1.20.2. ACCP recommends therapy with I.V. gammaglobulin (2 g/kg as a single dose) within 10 days of the onset of symptoms (Grade 1A).

1.21 Anticoagulation Therapy for Kawasaki Disease in Children With Giant Aneurysms

1.21.1. In children with giant coronary aneurysms following Kawasaki disease, ACCP suggests therapy with warfarin (target INR, 2.5; INR range, 2.0-3.0) in addition to low-dose aspirin (Grade 2C).

1.22 Sinovenous Thrombosis in Neonates

1.22.1. For neonates with CSVT, without large ischemic infarctions or ICH, ACCP suggests initial treatment with either UFH or LMWH followed by treatment with LMWH for 3 months (Grade 2C).

1.22.2. For neonates with CSVT, with large ischemic infarctions or ICH, ACCP suggests radiographic monitoring and the commencement of anticoagulation therapy if extension occurs (Grade 2C).

1.23 Sinovenous Thrombosis in Children

1.23.1. For children with CSVT, ACCP suggests treatment for 5-7 days with either UFH or LMWH followed by treatment with LMWH or VKAs (target INR, 2.5; INR range, 2.0-3.0) for 3-6 months even in the presence of a localized hemorrhagic infarction (Grade 2C).

1.24 Arterial Ischemic Stroke in Neonates

1.24.1. For neonates with noncardioembolic AIS, ACCP suggests that clinicians do **not** use anticoagulation or aspirin therapy (Grade 2C).

1.24.2. For neonates with cardioembolic AIS, ACCP suggests anticoagulation therapy with either UFH or LMWH for 3 months (Grade 2C).

1.25 Arterial Ischemic Stroke in Children

1.25.1. For children with AIS, ACCP suggests treatment with UFH or LMWH for 5-7 days and until cardioembolic stroke or vascular dissection has been excluded (Grade 2C).

1.25.2. For children with AIS and cardioembolic stroke or vascular dissection, ACCP suggests treatment for 5-7 days with UFH or LMWH followed by treatment with LMWH or VKAs for 3-6 months (Grade 2C).

ANTITHROMBOTIC THERAPY IN CHILDREN *(Continued)*

1.25.3. For all children with AIS, ACCP suggests treatment with 2-5 mg/kg/d aspirin after anticoagulation therapy has been discontinued (Grade 2C).

1.25.4. For children with sickle cell disease who are >2 years of age, ACCP recommends screening for stroke using transcranial Doppler imaging. If transcranial Doppler imaging is unavailable, ACCP recommends intermittent screening with MRI (Grade 1C).

1.25.5. For children with sickle cell disease who have ischemic stroke, ACCP recommends therapy with I.V. hydration and exchange transfusion to reduce hemoglobin S levels to <30% of total hemoglobin (Grade 1C).

1.25.6. For children with sickle cell disease who have ischemic stroke, after an initial exchange transfusion ACCP suggests a long-term transfusion program (Grade 2C).

1.26 Purpura Fulminans

1.26.1. For neonates with homozygous PC deficiency, ACCP recommends the administration of either 10-20 mL/kg FFP every 12 h or PC concentrate, when available, at a concentration of 20-60 units/kg until the clinical lesions resolve (Grade 1C+).

1.26.2. ACCP suggests long-term treatment with VKAs (Grade 2C), LMWH (Grade 2C), PC replacement (Grade 1C+), or liver transplantation (Grade 2C).

[1]The ACCP Consensus Conference on Antithrombotic Therapy uses grades of recommendations that are based on clarity of benefits versus risks of treatment (1 = clear risk/benefit, strong recommendation; 2 = unclear risk/benefit, weaker recommendation) and quality of the research methodology supporting the underlying evidence (A = randomized trials with consistent results; B = randomized trials with inconsistent results or with major weaknesses in methodology; C = observational studies and generalizations of randomized trials to another group of patients; C+ = observational studies with overwhelmingly compelling results or secure generalizations of randomized trials). The highest rating (1A) implies a strong recommendation; one that can be applied to most patients in most circumstances without reservations. The lowest rating (2C) implies a very weak recommendation; one in which other alternatives may be equally reasonable. For further information see Guyatt G, Schunemann HJ, Cook D, et al, "Applying the Grades of Recommendation for Antithrombotic and Thrombolytic Therapy: The Seventh ACCP Conference on Antithrombotic and Thrombolytic Therapy," *Chest*, 2004, 126(3 Suppl):179S-187S.

TOTAL BLOOD VOLUME

Age	Example Weight (kg) [age]	Approximate Total Blood Volume (mL/kg)[1]	Estimated Total Blood Volume (mL)
Premature infant	1.5	89-105	134-158
Term newborn	3.4	78-86	265-292
1-12 months	7.6 [6 months]	73-78	555-593
1-3 years	12.4 [2 years]	74-82	918-1017
4-6 years	18.2 [5 years]	80-86	1456-1565
7-18 years	45.5 [13 years]	83-90	3777-4095
Adults	70.0	68-88	4760-6160

[1]Approximate total blood volume information compiled from *Nathan and Oski's Hematology of Infancy and Childhood*, 5th ed, Nathan DG and Orkin SH, eds, Philadelphia, PA: WB Saunders, 1998.

ASSESSMENT OF LIVER FUNCTION

Child-Pugh Score

Component	Score Given for Observed Findings		
	1	2	3
Encephalopathy grade[1]	None	1-2	3-4
Ascites	None	Mild or controlled by diuretics	Moderate or refractory despite diuretics
Albumin (g/dL)	>3.5	2.8-3.5	<2.8
Total bilirubin (mg/dL) or Modified total bilirubin[2]	<2 (<34 micromoles/L) <4	2-3 (34-50 micromoles/L) 4-7	>3 (>50 micromoles/L) >7
Prothrombin time (seconds prolonged) or INR	<4 <1.7	4-6 1.7-2.3	>6 >2.3

[1]Encephalopathy Grades

Grade 0: Normal consciousness, personality, neurological examination, electroencephalogram

Grade 1: Restless, sleep disturbed, irritable/agitated, tremor, impaired handwriting, 5 cps waves

Grade 2: Lethargic, time-disoriented, inappropriate, asterixis, ataxia, slow triphasic waves

Grade 3: Somnolent, stuporous, place-disoriented, hyperactive reflexes, rigidity, slower waves

Grade 4: Unrousable coma, no personality/behavior, decerebrate, slow 2-3 cps delta activity

Alternative Encephalopathy Grades

Grade 1: Mild confusion, anxiety, restlessness, fine tremor, slowed coordination

Grade 2: Drowsiness, disorientation, asterixis

Grade 3: Somnolent but rousable, marked confusion, incomprehensible speech, incontinent, hyperventilation

Grade 4: Coma, decerebrate posturing, flaccidity

[2]Modified total bilirubin used to score patients who have Gilbert's syndrome or who are taking indinavir.

Child-Pugh Classification

Class A (mild hepatic impairment): Score 5-6
Class B (moderate hepatic impairment): Score 7-9
Class C (severe hepatic impairment): Score 10-15

References

Centers for Disease Control and Prevention, "Report of the NIH Panel to Define Principles of Therapy of HIV Infection and Guidelines for the Use of Antiretroviral Agents in HIV-Infected Adults and Adolescents," March 23, 2004, located at (URL) http://www.aidsinfo.nih.gov.

U.S. Department of Health and Human Services Food and Drug Administration, "Guidance for Industry, Pharmacokinetics in Patients With Impaired Hepatic Function: Study Design, Data Analysis, and Impact on Dosing and Labeling," May 2003, located at (URL) http://www.fda.gov/cder/guidance/3625fnl.pdf.

HOTLINE PHONE NUMBERS

AIDS Hotline	800-590-2437
AMA Foreign Drug	312-464-4575
AMA Library Answer Center	312-464-4818
American Association of Poison Control Centers (AAPCC) Poison Prevention	202-625-3333
American College of Clinical Pharmacy (ACCP)	816-531-2177
American Dental Association (ADA)	800-621-8099
American Medical Association (AMA)	312-464-5000
American Pharmaceutical Association (APhA)	202-628-4410
American Association of Health-System Pharmacists	301-657-3000
Animal Poison Care Hotline (24-hours)	800-548-2423
Canadian Pharmaceutical Association	613-523-7877
Center for Disease Control	1-800-311-3435
Use this number for the following departments also:	
CDC Disease Information	
CDC Epidemiology Program	
CDC Immunity Division	
CDC Influenza Branch	
CDC International Travelers Information	
CDC Parasitic Division	
CDC STDs	
CDC Tuberculosis Section	
FDA (Rare Diseases/Orphan Drugs)	800-300-7469
National Cancer Institute	301-496-1196
Asthma and Allergy Foundation of America	1-800-7-ASTHMA
Cancer Treatment (of NCI)	1-800-4-CANCER
Epilepsy Foundation of America	301-459-3700
National Council on Patient Information & Education	301-656-8565
National Institute of Health	301-496-4000
National Poison Center	202-362-3867
Emergency	800-222-1222
Parental Stress	800-632-8188
Pediatric Pharmacy Advocacy Group (PPAG) Membership and Drug Information	720-981-7356
Pesticides (Mon-Fri, 6:30 AM - 4:30 PM Pacific)	800-858-7378
Rocky Mountain Poison Control Information	800-525-6115

ENDOCARDITIS PROPHYLAXIS

Recommendations by the American Heart Association (*JAMA*, 1997, 277:1794-801)

Consensus Process – The recommendations were formulated by the writing group after specific therapeutic regimens were discussed. The consensus statement was subsequently reviewed by outside experts not affiliated with the writing group and by the Science Advisory and Coordinating Committee of the American Heart Association. These guidelines are meant to aid practitioners but are not intended as the standard of care or as a substitute for clinical judgment.

Table 1. Cardiac Conditions[1]

Endocarditis Prophylaxis Recommended

- High-Risk Category
  - Prosthetic cardiac valves, including bioprosthetic and homograft valves
  - Previous bacterial endocarditis
  - Complex cyanotic congenital heart disease (eg, single ventricle states, transposition of the great arteries, tetralogy of Fallot)
  - Surgically constructed systemic pulmonary shunts or conduits
- Moderate-Risk Category
  - Most other congenital cardiac malformations (other than above and below)
  - Acquired valvar dysfunction (eg, rheumatic heart disease)
  - Hypertrophic cardiomyopathy
  - Mitral valve prolapse with valvar regurgitation and/or thickened leaflets

Endocarditis Prophylaxis Not Recommended

- Negligible-Risk Category (no greater risk than the general population)
  - Isolated secundum atrial septal defect
  - Surgical repair of atrial septal defect, ventricular septal defect, or patent ductus arteriosus (without residua beyond 6 months)
  - Previous coronary artery bypass graft surgery
  - Mitral valve prolapse without valvar regurgitation
  - Physiologic, functional, or innocent heart murmurs
  - Previous Kawasaki disease without valvar dysfunction
  - Previous rheumatic fever without valvar dysfunction
  - Cardiac pacemakers (intravascular and epicardial) and implanted defibrillators

[1]This table lists selected conditions but is not meant to be all-inclusive.

Patient With Suspected Mitral Valve Prolapse

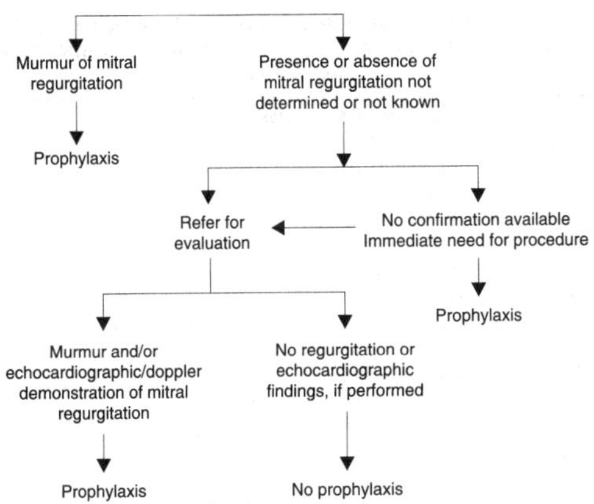

Table 2. Dental Procedures and Endocarditis Prophylaxis

Endocarditis Prophylaxis Recommended[1]
Dental extractions
Periodontal procedures including surgery, scaling and root planing, probing, and recall maintenance
Dental implant placement and reimplantation of avulsed teeth
Endodontic (root canal) instrumentation or surgery only beyond the apex
Subgingival placement of antibiotic fibers or strips
Initial placement of orthodontic bands but not brackets
Intraligamentary local anesthetic injections
Prophylactic cleaning of teeth or implants where bleeding is anticipated
Endocarditis Prophylaxis Not Recommended
Restorative dentistry[2] (operative and prosthodontic) with or without retraction cord[3]
Local anesthetic injections (nonintraligamentary)
Intracanal endodontic treatment; post placement and buildup[3]
Placement of rubber dams[3]
Postoperative suture removal
Placement of removable prosthodontic or orthodontic appliances
Taking of oral impressions[3]
Fluoride treatments
Taking of oral radiographs
Orthodontic appliance adjustment
Shedding of primary teeth

[1]Prophylaxis is recommended for patients with high- and moderate-risk cardiac conditions.

[2]This includes restoration of decayed teeth (filling cavities) and replacement of missing teeth.

[3]Clinical judgment may indicate antibiotic use in selected circumstances that may create significant bleeding.

ENDOCARDITIS PROPHYLAXIS *(Continued)*

Table 3. Recommended Standard Prophylactic Regimen for Dental, Oral, or Upper Respiratory Tract Procedures in Patients Who Are at Risk

Endocarditis Prophylaxis Recommended

- Respiratory Tract
  - Tonsillectomy and/or adenoidectomy
  - Surgical operations that involve respiratory mucosa
  - Bronchoscopy with a rigid bronchoscope
- Gastrointestinal Tract[1]
  - Sclerotherapy for esophageal varices
  - Esophageal stricture dilation
  - Endoscopic retrograde cholangiography with biliary obstruction
  - Biliary tract surgery
  - Surgical operations that involve intestinal mucosa
- Genitourinary Tract
  - Prostatic surgery
  - Cystoscopy
  - Urethral dilation

Endocarditis Prophylaxis Not Recommended

- Respiratory Tract
  - Endotracheal intubation
  - Bronchoscopy with a flexible bronchoscope, with or without biopsy[2]
  - Tympanostomy tube insertion
- Gastrointestinal Tract
  - Transesophageal echocardiography[2]
  - Endoscopy with or without gastrointestinal biopsy[2]
- Genitourinary Tract
  - Vaginal hysterectomy[2]
  - Vaginal delivery[2]
  - Cesarean section
  - In uninfected tissues:
    - Urethral catheterization
    - Uterine dilatation and curettage
    - Therapeutic abortion
    - Sterilization procedures
    - Insertion or removal of intrauterine devices
- Other
  - Cardiac catheterization, including balloon angioplasty
  - Implanted cardiac pacemakers, implanted defibrillators, and coronary stents
  - Incision or biopsy or surgically scrubbed skin
  - Circumcision

[1]Prophylaxis is recommended for high-risk patients, optional for medium-risk patients.

[2]Prophylaxis is optional for high-risk patients.

Table 4. Endocarditis Prophylaxis[1]

	Dosage for Adults	Dosage for Children[2]
DENTAL AND UPPER RESPIRATORY PROCEDURES		
Oral[3]		
Amoxicillin[4]	2 g 1 h before procedure	50 mg/kg 1 h before procedure
Penicillin allergy:		
Clindamycin or	600 mg 1 h before procedure	20 mg/kg 1 h before procedure
Cephalexin or	2 g 1 h before procedure	50 mg/kg 1 h before procedure
Azithromycin or Clarithromycin	500 mg 1 h before procedure	15 mg/kg 1 h before procedure
Parenteral[3]		
Ampicillin	2 g I.M. or I.V. 30 minutes before procedure	50 mg/kg I.M. or I.V. 30 minutes before procedure
Penicillin allergy:		
Clindamycin or	600 mg I.V. 30 minutes before procedure	20 mg/kg I.V. 30 minutes before procedure
Cefazolin (not to be used in individuals with immediate-type hypersensitivity reaction to penicillins)	1 g I.M. or I.V. 30 minutes before procedure	25 mg/kg I.M. or I.V. 30 minutes before procedure
GASTROINTESTINAL AND GENITOURINARY PROCEDURES[5]		
Oral[3]		
Amoxicillin for moderate risk patients	2 g 1 h before procedure	50 mg/kg 1 h before procedure
Parenteral[3]		
Ampicillin for moderate risk patients	2 g I.M. or I.V. 30 minutes before procedure	50 mg/kg I.M. or I.V. 30 minutes before procedure
Ampicillin **plus**	2 g I.M. or I.V. 30 minutes before procedure; ampicillin 1 g I.M./I.V. or amoxicillin 1 g P.O. 6 h later	50 mg/kg I.M. or I.V. 30 minutes before procedure and 25 mg/kg I.M./I.V. or amoxicillin 25 mg/kg P.O. 6 h later
Gentamicin for high-risk patients	1.5 mg/kg (max: 120 mg) I.M. or I.V. 30 minutes before procedure	1.5 mg/kg I.M. or I.V. 30 minutes before procedure

ENDOCARDITIS PROPHYLAXIS *(Continued)*

Table 4. Endocarditis Prophylaxis[1] *(continued)*

	Dosage for Adults	Dosage for Children[2]
Penicillin allergy:		
Vancomycin for moderate-risk patients	1 g I.V. infused **slowly over 1 h**; complete infusion within 30 minutes before procedure	20 mg/kg I.V. infused **slowly over 1 h**; complete infusion within 30 minutes before procedure
Vancomycin **plus**	1 g I.V. infused slowly over 1 h; complete infusion within 30 minutes before procedure	20 mg/kg I.V. infused slowly over 1 h; complete infusion within 30 minutes before procedure
Gentamicin for high-risk patients	1.5 mg/kg (max: 120 mg) I.M. or I.V. 30 minutes before procedure	1.5 mg/kg I.M. or I.V. 30 minutes before procedure

[1]Endocarditis prophylaxis recommended

High-risk category:

Prosthetic cardiac valves

Previous bacterial endocarditis

Complex cyanotic congenital heart disease (eg, single ventricle states, transposition of the great arteries, tetralogy of Fallot)

Surgically constructed systemic pulmonary shunts or conduits

Moderate-risk category:

Most other congenital cardiac malformations (other than high-risk category)

Acquired valvar dysfunction (eg, rheumatic heart disease)

Hypertrophic cardiomyopathy

Mitral valve prolapse with valvar regurgitation and/or thickened leaflets

[2]Children's dose should not exceed adult dosage.

[3]Oral regimens are more convenient and safer. Parenteral regimens are more likely to be effective; they are recommended especially for patients with prosthetic heart valves, those who have had endocarditis previously, or those taking continuous oral penicillin for rheumatic fever prophylaxis.

[4]Amoxicillin is recommended because of its excellent bioavailability and good activity against streptococci and enterococci.

[5]For a review of the risk of bacteremia and endocarditis with various procedures, see Mandell GL, Bennett JE, Dolin R, eds, *Principles and Practice of Infectious Diseases*, 4th ed, New York, NY: Churchill Livingstone, 1995, 794.

References

Dajani AS, Taubert KA, Wilson W, et al, "Prevention of Bacterial Endocarditis. Recommendations by the American Heart Association," *JAMA*, 1997, 277(22):1794-1801.

PEDIATRIC HIV

Selected tables from the Centers for Disease Control and Prevention, "Guidelines for the Use of Antiretroviral Agents in Pediatric HIV Infection," first published in *MMWR*, 1998:47(No.RR-4), April 17, 1998, updated as a "Living Document", March 24, 2005, located at (URL) http://www.aidsinfo.nih.gov.

1994 Revised Human Immunodeficiency Virus Pediatric Classification System: Immune Categories Based on Age-specific CD4+ T cell and Percentage[1]

Immune Category	<12 mo		1-5 y		6-12 y	
	No./mm³	%	No./mm³	%	No./mm³	%
Category 1 no suppression	≥1500	≥25	≥1000	≥25	≥500	≥25
Category 2 moderate suppression	750-1499	15-24	500-999	15-24	200-499	15-24
Category 3 severe suppression	<750	<15	<500	<15	<200	<15

[1]Modified from: CDC,"1994 Revised Classification System for Human Immunodeficiency Virus Infection in Children Less Than 13 Years of Age," *MMWR*, 1994, 43(RR-12):1-10.

1994 Revised Human Immunodeficiency Virus Pediatric Classification System: Clinical Categories[1]

Category N: Not Symptomatic

Children who have no signs or symptoms considered to be the result of HIV infection or who have only **one** of the conditions listed in category A

Category A: Mildly Symptomatic

Children with **two** or more of the following conditions, but none of the conditions listed in categories B and C:

- Lymphadenopathy (≥0.5 cm at more than two sites; bilateral = one site)
- Hepatomegaly
- Splenomegaly
- Dermatitis
- Parotitis
- Recurrent or persistent upper respiratory infection, sinusitis, or otitis media

Category B: Moderately Symptomatic

Children who have symptomatic conditions, other than those listed for category A or category C, that are attributed to HIV infection. Examples of conditions in clinical category B include but are not limited to the following:

- Anemia (<8 g/dL), neutropenia (<1000/mm^3), or thrombocytopenia (<100,000/mm^3) persisting ≥30 days
- Bacterial meningitis, pneumonia, or sepsis (single episode)
- Candidiasis, oropharyngeal (ie, thrush) persisting for >2 months in children aged >6 months
- Cardiomyopathy
- Cytomegalovirus infection with onset before age 1 month
- Diarrhea, recurrent or chronic
- Hepatitis
- Herpes simplex virus (HSV) stomatitis, recurrent (ie, more than two episodes within 1 year)

PEDIATRIC HIV *(Continued)*

- HSV bronchitis, pneumonitis, or esophagitis with onset before age 1 month
- Herpes zoster (ie, shingles) involving at least two distinct episodes or more than one dermatome
- Leiomyosarcoma
- Lymphoid interstitial pneumonia (LIP) or pulmonary lymphoid hyperplasia complex
- Nephropathy
- Nocardiosis
- Fever lasting >1 month
- Toxoplasmosis with onset before age 1 month
- Varicella, disseminated (ie, complicated chickenpox)

Category C: Severely Symptomatic

Children who have any condition listed in the 1987 surveillance case definition for acquired immunodeficiency syndrome, with the exception of LIP (which is a category B condition).

[1]Centers for Disease Control and Prevention, "1994 Revised Classification System for Human Immunodeficiency Virus Infection in Children Less Than 13 Years of Age," *MMWR*, 1994, 43(RR-12):1-10.

Indications for Initiation of Antiretroviral Therapy in Children <12 Months of Age Infected With Human Immunodeficiency Virus (HIV) Infection

This table provides general guidance rather than absolute recommendations for an individual patient. Factors to be considered in decisions about initiation of therapy include the risk of disease progression as determined by CD4+ percentage, the potential benefits and risks of therapy, and the ability of the caregiver to adhere to administration of the therapeutic regimen. Issues associated with adherence should be fully assessed, discussed, and addressed with the caregivers for the HIV-infected infant before the decision to initiate therapy is made.

Clinical Category		CD4+ Cell Percentage	Plasma HIV RNA Copy Number[1]	Recommendation
Symptomatic (clinical category A, B, or C)	or	<25% (immune category 2 or 3)	Any value	Treat
Asymptomatic (clinical category N)	and	≥25% (immune category 1)	Any value	Consider treatment[2]

[1]Plasma HIV RNA levels are higher in HIV-infected infants than older infected children and adults. Because overall HIV RNA levels are high and overlap between infants who have and those who do not have rapid disease progression, HIV RNA levels may be difficult to interpret in infants <12 months of age.

[2]Because HIV infection progresses more rapidly in infants than older children or adults, some experts would treat all HIV-infected infants <6 months or <12 months of age, regardless of clinical, immunologic, or virologic parameters.

Indications for Initiation of Antiretroviral Therapy in Children ≥1 Year of Age Infected With Human Immunodeficiency Virus (HIV)

This table provides general guidance rather than absolute recommendations for an individual patient. Factors to be considered in decisions about initiation of therapy include the risk of disease progression as determined by $CD4^+$ percentage and plasma HIV RNA copy number, the potential benefits and risks of therapy, and the ability of the caregiver to adhere to administration of the therapeutic regimen. Issues associated with adherence should be fully assessed, discussed, and addressed with the child, if age-appropriate, and caregiver before the decision to initiate therapy is made.

Clinical Category		$CD4^+$ Cell Percentage		Plasma HIV RNA Copy Number	Recommendation
AIDS (clinical category C)	**or**	<15% (immune category 3)		Any value	Treat
Mild-moderate symptoms (clinical category A or B)	**or**	15%-25%[1] (immune category 2)	**or**	≥100,000 copies/mL[2]	Consider treatment
Asymptomatic (clinical category N)	**and**	>25% (immune category 1)	**and**	<100,000 copies/mL[2]	Many experts would defer therapy and closely monitor clinical, immune, and viral parameters

[1]Many experts would initiate therapy if $CD4^+$ cell percentage is between 15% to 20%, and defer therapy with increased monitoring frequency in children with $CD4^+$ cell percentage 21% to 25%.

[2]There is controversy among pediatric HIV experts regarding the plasma HIV RNA threshold warranting consideration of therapy in children in the absence of clinical or immune abnormalities; some experts would consider initiation of therapy in asymptomatic children if plasma HIV RNA levels were between 50,000 to 100,000 copies/mL.

PEDIATRIC HIV *(Continued)*

Recommended Antiretroviral Regimens for Initial Therapy for Human Immunodeficiency Virus (HIV) Infection in Children

Protease Inhibitor-Based Regimens	
Strongly recommended	Two NRTIs[1] ***plus*** lopinavir/ritonavir ***or*** nelfinavir ***or*** ritonavir
Alternative	Two NRTIs[1] ***plus*** amprenavir (children ≥4 years old)[2] ***or*** indinavir
Non-nucleoside Reverse Transcriptase Inhibitor-Based Regimens	
Strongly recommended	Children >3 years: Two NRTIs[1] ***plus*** efavirenz[3] (with or without nelfinavir)
	Children ≤3 years or who can't swallow capsules: Two NRTIs[1] ***plus*** nevirapine[3]
Alternative	Two NRTIs[1] ***plus*** nevirapine[3] (children >3 years)
Nucleoside Analogue-Based Regimens	
Strongly recommended	None
Alternative	Zidovudine ***plus*** lamivudine ***plus*** abacavir
Use in special circumstances	Two NRTIs[1]
Regimens That Are Not Recommended	
Monotherapy[4]	
Certain two NRTI combinations[1]	
Two NRTIs ***plus*** saquinavir soft or hard gel capsule as a sole protease inhibitor[5]	
Insufficient Data to Recommend	
Two NRTIs[1] ***plus*** delavirdine	
Dual protease inhibitors, including saquinavir soft or hard gel capsule with low dose ritonavir, with the exception of lopinavir/ritonavir[4]	
NRTI **plus** NNRTI **plus** protease inhibitor[6]	
Tenofovir-containing regimens	
Enfuvirtide (T-20)-containing regimens	
Emtricitabine (FTC)-containing regimens	
Atazanavir-containing regimens	
Fosamprenavir-containing regimens	

NRTI = nucleoside analogue reverse transcriptase inhibitor.

NNRTI = non-nucleoside analogue reverse transcriptase inhibitor.

[1]Dual NRTI combination recommendations:

Strongly recommended choices: Zidovudine plus didanosine or lamivudine; or stavudine plus lamivudine.

Alternative choices: Abacavir plus zidovudine or lamivudine; or didanosine plus lamivudine.

Use in special circumstances: Stavudine plus didanosine; or zalcitabine plus zidovudine.

Insufficient data: Tenofovir- or emtricitabine-containing regimens.

Not recommended: Zalcitabine plus didanosine, stavudine, or lamivudine; or zidovudine plus stavudine.

[2]Amprenavir should not be administered to children <4 years of age due to the propylene glycol and vitamin E content of the oral liquid preparation and lack or pharmacokinetic data in this age group.

[3]Efavirenz is currently available only in capsule form, although a liquid formulation is currently under study to determine appropriate dosage in HIV-infected children <3 years of age; nevirapine would be the preferred NNRTI for children <3 years of age or who require a liquid formulation.

[4]Except for zidovudine chemoprophylaxis administered to HIV-exposed infants during the first 6 weeks of life to prevent perinatal HIV transmission; if an infant is confirmed as HIV-infected while receiving zidovudine prophylaxis, therapy should either be discontinued or changed to a combination antiretroviral drug regimen.

[5]With the exception of lopinavir/ritonavir, data on the pharmacokinetics and safety of dual protease inhibitor combinations (eg, low dose ritonavir pharmacologic boosting of saquinavir, indinavir, or nelfinavir) are limited, use of dual protease inhibitors as a component of initial therapy is not recommended, although such regimens may have utility as secondary treatment regimens for children who have failed initial therapy. Saquinavir soft and hard gel capsule require low dose ritonavir boosting to achieve adequate levels in children, but pharmacokinetic data on appropriate dosing not yet available.

[6]With the exception of efavirenz plus nelfinavir plus 1 or 2 NRTIs, which has been studied in HIV-infected children and shown to have virologic and immunologic efficacy in a clinical trial.

Considerations for Changing Antiretroviral Therapy for Human Immunodeficiency Virus (HIV)-Infected Children

Virologic Considerations[1]

- Less than a minimally acceptable virologic response after 8-12 weeks of therapy. For children receiving aggressive antiretroviral therapy, such a response is defined as a less than tenfold (1.0 $\log_{10}$) decrease from baseline HIV RNA levels.
- HIV RNA not suppressed to undetectable levels after 4-6 months of antiretroviral therapy.[2]
- Repeated detection of HIV RNA in children who initially had undetectable levels in response to antiretroviral therapy.[3]
- A reproducible increase in HIV RNA copy number among children who have had a substantial HIV RNA response, but still have low levels of detectable HIV RNA. Such an increase would warrant change in therapy if, after achieving a virologic nadir, a greater than threefold (>0.5 $\log_{10}$) increase in copy number for children ≥2 years of age and greater than fivefold (>0.7 $\log_{10}$) increase is observed for children <2 years of age.

Immunologic Considerations

- Change in immunologic classification.[4]
- For children with $CD4^+$ T-cell percentages of <15% (ie, those in immune category 3), a persistent decline of 5 percentiles or more in $CD4^+$ T-cell percentage (eg, from 15% to 10%).
- A rapid and substantial decrease in absolute $CD4^+$ T-cell count (ie, a >30% decline in <6 months).

Clinical Considerations

- Progressive neurodevelopmental deterioration.
- Growth failure defined as persistent decline in weight-growth velocity despite adequate nutritional support and without other explanation.
- A disease progression defined as advancement from one pediatric clinical category to another (ie, from clinical category A to clinical category B).[5]

[1]At least two measurements (taken 1 week apart) should be performed before considering a change in therapy.

[2]The initial HIV RNA level of the child at the start of therapy and the level achieved with therapy should be considered when contemplating potential drug changes. For example, an immediate change in therapy may not be warranted if there is a sustained 1.5-2.0 $\log_{10}$ decrease in HIV RNA copy number, even if RNA remains detectable at low levels.

[3]Continued observation with more frequent evaluation of HIV RNA levels should be considered if the HIV RNA increase is limited (ie, <5000 copies/mL). The presence of repeatedly detectable or increasing RNA levels suggests the development of resistance mutations.

[4]Minimal changes in $CD4^+$ T-cell percentile that may result in change in immunologic category (ie, from 26% to 24%, or 16% to 14%) may not be as concerning as a rapid substantial change in $CD4^+$ T-cell percentile within the same immunologic category (ie, a drop from 35% to 25%).

[5]In patients with stable immunologic and virologic parameters, progression from one clinical category to another may not represent an indication to change therapy. Thus, in patients whose disease progression is not associated with neurologic deterioration or growth failure, virologic and immunologic considerations are important in deciding whether to change therapy.

PEDIATRIC HIV *(Continued)*

Strategies to Improve Adherence With Antiretroviral Medications

Initial Intervention Strategies

- Establish trust and identify mutually acceptable goals for care.
- Obtain explicit agreement on need for treatment and adherence.
- Identify depression, low self-esteem, or drug use that may decrease adherence. Treat prior to starting therapy, if possible.
- Identify family, friends, health team members, or others who can help with adherence support.
- Educate patient and family about the critical role of adherence in therapy outcome.
- Identify the adherence target: 95% of prescribed doses.
- Educate patient and family about the relationship between partial adherence and resistance.
- Educate patient and family about resistance and constraint of later choices of antiretroviral drug (ie, explain that while a failure of adherence may be temporary, the effects on treatment choice may be permanent).
- Develop a treatment plan that the patient and family understand and to which they feel committed.
- Establish readiness to take medication by practice sessions or other means.
- Consider a brief period of hospitalization at start of therapy in selected circumstances, for patient education and to assess tolerability of medications chosen.

Medication Strategies

- Choose the simplest regimen possible, reducing dosing frequency and number of pills.
- Choose a regimen with dosing requirements that best conform to the daily and weekly routines and variations in patient and family activities.
- Choose the best-tasting liquid medicine possible.
- Choose drugs with the fewest side effects; inform patient regarding medication side effects; anticipate and treat side effects.
- Simplify food requirements for medication administration.
- Prescribe drugs carefully to avoid adverse drug-drug interactions.

Follow-up Intervention Strategies

- Monitor adherence at each visit, and in between visits by telephone or letter as needed.
- Provide ongoing support, encouragement, and understanding of the difficulties of the demands of trying to be >95% adherent with medication doses.
- Use patient education aids including pictures, calendars, stickers.
- Use pillboxes, reminders, alarms, pagers, timers.
- Provide nurse, social worker, or other practitioner adherence clinic visits or telephone calls.
- Provide access to support groups or one-on-one counseling for patients with depression or drug use issues that are known to decrease adherence.
- Provide pharmacist-based adherence clinics.
- Consider gastrostomy tube use in selected circumstances.
- Consider a brief period of hospitalization during therapy in selected circumstances of apparent virologic failure to assess adherence and reinforce that medication adherence is fundamental to successful antiretroviral therapy.

ADULT AND ADOLESCENT HIV

Selected tables from the Centers for Disease Control and Prevention, "Report of the NIH Panel to Define Principles of Therapy of HIV Infection and Guidelines for the Use of Antiretroviral Agents in HIV-Infected Adults and Adolescents," first published in *MMWR,* 1998:47(No. RR-5), April 24, 1998, updated as a "Living Document," April 7, 2005, located at (URL) http://www.aidsinfo.nih.gov.

Indications for Plasma HIV RNA Testing[1]

Clinical Indication	Information	Use
Syndrome consistent with acute HIV infection	Establishes diagnosis when HIV antibody test is negative or indeterminate	Diagnosis[2]
Initial evaluation of newly diagnosed HIV infection	Baseline viral load "set point"	Use in conjunction with $CD4^+$ T-cell count for decision to start or defer therapy
Every 3-4 months in patients not on therapy	Changes in viral load	Use in conjunction with $CD4^+$ T-cell count for decision to start therapy
2-8 weeks after initiation of or change in antiretroviral therapy	Initial assessment of drug efficacy	Decision to continue or change therapy
3-4 months after start of therapy	Assessment of virologic effect of therapy	Decision to continue or change therapy
Every 3-4 months in patients on therapy	Durability of antiretroviral effect	Decision to continue or change therapy
Clinical event or significant decline in $CD4^+$ T cells	Association with changing or stable viral load	Decision to continue, initiate, or change therapy

[1]Acute illness (eg, bacterial pneumonia, tuberculosis, herpes simplex virus, *Pneumocystis jiroveci* pneumonia), and vaccinations can cause an increase in plasma HIV RNA for 2-4 weeks; viral load testing should not be performed during this time. Plasma HIV RNA results should usually be verified with a repeat determination before starting or making changes in therapy.

[2]Diagnosis of HIV infection made by HIV RNA testing should be confirmed by standard methods (ie, ELISA and Western blot testing) performed 2-4 months after the initial indeterminate or negative test.

Recommendations for Using Drug-Resistance Assays

Clinical Setting / Recommendation	Rationale
Drug-Resistance Assay Recommended	
Virologic failure during combination antiretroviral therapy	Determine the role of resistance in drug failure and maximize the number of active drugs in the new regimen, if indicated.
Suboptimal suppression of viral load after antiretroviral therapy initiation	Determine the role of resistance and maximize the number of active drugs in the new regimen, if indicated.
Acute human immunodeficiency virus (HIV) infection, if decision is made to initiate therapy	Determine if drug-resistant virus was transmitted to help design an initial regimen or to change regimen accordingly (if therapy was initiated prior to test results).
Drug-Resistance Assay Should Be Considered	
Chronic HIV infection before therapy initiation	Available assays may not detect minor drug-resistant species. However, should consider if significant probability that patient was infected with drug-resistant virus (ie, if the patient is thought to have been infected by a person receiving antiretroviral drugs).
Drug-Resistance Assay Not Usually Recommended	
After discontinuation of drugs	Drug-resistance mutations may become minor species in the absence of selective drug pressure, and available assays may not detect minor drug-resistant species. If testing is performed in this setting, the detection of drug resistance may be of value, but its absence does not rule out the presence of minor drug-resistant species.
Plasma viral load <1000 HIV RNA copies/mL	Resistance assays cannot be consistently performed because of low copy number of HIV RNA; patients/providers may incur charges and not receive results.

ADULT AND ADOLESCENT HIV *(Continued)*

Goals of HIV Therapy and Strategies to Achieve Them

Goals of Therapy

- Maximal and durable suppression of viral load
- Restoration and/or preservation of immunologic function
- Improvement of quality of life
- Reduction of HIV-related morbidity and mortality

Strategies to Achieve Goals of Therapy

- Maximize adherence to the antiretroviral regimen
- Rational sequencing of drugs
- Preservation of future treatment options
- Selection of appropriate combination therapy

Indications for Initiating Antiretroviral Therapy for the Chronically HIV-1-Infected Patient

The optimal time to initiate therapy is unknown among persons with asymptomatic disease and $CD4^+$ T-cell count of >200 cells/mm^3. This table provides general guidance rather than absolute recommendations for an individual patient. All decisions regarding initiating therapy should be made on the basis of prognosis as determined by the $CD4^+$ T-cell count and level of plasma HIV RNA, the potential benefits and risks of therapy, and the willingness of the patient to accept therapy.

Clinical Category	$CD4^+$ T-Cell Count	Plasma HIV RNA	Recommendation
AIDS-defining illness or severe symptoms[1]	Any value	Any value	Treat
Asymptomatic[2]	<200/mm^3	Any value	Treat
Asymptomatic	>200/mm^3 but ≤350/mm^3	Any value	Treatment should be offered following full discussion of pros and cons with each patient
Asymptomatic	>350/mm^3	≥100,000	Most clinicians recommend deferring therapy, but some clinicians will treat
Asymptomatic	>350/mm^3	<100,000	Defer therapy

[1]AIDS-defining illness per Centers for Disease Control, 1993. Severe symptoms include unexplained fever or diarrhea >2-4 weeks, oral candidiasis, or >10% unexplained weight loss.

[2]Clinical benefit has been demonstrated in controlled trials only for patients with $CD4^+$ T cells <200/mm^3; however, the majority of clinicians would offer therapy at a $CD4^+$ T-cell threshold <350/mm^3. A collaborative analysis of data from 13 cohort studies from Europe and North America found that lower CD4 count, higher HIV viral load, injection drug use, and age >50 were all predictors of progression to AIDS or death in antiretroviral naive patients beginning combination antiretroviral therapy. These data indicate that the prognosis is better for patients who initiate therapy at >200 cells/mm^3, but risk after initiation of therapy does not vary considerably at >200 cells/mm^3.

Antiretroviral Regimens Recommended for Treatment of HIV-1 Infection in Antiretroviral Naive Patients

Regimens should be individualized based on the advantages and disadvantages of each combination such as pill burden, dosing frequency, toxicities, drug-drug interaction potential, comorbid conditions, and level of plasma HIV-RNA. Preferred regimens are in bold type; regimens are designated as "preferred" for use in treatment-naive patients when clinical trial data suggest optimal and durable efficacy with acceptable tolerability and ease of use. Alternative regimens are those where clinical trial data show efficacy, but it is considered alternative due to disadvantages compared to the preferred agent, such as antiviral activity, durability, tolerability, drug interaction potential, or ease of use. In some cases, based on individual patient characteristics, a regimen listed as an alternative regimen in this table may actually be the preferred regimen for a selected patient. Clinicians initiating antiretroviral regimens in the HIV-1-infected pregnant patient should refer to "Recommendations for Use of Antiretroviral Drugs in Pregnant HIV-1-Infected Women for Maternal Health and Interventions to Reduce Perinatal HIV-1 Transmission in the United States," at **http://aidsinfo.nih.gov/guidelines**.

	Preferred Regimens
NNRTI-Based	**Efavirenz + (lamivudine or emtricitabine) + (zidovudine or tenofovir DF)** [**Note:** Efavirenz is not recommended for use in first trimester of pregnancy or in women with high pregnancy potential[1]]
PI-Based	**Lopinavir/ritonavir (coformulation) + (lamivudine or emtricitabine) + zidovudine**
	Alternative Regimens
NNRTI-Based	**Efavirenz** + (lamivudine or emtricitabine) + (abacavir or didanosine or stavudine) [**Note:** Efavirenz is not recommended for use in first trimester of pregnancy or in women with high pregnancy potential[1]]
	Nevirapine + (lamivudine or emtricitabine) + (zidovudine or stavudine or didanosine or abacavir or tenofovir) [**Note:** High incidence (11%) of symptomatic hepatic events was observed in women with pre-nevirapine $CD4^+$ T-cell counts >250 cells/mm^3 and men with $CD4^+$ T-cell counts >400 cells/mm^3 (6.3%). Nevirapine should not be initiated in these patients unless the benefit clearly outweighs the risk.
PI-Based	**Atazanavir** + (lamivudine or emtricitabine) + (zidovudine or stavudine or abacavir or didanosine) or (tenofovir + ritonavir 100 mg/d)
	Fosamprenavir + (lamivudine or emtricitabine) + (zidovudine or stavudine or abacavir or tenofovir or didanosine)
	Fosamprenavir/ritonavir[2]+ (lamivudine or emtricitabine) + (zidovudine or stavudine or abacavir or tenofovir or didanosine)
	Indinavir/ritonavir[2]+ (lamivudine or emtricitabine) + (zidovudine or stavudine or abacavir or tenofovir or didanosine)
	Lopinavir/ritonavir + (lamivudine or emtricitabine) + (stavudine or abacavir or tenofovir or didanosine)
	Nelfinavir + (lamivudine or emtricitabine) + (zidovudine or stavudine or abacavir or tenofovir or didanosine)
	Saquinavir (soft or hard gel capsule or tablets)/**ritonavir**[2] + (lamivudine or emtricitabine) + (zidovudine or stavudine or abacavir or tenofovir or didanosine)
3 NRTI-Based	**Abacavir** + zidovudine + lamivudine – **only when a preferred or an alternative NNRTI- or a PI-based regimen cannot or should not be used**

[1]Women with childbearing potential implies women who want to conceive or those who are not using effective contraception.

[2]Low-dose (100-400 mg) ritonavir per day.

ADULT AND ADOLESCENT HIV *(Continued)*

Antiretroviral Drugs and Components Not Recommended as Initial Therapy

Drugs / Components	Reasons for Not Recommending as Initial Therapy
Amprenavir (unboosted or ritonavir boosted)	• High pill burden
Delavirdine	• Inferior virologic efficacy • Inconvenient dosing (3 times/day)
Enfuvirtide	• No clinical trial experience in treatment-naive patients • Requires twice daily subcutaneous injections
Indinavir (unboosted)	• Inconvenient dosing (3 times/day with meal restrictions)
Ritonavir as sole PI	• High pill burden • Gastrointestinal intolerance
Saquinavir soft gel capsule (unboosted)	• High pill burden • Inferior virologic efficacy
Zalcitabine + zidovudine	• Inferior virologic efficacy • Higher rate of adverse effects than other 2-NRTI alternatives

Antiretroviral Regimens or Components That Should Not Be Offered at Any Time

	Rationale	Exception
Antiretroviral Regimens Not Recommended		
Monotherapy	• Rapid development of resistance • Inferior antiretroviral activity when compared to combination with three or more antiretrovirals	Pregnant women with pretreatment HIV-RNA <1000 copies/mL using zidovudine monotherapy for prevention of perinatal HIV transmission and not for HIV treatment for the mother[1]; however, combination therapy is generally preferred
2-NRTI regimens	• Rapid development of resistance • Inferior antiretroviral activity when compared to combination with three or more antiretrovirals	For patients currently on this treatment, some clinicians may continue if virologic goals are achieved
Abacavir + tenofovir + lamivudine (or emtricitabine) as a triple-NRTI regimen	High rate of early virologic nonresponse seen when this triple NRTI combination was used as initial regimen in treatment naive patients	No exception
Tenofovir + didanosine + lamivudine (or emtricitabine) combination as a triple-NRTI regimen	High rate of early virologic nonresponse seen when this triple NRTI combination was used as initial regimen in treatment naive patients	No exception

Antiretroviral Regimens or Components That Should Not Be Offered at Any Time *(continued)*

	Rationale	Exception
Antiretroviral Components Not Recommended as Part of Antiretroviral Regimen		
Amprenavir oral solution in: • pregnant women • children <4 y • patients with renal or hepatic failure • patients on metronidazole or disulfiram	Oral liquid contains large amount of the excipient propylene glycol, which may be toxic in the patients at risk	No exception
Amprenavir + fosamprenavir	Amprenavir is the active antiviral for both drugs, combined use have no benefit and may increase toxicities	No exception
Amprenavir oral solution + ritonavir oral solution	The large amount of propylene glycol used as a vehicle in amprenavir oral solution may compete with ethanol (the vehicle in oral ritonavir solution) for the same metabolic pathway for elimination. This may lead to accumulation of either one of the vehicles.	No exception
Atazanavir + indinavir	Potential additive hyperbilirubinemia	No exception
Didanosine + stavudine	• High incidence of toxicities – peripheral neuropathy, pancreatitis, and hyperlactatemia • Reports of serious, even fatal, cases of lactic acidosis with hepatic steatosis with or without pancreatitis in pregnant women[1]	When no other antiretroviral options are available and potential benefits outweigh the risks[1]
Didanosine + zalcitabine	Additive peripheral neuropathy	No exception
Efavirenz in first trimester of pregnancy or in women with significant childbearing potential[1]	Teratogenic in nonhuman primates	When no other antiretroviral options are available and potential benefits outweigh the risks[1]
Emtricitabine + lamivudine	• Similar resistance profile • No potential benefit	No exception
Lamivudine + zalcitabine	*In vitro* antagonism	No exception
Nevirapine initiation in women with CD4 >250 cells/mm^3 or men with CD4 >400 cells/mm^3	Higher incidence of symptomatic (including serious and even fatal) hepatic events in these patient groups	Only if the benefit clearly outweighs the risk
Saquinavir hard gel capsule (Invirase®) as **single** protease inhibitor	• Poor oral bioavailability (4%) • Inferior antiretroviral activity when compared to other protease inhibitors	No exception
Stavudine + zalcitabine	Additive peripheral neuropathy	No exception
Stavudine + zidovudine	Antagonistic effect on HIV-1	No exception

[1]When constructing an antiretroviral regimen for an HIV-infected pregnant woman, please consult "Public Health Service Task Force Recommendations for the Use of Antiretroviral Drugs in Pregnant HIV-1-Infected Women for Maternal Health and Interventions to Reduce Perinatal HIV-1 Transmission in the United States" in **http://www.aidsinfo.nih.gov/guidelines**.

ADULT AND ADOLESCENT HIV *(Continued)*

Summary of Guidelines for Changing an Antiretroviral Regimen for Suspected Treatment Regimen Failure

Patient Assessment

- Review antiretroviral treatment history.
- Assess for evidence of clinical progression (eg, physical exam, laboratory and/or radiologic tests)
- Assess adherence, tolerability, and pharmacokinetic issues.
- Distinguish between limited, intermediate, and extensive prior therapy and drug resistance.
- Perform resistance testing while patient is taking therapy (or within 4 weeks after regimen discontinuation).
- Identify active drugs and drug classes to use in designing new regimen.

Patient Management: Specific Clinical Scenarios

- **Limited or intermediate prior treatment with low (but not suppressed) HIV RNA level (eg, up to 5000 copies/mL):** The goal of treatment is to resuppress HIV RNA to below level of assay detection. Consider intensifying with one drug (eg, tenofovir) or pharmacokinetic enhancement (use of ritonavir boosting of a protease inhibitor), perform resistance testing if possible, or most aggressively, change two or more drugs in the regimen. If continuing the same treatment regimen, HIV RNA levels should be followed closely because ongoing viral replication will lead to accumulation of additional resistance mutations.
- **Limited or intermediate prior treatment with resistance to one drug:** Consider changing the one drug, pharmacokinetic enhancement (few data available), or, most aggressively, change two or more drugs in the regimen.
- **Limited or intermediate prior treatment resistance to more than one drug:** The goal of treatment is to suppress viremia to prevent further selection of resistance mutations. Consider optimizing the regimen by changing classes (eg, PI-based to NNRTI-based and vice versa) and/or adding new active drugs. (See table **Treatment Options Following Virologic Failure on Initial Recommended Therapy Regimens**.)
- **Prior treatment with no resistance identified:** Consider the timing of the drug resistance test (eg, was the patient off antiretroviral medications?) and/or nonadherence. Consider resuming the same regimen or starting a new regimen and then repeating genotypic testing early (eg, 2-4 weeks) to determine if a resistant virus becomes evident.
- **Extensive prior treatment and drug resistance:** It is reasonable to continue the same antiretroviral regimen if there are few or no treatment options. In general, avoid adding a single active drug because of the risk for the rapid development of resistance to that drug. In advanced HIV disease with a high likelihood of clinical progression (eg, CD4 cell count <100 cells/mm^3), adding a single drug may reduce the risk of immediate clinical progression. In this complicated scenario, expert advise should be sought.

Treatment Options Following Virologic Failure on Initial Recommended Therapy Regimens

Regimen Class	Initial Regimen	Recommended Change
NNRTI	2 NRTIs + NNRTI	• 2 NRTIs (based on resistance testing) + PI (with or without low-dose ritonavir)
PI	2 NRTIs + PI (with or without low-dose ritonavir)	• 2 NRTIs (based on resistance testing) + NNRTI
Triple nucleosides	3 nucleosides	• 2 NRTIs (based on resistance testing) + NNRTI or PI (with or without low-dose ritonavir) • NNRTI + PI (with or without low-dose ritonavir) • Nucleoside(s) (based on resistance testing) + NNRTI + PI (with or without low-dose ritonavir)

Associated Signs and Symptoms of Acute Retroviral Syndrome and Percentage of Expected Frequency

- Fever (96%)
- Lymphadenopathy (74%)
- Pharyngitis (70%)
- Rash (70%)
  - Erythematous maculopapular with lesions on face and trunk and sometimes extremities, including palms and soles
  - Mucocutaneous ulceration involving mouth, esophagus, or genitals
- Myalgia or arthralgia (54%)
- Diarrhea (32%)
- Headache (32%)
- Nausea and vomiting (27%)
- Hepatosplenomegaly (14%)
- Weight loss (13%)
- Thrush (12%)
- Neurologic symptoms (12%)
  - Meningoencephalitis or aseptic meningitis
  - Peripheral neuropathy or radiculopathy
  - Facial palsy
  - Guillain-Barré syndrome
  - Brachial neuritis
  - Cognitive impairment or psychosis

Reference

Niu MT, Stein DS, and Schnittman SM, "Primary Human Immunodeficiency Virus Type 1 Infection: Review of Pathogenesis and Early Treatment Intervention in Humans and Animal Retrovirus Infections," *J Infect Dis*, 1993, 168(6):1490-501.

PERINATAL HIV

Selected tables from the Perinatal HIV Guidelines Working Group, Public Health Service Task Force, "Recommendations for Use of Antiretroviral Drugs in Pregnant HIV-1-Infected Women for Maternal Health and Interventions to Reduce Perinatal HIV-1 Transmission in the United States," February 24, 2005, located at (URL) http://www.aidsinfo.nih.gov.

Pediatric AIDS Clinical Trials Group (PACTG) 076 Zidovudine (ZDV) Regimen

ZDV Perinatal Transmission Prophylaxis Regimen

Time of ZDV Administration	Regimen
Antepartum	Oral administration (to the pregnant woman) of 100 mg ZDV 5 times daily,[1] initiated at 14-34 weeks gestation and continued throughout the pregnancy.
Intrapartum	During labor, intravenous administration (to the pregnant women) of ZDV in a 1-hour initial dose of 2 mg/kg body weight, followed by a continuous infusion of 1 mg/kg body weight/hour until delivery.
Postpartum	Oral administration of ZDV to the newborn infant (ZDV syrup at 2 mg/kg body weight/dose every 6 hours) for the first 6 weeks of life, beginning at 8-12 hours after birth.[2]

[1]Oral ZDV administered as 200 mg 3 times daily or 300 mg twice daily is currently used in general clinical practice and is an acceptable alternative regimen to 100 mg orally 5 times daily.

[2]Intravenous dosage for full-term infants who cannot tolerate oral intake is 1.5 mg/kg body weight intravenously every 6 hours. ZDV dosing for infants <35 weeks gestation at birth is 1.5 mg/kg/dose intravenously, or 2 mg/kg/dose orally, every 12 hours, advancing to every 8 hours at 2 weeks of age if >30 weeks gestation at birth or at 4 weeks of age if <30 weeks gestation at birth.

Clinical Scenarios and Recommendations for the Use of Antiretroviral Drugs to Reduce Perinatal Human Immunodeficiency Virus Type (HIV-1) Transmission

SCENARIO #1
HIV-1-infected pregnant women who have not received prior antiretroviral therapy

- Pregnant women with HIV-1 infection must receive standard clinical, immunologic, and virologic evaluation. Recommendations for initiation and choice of antiretroviral therapy should be based on the same parameters used for persons who are not pregnant, although the known and unknown risks and benefits of such therapy during pregnancy must be considered and discussed.
- The three-part ZDV chemoprophylaxis regimen, initiated after the first trimester, is recommended for all pregnant women with HIV-1 regardless of antenatal HIV RNA copy number to reduce the risk for perinatal transmission.
- The combination of ZDV chemoprophylaxis with additional antiretroviral drugs for treatment of HIV-1 infection is recommended for infected women whose clinical, immunologic, or virologic status requires treatment or who have HIV-1 RNA over 1000 copies/mL regardless of clinical or immunologic status, and can be considered for women with HIV-1 RNA <1000 copies/mL.
- Women who are in the first trimester of pregnancy may consider delaying initiation of therapy until after 10-12 weeks' gestation.

SCENARIO #2
HIV-1-infected women receiving antiretroviral therapy during the current pregnancy

- HIV-1-infected women receiving antiretroviral therapy in whom pregnancy is identified after the first trimester should continue therapy. ZDV should be a component of the antenatal antiretroviral treatment regimen after the first trimester whenever possible, although this may not always be feasible.
- For women receiving antiretroviral therapy in whom pregnancy is recognized during the first trimester, the woman should be counseled regarding the benefits and potential risks of antiretroviral administration during this period, and continuation of therapy should be considered. If therapy is discontinued during the first trimester, all drugs should be stopped and reintroduced simultaneously to avoid the development of drug resistance.
- Regardless of the antepartum antiretroviral regimen, ZDV administration is recommended during the intrapartum period and for the newborn.

SCENARIO #3
HIV-1-infected women in labor who have had no prior therapy

Several effective regimens are available (see Comparison of Intrapartum / Postpartum Regimens). These include:

- intrapartum intravenous ZDV followed by 6 weeks of ZDV for the newborn
- oral ZDV and 3TC during labor, followed by 1 week of oral ZDV-3TC for the newborn
- a single-dose nevirapine at the onset of labor followed by a single dose of nevirapine for the newborn at age 48 hours, and
- the two-dose nevirapine regimen combined with intrapartum intravenous ZDV and 6-week ZDV for the newborn

In the immediate postpartum period, the woman should have appropriate assessments (eg, $CD4^+$ count and HIV-1 RNA copy number) to determine whether antiretroviral therapy is recommended for her own health.

SCENARIO #4
Infants born to mothers who have received no antiretroviral therapy during pregnancy or intrapartum

- The 6-week neonatal ZDV component of the ZDV chemoprophylactic regimen should be discussed with the mother and offered for the newborn.
- ZDV should be initiated as soon as possible after delivery – preferably within 6-12 hours of birth.
- Some clinicians may choose to use ZDV in combination with other antiretroviral drugs, particularly if the mother is known or suspected to have ZDV-resistant virus. However, the efficacy of this approach for prevention of transmission has not been proven in clinical trials, and appropriate dosing regimens for neonates are incompletely defined for many drugs.
- In the immediate postpartum period, the woman should undergo appropriate assessments (eg, $CD4^+$ count and HIV-1 RNA copy number) to determine whether antiretroviral therapy is required for her own health. The infant should undergo early diagnostic testing so that if HIV-1-infected, treatment can be initiated as soon as possible.

PERINATAL HIV *(Continued)*

Note: Discussion of treatment options and recommendations should be noncoercive, and the final decision regarding the use of antiretroviral drugs is the responsibility of the woman. A decision to not accept treatment with ZDV or other drugs should not result in punitive action or denial of care. Use of ZDV should not be denied to a woman who wishes to minimize exposure of the fetus to other antiretroviral drugs and who, therefore, chooses to receive only ZDV during pregnancy to reduce the risk for perinatal transmission.

Comparison of Intrapartum / Postpartum Regimens for HIV-1-Infected Women in Labor Who Have Had No Prior Antiretroviral Therapy (Scenario #3)

ZDV

Source of Evidence: Epidemiologic data, U.S.; compared to no ZDV treatment

Maternal Intrapartum: 2 mg/kg intravenous bolus, followed by continuous infusion of 1 mg/kg/h until delivery

Infant Postpartum: 2 mg/kg orally every 6 hours for 6 weeks[1]

Data on Transmission: Transmission 10% with ZDV compared to 27% with no ZDV treatment, a 62% reduction (95% CI, 19% to 82%)

Advantages: Has been standard recommendation

Disadvantages:

- Requires intravenous administration and availability of ZDV intravenous formulation
- Adherence to 6-week infant regimen
- Reversible, mild anemia with 6-week infant ZDV regimen

ZDV / 3TC

Source of Evidence: Clinical trial, Africa; compared to placebo

Maternal Intrapartum: ZDV 600 mg orally at onset of labor, followed by 300 mg orally every 3 hours until delivery **and** 3TC 150 mg orally at onset of labor, followed by 150 mg orally every 12 hours until delivery

Infant Postpartum: ZDV 4 mg/kg orally every 12 hours **and** 3TC 2 mg/kg orally every 12 hours for 7 days

Data on Transmission: Transmission at 6 weeks 9% with ZDV-3TC vs 15% with placebo, a 42% reduction

Advantages: Oral regimen; adherence easier than 6 weeks of ZDV

Disadvantages: Requires administration of two drugs

Nevirapine

Source of Evidence: Clinical trial, Africa; compared to oral ZDV given intrapartum and for 1 week to the infant

Maternal Intrapartum: Single 200 mg oral dose at onset of labor

Infant Postpartum: Single 2 mg/kg oral dose at age 48-72 hours[2]

Data on Transmission: Transmission at 6 weeks 12% with nevirapine compared to 21% with ZDV, a 47% reduction (95% CI,[1] 20% to 64%)

Advantages: Inexpensive; oral regimen; simple, easy to administer; can give directly observed treatment

Disadvantages:

- Unknown efficacy if mother has nevirapine-resistant virus
- Transient nevirapine resistance mutations detected at 6 weeks postpartum in 19% of women receiving single-dose intrapartum nevirapine, and 46% of infants who became infected despite receiving nevirapine

ZDV-Nevirapine

Source of Evidence: Theoretical

Maternal Intrapartum: ZDV 2 mg/kg intravenous bolus, followed by continuous infusion of 1 mg/kg/h until delivery **and** nevirapine single 200 mg oral dose at onset of labor

Infant Postpartum: ZDV 2 mg/kg orally every 6 hours for 6 weeks **and** nevirapine single 2 mg/kg oral dose at age 48-72 hours[2]

Data on Transmission: No data

Advantages: Potential benefit if maternal virus is resistant to either nevirapine or ZDV; synergistic inhibition of HIV replication with combination *in vitro*

Disadvantages:

- Requires intravenous administration and availability of ZDV intravenous formulation
- Adherence to 6-week infant ZDV regimen
- Unknown if additive efficacy with combination
- Transient nevirapine resistance mutations detected at 6 weeks postpartum in 15%-25% of women receiving single-dose intrapartum nevirapine with ZDV or other antiretroviral drugs

ZDV = zidovudine, CI = confidence interval, 3TC = lamivudine.

Footnotes

[1]ZDV dosing for infants <35 weeks gestation at birth is 1.5 mg/kg/dose intravenously, or 2 mg/kg/dose orally, every 12 hours, advancing to every 8 hours at 2 weeks of age if ≥30 weeks gestation at birth or at 4 weeks of age if <30 weeks gestation at birth.

[2]If the mother received nevirapine <1 hour prior to delivery, the infant should be given 2 mg/kg oral nevirapine as soon as possible after birth and again at 48-72 hours.

Recommendations Related to Antiretroviral Drug Resistance and Drug Resistance Testing for Pregnant Women With HIV-1 Infection

- All pregnant HIV-1-infected women should be offered highly active antiretroviral therapy to maximally suppress viral replication, reduce the risk of perinatal transmission, and minimize the risk of development of resistant virus.
- For women for whom combination antiretroviral therapy would be considered optional (HIV-1 RNA <1000 copies/mL) and who wish to restrict their exposure to antiretroviral drugs during pregnancy, monotherapy with the three-part zidovudine (ZDV) prophylaxis regimen (or in selected circumstances, dual nucleosides) should be offered. In these circumstances, the development of resistance should be minimized by limited viral replication (assuming HIV-1 RNA levels remain low) and the time-limited exposure to ZDV. Monotherapy with ZDV does not suppress HIV-1 replication to undetectable levels in most cases, theoretically, such therapy might select for ZDV-resistant viral variants, potentially limiting future treatment options. These considerations should be discussed with the pregnant woman.
- Recommendations for resistance testing for HIV-1-infected pregnant women are the same as for nonpregnant patients: Acute HIV-1 infection, virologic failure, suboptimal viral suppression after initiation of antiretroviral therapy, or high likelihood of exposure to resistant virus based on community prevalence or source characteristics.
- Women who have a history of presumed or documented ZDV resistance and are on antiretroviral regimens that do not include ZDV for their own health should still receive intravenous ZDV intrapartum and oral ZDV for their infants according to the PACTG 076 protocol whenever possible. A key mechanism by which ZDV reduce perinatal transmission is likely through pre- and

PERINATAL HIV *(Continued)*

postexposure prophylaxis of the infant, which may be less dependent on drug sensitivity than is reduction of viral replication. However, these women are not good candidates for ZDV alone.

- Optimal antiretroviral prophylaxis of the infant born to a woman with HIV-1 known to be resistant to ZDV or other agents should be determined in consultation with pediatric infectious disease specialists, taking into account resistance patterns, available drug formulations, and infant pharmacokinetic data, when available.
- If women receiving combination therapy require temporary discontinuation for any reason during pregnancy, all drugs should be stopped and reintroduced simultaneously to reduce the potential for emergence of resistance.
- Optimal adherence to antiretroviral medications is a key part of the strategy to reduce the development of resistance.
- Because the prevalence of drug-resistant virus is an evolving phenomenon, surveillance is needed to monitor the prevalence of drug-resistant virus in pregnant women over time and the risk of transmission of resistant viral strains.

Clinical Scenarios and Recommendations Regarding Mode of Delivery to Reduce Perinatal Human Immunodeficiency Virus Type (HIV-1) Transmission

SCENARIO A

HIV-1-infected women presenting in late pregnancy (after about 36 weeks of gestation), known to be HIV-1-infected but not receiving antiretroviral therapy, and who have HIV-1 RNA level and lymphocyte subsets pending but unlikely to be available before delivery.

Recommendations

Therapy options should be discussed in detail. The woman should be started on antiretroviral therapy including at least the PACTG 076 ZDV regimen. The woman should be counseled that scheduled cesarean section is likely to reduce the risk of transmission to her infant. She should also be informed of the increased risks to her of cesarean section, including increased rates of postoperative infection, anesthesia risks, and other surgical risks.

If cesarean section is chosen, the procedure should be scheduled at 38 weeks of gestation based on the best available clinical information. When scheduled cesarean section is performed, the woman should receive continuous intravenous ZDV infusion beginning 3 hours before surgery and her infant should receive 6 weeks of ZDV therapy after birth. Options for continuing or initiating combination antiretroviral therapy after delivery should be discussed with the woman as soon as her viral load and lymphocyte subset results are available.

SCENARIO B

HIV-1-infected women who initiated prenatal care early in the third trimester, are receiving highly active combination antiretroviral therapy, and have an initial virologic response, but have HIV-1 RNA levels that remain substantially over 1000 copies/mL at 36 weeks of gestation.

Recommendations

The current combination antiretroviral regimen should be continued as the HIV-1 RNA level is dropping appropriately. The woman should be counseled that although she is responding to the antiretroviral therapy, it is unlikely that her HIV-1

RNA level will fall below 1000 copies/mL before delivery. Therefore, scheduled cesarean section may provide additional benefit in preventing intrapartum transmission of HIV-1. She should also be informed of the increased risks to her of cesarean section, including increased rates of postoperative infection, anesthesia risks, and surgical risks.

If she chooses scheduled cesarean section, it should be performed at 38 weeks' gestation according to the best available dating parameters, and intravenous ZDV should be begun at least 3 hours before surgery. Other antiretroviral medications should be continued on schedule as much as possible before and after surgery. The infant should receive oral ZDV for 6 weeks after birth. The importance of adhering to therapy after delivery for her own health should be emphasized.

SCENARIO C

HIV-1-infected women on highly active combination antiretroviral therapy with an undetectable HIV-1 RNA level at 36 weeks of gestation.

Recommendations

The woman should be counseled that her risk of perinatal transmission of HIV-1 with a persistently undetectable HIV-1 RNA level is low, probably 2% or less, even with vaginal delivery. There is currently no information to evaluate whether performing a scheduled cesarean section will lower her risk further.

Cesarean section has an increased risk of complications for the woman compared to vaginal delivery, and these risks must be balanced against the uncertain benefit of cesarean section in this case.

SCENARIO D

HIV-1-infected women who have elected scheduled cesarean section but present in early labor or shortly after rupture of membranes.

Recommendations

Intravenous ZDV should be started immediately since the woman is in labor or has ruptured membranes.

If labor is progressing rapidly, the woman should be allowed to deliver vaginally. If cervical dilatation is minimal and a long period of labor is anticipated, some clinicians may choose to administer the loading dose of intravenous ZDV and proceed with cesarean section to minimize the duration of membrane rupture and avoid vaginal delivery. Others might begin Pitocin® augmentation to enhance contractions and potentially expedite delivery.

If the woman is allowed to labor, scalp electrodes and other invasive monitoring and operative delivery should be avoided if possible. The infant should be treated with 6 weeks of ZDV therapy after birth.

IMMUNIZATION GUIDELINES

Standards for Pediatric Immunization Practices

Standard 1.	Immunization services are readily available.
Standard 2.	There are no barriers or unnecessary prerequisites to the receipt of vaccines.
Standard 3.	Immunization services are available free or for a minimal fee.
Standard 4.	Providers utilize all clinical encounters to screen and, when indicated, immunize children.
Standard 5.	Providers educate parents and guardians about immunizations in general terms.
Standard 6.	Providers question parents or guardians about contraindications and, before immunizing a child, inform them in specific terms about the risks and benefits of the immunizations their child is to receive.
Standard 7.	Providers follow only true contraindications.
Standard 8.	Providers administer simultaneously all vaccine doses for which a child is eligible at the time of each visit.
Standard 9.	Providers use accurate and complete recording procedures.
Standard 10.	Providers co-schedule immunization appointments in conjunction with appointments for other child health services.
Standard 11.	Providers report adverse events following immunization promptly, accurately, and completely.
Standard 12.	Providers operate a tracking system.
Standard 13.	Providers adhere to appropriate procedures for vaccine management.
Standard 14.	Providers conduct semiannual audits to assess immunization coverage levels and to review immunization records in the patient populations they serve.
Standard 15.	Providers maintain up-to-date, easily retrievable medical protocols at all locations where vaccines are administered.
Standard 16.	Providers operate with patient-oriented and community-based approaches.
Standard 17.	Vaccines are administered by properly trained individuals.
Standard 18.	Providers receive ongoing education and training on current immunization recommendations.

Recommended by the National Vaccine Advisory Committee, April 1992.
Modified by the United States Public Health Service, 1993.
Endorsed by the American Academy of Pediatrics, May 1992.

The Standards represent the consensus of the National Vaccine Advisory Committee (NVAC) and of a broad group of medical and public health experts about what constitutes the most desirable immunization practices. It is recognized by the NVAC that not all of the current immunization practices of public and private providers are in compliance with the Standards. Nevertheless, the Standards are expected to be useful as a means of helping providers to identify needed changes, to obtain resources if necessary, and to actually implement the desirable immunization practices in the future.

Table 1. Dosage and Administration Guidelines for Vaccines Available in the United States

Vaccine	Dosage	Route of Administration	Type
DT[1]	0.5 mL	I.M.; do not give SubQ	Toxoids
Td[1]	0.5 mL	I.M.; do not give SubQ	Toxoids
DTaP (Tripedia®, Infanrix®)[2]	0.5 mL	I.M.; do not give SubQ	Diphtheria and tetanus toxoids with inactivated acellular pertussis
DTaP-PRP-T (Tripedia®/ActHIB®, TriHIBit®)	0.5 mL	I.M.; do not give SubQ	Polysaccharide-protein conjugate with toxoids and inactivated bacteria
DTaP and hepatitis B (recombinant) and inactivated poliovirus vaccine combined (Pediarix™)	0.5 mL	I.M.; do not give SubQ	Diphtheria and tetanus toxoids with inactivated acellular pertussis, recombinant – derived inactivated viral antigen and inactivated virus
Haemophilus B conjugate vaccine	0.5 mL	I.M. PRP-D, HbOC, or PRP-T can be given SubQ in individuals at risk of hemorrhage	Polysaccharide protein conjugate
HibTITER® (HbOC),[3] manufactured by Lederle Laboratories	0.5 mL	I.M.	Oligosaccharide (diphtheria CRM_{197} protein conjugate)
PedvaxHIB® (PRP-OMP),[4] manufactured by MSD	0.5 mL	I.M.; do not give SubQ	Polysaccharide (meningococcal protein conjugate)
ActHIB® (PRP-T), manufactured by Pasteur Merieux Serums & Vaccines	0.5 mL	I.M.	Tetanus toxoid protein conjugate
Haemophilus b conjugate – PRP-OMP and hepatitis B (recombinant) (Comvax®)	0.5 mL	I.M.; do not give SubQ	Polysaccharide-protein conjugate with inactivated virus
Hepatitis A vaccine, inactivated		I.M.; do not give SubQ	Inactivated virus
Havrix®			
Children 2-18 y:	0.5 mL (720 ELISA units) with 2nd dose given 6-12 mo later		
Children >18 y and adults:	1 mL (1440 ELISA units) with 2nd dose given 6-12 mo later		
VAQTA®			
Children 2-17 y:	0.5 mL (25 units) with 2nd dose given 6-18 mo later		
Children >17 y and adults:	1 mL (50 units) with 2nd dose given 6 mo later		

IMMUNIZATION GUIDELINES *(Continued)*

Table 1. Dosage and Administration Guidelines for Vaccines Available in the United States *(continued)*

Vaccine	Dosage	Route of Administration	Type
Hepatitis B[5]		I.M. in the anterolateral thigh or in the deltoid muscle[7]	Yeast recombinant-derived inactivated viral antigen
Infants born to HB_sAg-negative mothers, children, and adolescents <20 y[6]			
Recombivax HB® (MSD)	5 mcg (0.5 mL)		
Engerix-B® (SKF)	10 mcg (0.5 mL)		
Infants born to HB_sAg-positive mothers (both immunization with hepatitis B and administration of 0.5 mL hepatitis B immune globulin is recommended for **infants** born to HB_sAg-positive mothers using different administration sites) within 12 hours of birth; administer vaccine at birth; repeat vaccine dose at 1 and 6 months following the initial dose			
Recombivax HB® (MSD)	5 mcg (0.5 mL)		
Engerix-B® (SKF)	10 mcg (0.5 mL)		
Adolescents 11-15 y			
Recombivax HB® (MSD)	10 mcg (1 mL) 2nd dose given 4-6 mo after the first dose (alternate two-dose hepatitis B vaccination schedule)		
Adults ≥20 y			
Recombivax HB® (MSD)	10 mcg (1 mL)		
Engerix-B® (SKF)	20 mcg (1 mL)		
Dialysis patients and immunosuppressed patients			
Recombivax HB® (MSD)	<20 y: 20 mcg (0.5 mL); ≥20 y, 40 mcg (1 mL) using special dialysis formulation		
Engerix-B® (SKF)[8]	<20 y, 20 mcg (1 mL); ≥20 y, 40 mcg (2 mL), give as two 1 mL doses at different sites		
Influenza		I.M. (2 doses 4+ weeks apart in children <9 years of age not previously immunized; only 1 dose needed for annual updates)	Inactivated virus subvirion (split) (contraindicated in patients allergic to chicken eggs)
Split virus only in pediatric patients			
6-35 mo	0.25 mL (1 or 2 doses)		
3-8 y	0.5 mL (1 or 2 doses)		

Table 1. Dosage and Administration Guidelines for Vaccines Available in the United States *(continued)*

Vaccine	Dosage	Route of Administration	Type
≥9 y	0.5 mL (1 dose)		
Measles	0.5 mL	SubQ	Live virus (contraindicated in patients with anaphylactic allergy to neomycin)
Most areas: Two doses (1st dose at 15 months with MMR; 2nd dose at 4-6 years or 11-12 years, depending on local school entry requirements)			
High-risk area: Two doses (1st dose at 12 months with MMR; 2nd dose as above)			
Children 6-15 months in epidemic situations: Dose is given at the time of first contact with a health care provider; children <1 year of age should receive single antigen measles vaccine. If vaccinated before 1 year, revaccinate at 15 months with MMR. A 3rd dose is administered at 4-6 years or 11-12 years, depending on local school entry requirements.			
Meningococcal			
Menactra™			Polysaccharide diphtheria toxoid conjugate
Adolescents and adults (11-55 y)	0.5 mL	I.M.	
Menomune®-A/C/Y/W-135			
Children ≥2 y and adults	0.5 mL[9]	SubQ	Polysaccharide
MMR[10]	0.5 mL	SubQ	Live virus
MR	0.5 mL	SubQ	Live virus
Mumps	0.5 mL	SubQ	Live virus
Pneumococcal heptavalent (Prevnar®)[11]	0.5 mL	I.M.	Protein-conjugated polysaccharide
Pneumococcal polyvalent[12]	0.5 mL (≥2 y)	I.M. or SubQ (I.M. preferred)	Polysaccharide
Poliovirus (OPV) trivalent	0.5 mL	Oral	Live virus
Poliovirus (IPV)[13] trivalent	0.5 mL	SubQ or I.M.	Inactivated virus
Rabies			
Human diploid cell vaccine (Imovax®)	1 mL	I.M.[14] or	Inactivated virus
(HDCV)	0.1 mL	I.D.[15]	
Rabies vaccine adsorbed (RVA)	1 mL	I.M.[14]	Inactivated virus
Purified chick embryo cell (PCEC) (RabAvert™)	1 mL	I.M.[14]	Inactivated virus
Rubella	0.5 mL (≥12 mo)[16]	SubQ	Live virus
Tetanus (adsorbed)[17]	0.5 mL	I.M.	Toxoid
Tetanus (fluid)	0.5 mL	I.M., SubQ	Toxoid
Typhoid			
Injection, suspension (AKD and HP)		SubQ	Inactivated bacteria

IMMUNIZATION GUIDELINES *(Continued)*

Table 1. Dosage and Administration Guidelines for Vaccines Available in the United States *(continued)*

Vaccine	Dosage	Route of Administration	Type
Children 6 mo - 10 y: 0.25 mL; repeat dose in ≥4 weeks. Booster: 0.25 mL every 3 years.			
Children >10 y and adults: 0.5 mL; repeat dose in ≥4 weeks. Booster: 0.5 mL every 3 years.			
Oral (Vivotif® Berna)		P.O.	Live bacteria
Adults: Primary immunization: 1 capsule qod (days 1, 3, 5, and 7). Booster: Repeat primary immunization series every 5 years.			
Varicella (Varivax®)	0.5 mL	SubQ	Live virus
Children 12 mo - 12 y: Single 0.5 mL dose			
Adolescents ≥13 y and adults: 0.5 mL dose x 2 (second 0.5 mL dose is administered 4 to 8 weeks later)			
Yellow fever	0.5 mL[18]	SubQ	Live attenuated virus

[1]DT for use in children <7 years of age. Td contains same amount of tetanus toxoid as DT & DTP, but a reduced dose of diphtheria toxoid. Td for use in children ≥7 years of age.

[2]DTaP is the recommended vaccine for primary vaccination against diphtheria, tetanus, and pertussis; including completion of the series in children who have received 1 or more doses of whole-cell DTP. The occurrence of fever and local reactions is lower with acellular pertussis vaccine than with whole-cell DTP.

[3]The conjugate (HbCV) vaccine is preferred over the polysaccharide (HbPV) vaccine. In children with a high risk for *Haemophilus influenzae* type b disease and HbCV is unavailable, an acceptable alternate is to give HbPV at 18 months of age with a 2nd dose at 24 months of age. Children <5 years of age who were previously vaccinated with HbPV between 18-23 months of age should be revaccinated with a single dose of HbCV at least 2 months after the initial dose of HbPV. Either HbCV or HbPV can be administered up to the 5th birthday. However, they are generally not recommended for children >5 years of age.

[4]PRP-OMP (PedvaxHIB®) manufactured by Merck, Sharp & Dohme is initiated at 2 months of age for 3 doses (2 months, 4 months and 12 months). If initiated at 7-11 months of age, 3 doses are administered (initial 2 doses at 2-month intervals, 3rd dose at 15-18 months of age); if initiated at 12-14 months of age, 2 doses are administered at 2- to 3-month intervals between doses; if initiated at 15-59 months of age, 1 dose is administered.

[5]Hepatitis B vaccine can be given at the same time with DTP, HbOC, polio, and/or MMR; administer 3 doses at 0, 1, and 6 months).

[6]Administer to newborns at 0-2 days of age before hospital discharge; repeat at 1-2 months and 6-18 months following the initial dose. If not vaccinated at birth, administer at 2, 4, and 6-18 months of age.

[7]Aluminum-absorbed vaccines must be injected deep in the muscle mass and not SubQ because they can cause local irritation, inflammation, granuloma formation, and necrosis. Only patients (ie, hemophiliacs) who are at risk of hemorrhage following I.M. injections should receive hepatitis B vaccine SubQ

[8]Engerix-B® — an alternate schedule for postexposure prophylaxis or more rapid induction using 4 doses at 0, 1, 2, and 12 months of age is recommended.

[9]Indicated in children ≥2 years of age at risk (anatomic or functional asplenia, those with terminal complement component or properdin deficiencies), in epidemic or highly endemic areas. The American College Health Association recommends immunization of college students.

[10]See measles.

[11]Routine administration to all children ≤23 months at 2, 4, 6, and 12-15 months. Initial dose should be given no earlier than at 6 weeks of age. Recommended for children 24-59 months who are at high risk for invasive pneumococcal infection.

[12]Indicated for children with sickle cell disease; asplenia; nephrotic syndrome or chronic renal failure; conditions associated with immunosuppression; CSF leaks; HIV infection. Advisory Committee on Immunization Practices (ACIP) also recommends that patients ≥2 years of age with chronic cardiovascular disease, chronic pulmonary disease, diabetes mellitus, or chronic liver disease receive pneumococcal immunization. Patients ≥2 years of age living in special environments in which the risk of invasive pneumococcal disease is high (ie, Alaskan native and certain American Indian populations) should receive pneumococcal immunization.

[13]The primary series consists of 3 doses. The first 2 doses should be administered at an interval of 8 weeks beginning at 2 months of age (minimum age of 6 weeks). The 3rd dose should be given at 6-18 months of age. A booster dose of 0.5 mL should be given to all children who have completed the primary series, before entering school. However, if the 3rd dose of the primary series is given on

or after the 4th birthday, a 4th dose is not required before entering school. When polio vaccine is given to persons >18 years of age, IPV should be given.

[14]In infants and small children, I.M. injection can be given into the midlateral aspect of the thigh; in older children and adults, I.M. injection can be given into the deltoid muscle. For postexposure prophylaxis, repeat doses are given on days 3, 7, 14, and 28 after the first dose. Initiate and complete immunization series with one vaccine product. Intradermal vaccine is not advised for postexposure prophylaxis.

[15]For pre-exposure prophylaxis against rabies for high-risk individuals, 1 mL I.M. or 0.1 mL intradermal is administered on days 0, 7, and 21 (or 28). Both I.M. and I.D. dosage forms are available. Preferred site for intradermal administration is the skin in the deltoid area. Patients taking chloroquine or mefloquine should only receive rabies vaccine by the I.M. route. Do **not** administer intradermally to minimize potential for vaccine failure.

[16]As MMR in a 2-dose schedule.

[17]Adsorbed preferred to fluid toxoid because of longer lasting immunity.

[18]≥9 months of age living in or traveling to endemic areas. Contraindicated in infants <4 months of age and in patients who have had an anaphylactic reaction to eggs. Increased risk of encephalitis associated with use of yellow fever vaccine in infants <9 months of age.

Note: For each vaccine, check the manufacturer's package insert for specific product information since preparations may change from time to time.

References

Advisory Committee on Immunization Practices, Measles Prevention, Recommendations of the Immunization Practices Advisory Committee, *MMWR Morb Mortal Wkly Rep*, 1989, 38(5-9):1-18.

American Academy of Pediatrics, Report of the Committee on Infectious Diseases (Red Book), 25th ed, 2000.

American Academy of Pediatrics, Committee on Infectious Diseases, "Acellular Pertussis Vaccines: Recommendations for Use as the Fourth and Fifth Doses," *Pediatrics*, 1992, 90:121-3.

American Academy of Pediatrics, Committee on Infectious Diseases, "Universal Hepatitis B Immunization," *Pediatrics*, 1992, 89(4 Pt 2):795-800.

American Academy of Pediatrics, Committee on Infectious Diseases, "Recommendations for the Use of Live Attenuated Varicella Vaccine," *Pediatrics*, 1995, 95(5):791-6.

American Academy of Pediatrics, Committee on Infectious Diseases, "Policy Statement: Recommendations for the Prevention of Pneumococcal Infections, Including the Use of Pneumococcal Conjugate Vaccine (Prevnar®), Pneumococcal Polysaccharide Vaccine, and Antibiotic Prophylaxis," *Pediatrics*, 2000, 106(2 Pt 1): 362-6.

American Academy of Pediatrics, Committee on Infectious Diseases, "Recommended Childhood and Adolescent Immunization Schedule – United States, 2005," *Pediatrics*, 2005, 115(1):182-6.

CDC, "Notice to Readers: Alternate Two-Dose Hepatitis B Vaccination Schedule for Adolescents Aged 11-15 Years," *MMWR Morb Mortal Wkly Rep*, 2000, 49(12):261.

CDC, "Recommended Childhood and Adolescent Immunization Schedule – United States, 2005," *MMWR*, 2005, 53(51 & 52):Q1-3.

IMMUNIZATION GUIDELINES *(Continued)*

Table 2. Currently Recommended Regimens for Routine *Haemophilus influenzae* Type b Conjugate Immunization for Children Immunized Beginning at 2-6 Months of Age[1]

Vaccine Product at Initiation	Total No. of Doses to Be Administered	Recommended Regimens
HbOC or PRP-T	4	3 doses at 2-month intervals initially; fourth dose at 12-15 months of age; any conjugate vaccine for dose 4[2]
PRP-OMP	3	2 doses at 2-month intervals initially; when feasible, same vaccine for doses 1 and 2; third dose at 12-15 months of age; any conjugate vaccine for dose 3[2]

[1]These vaccines may be given in combination products or as reconstituted products with DTaP or DTP, provided the combination or reconstituted vaccine is approved by the U.S. Food and Drug Administration for the child's age and the administration of the other vaccine component(s) also is justified.

[2]The safety and efficacy of PRP-OMP, PRP-T, HbOC, and PRP-D are likely to be equivalent for children ≥12 months of age. If a different product is given for dose 2, then the recommendations for that product (eg, HbOC or PRP-T) apply.

Adapted from "Report of the Committee on Infectious Diseases," *2000 Red Book®*, 25th ed, 268.

Table 3. Recommendations for Pneumococcal Conjugate Vaccine Use Among Healthy Children During Moderate and Severe Shortages

Age at First Vaccination (mo)	No Shortage[1]	Moderate Shortage	Severe Shortage
<6	2, 4, 6, and 12-15 months	2, 4, and 6 months (defer fourth dose)	2 doses at 2-month interval in first 6 months of life (defer third and fourth doses)
7-11	2 doses at 2-month interval; 12-15 month dose	2 doses at 2-month interval; 12-15-month dose	2 doses at 2-month interval (defer third dose)
12-23	2 doses at 2-month interval	2 doses at 2-month interval	1 dose (defer second dose)
>24	1 dose should be considered	No vaccination	No vaccination
Reduction in vaccine doses used[2]		21%	46%

[1]The vaccine schedule for no shortage is included as a reference. Providers should not use the no shortage schedule regardless of their vaccine supply until the national shortage is resolved.

[2]Assumes that approximately 85% of vaccine is administered to healthy infants beginning at age <7 months; approximately 5% is administered to high-risk infants beginning at age <7 months; and approximately 10% is administered to healthy children beginning at age 7-24 months. Actual vaccine savings will depend on a provider's vaccine use.

Adapted from the Advisory Committee on Immunization Practices, "Updated Recommendations on Use of Pneumococcal Conjugate Vaccine in a Setting of Vaccine Shortage," *MMWR Morb Mortal Wkly Rep*, 2001, 50(50):1140-2.

Table 4. Recommended Regimens for Pneumococcal Conjugate Vaccine Among Children With a Late Start or Lapse in Vaccine Administration

Age at Examination (mo)	Previous Pneumococcal Conjugate Vaccination History	Recommended Regimen[1]
2-6	0 doses	3 doses 2 months apart, 4th dose at 12-15 months
	1 dose	2 doses 2 months apart, 4th dose at 12-15 months
	2 doses	1 dose, 4th dose at 12-15 months
7-11	0 doses	2 doses 2 months apart, 3rd dose at 12-15 months
	1 or 2 doses before age 7 months	1 dose at 7-11 months, with another dose at 12-15 months (≥2 months later)
12-23	0 doses	2 doses ≥2 months apart
	1 dose before age 12 months	2 doses ≥2 months apart
	1 dose at ≥12 months	1 dose ≥2 months after the most recent dose
	2 or 3 doses before age 12 months	1 dose ≥2 months after the most recent dose
24-59		
Healthy children[2]	Any incomplete schedule	Consider 1 dose ≥2 months after the most recent dose
High risk[3]	<3 doses	1 dose ≥2 months after the most recent dose and another dose ≥2 months later
	3 doses	1 dose ≥2 months after the most recent dose

[1]For children vaccinated at age <1 year, the minimum interval between doses is 4 weeks. Doses administered at ≥12 months should be at least 8 weeks apart.

[2]Providers should consider 1 dose for healthy children 24-59 months, with priority to children 24-35 months, American Indian/Alaska native and black children, and those who attend group child care centers.

[3]Children with sickle cell disease, asplenia, human immunodeficiency virus infection, chronic illness, cochlear implant, or immunocompromising condition.

Adapted from "CDC. Notice to Readers: Pneumococcal Conjugate Vaccine Shortage Resolved," *MMWR Morb Mortal Wkly Rep*, 2003, 52(19):446-7.

IMMUNIZATION GUIDELINES *(Continued)*

Table 5. Persons Who Should Receive Pre-exposure Hepatitis B Immunization

- All infants
- Children at high risk for early childhood HBV infection
- Adolescents: Hepatitis B vaccination should be given by or before 11-12 years of age. Special efforts should be made to vaccinate all adolescents, not only those at high risk
- Hemophiliac patients and other recipients of certain blood products
- Intravenous drug abusers
- Heterosexual persons who have had more than one sex partner in the previous 6 months and/or those with a recent episode of a sexually transmitted disease
- Sexually active men who have sex with men
- Household and sexual contacts of HB_sAg-positive persons
- Members of households with adoptees who are hepatitis B surface antigen-positive
- Children and other household contacts in populations of high HBV endemicity
- Staff and residents of institutions for the developmentally disabled
- Staff of nonresidential day care and school programs for developmentally disabled if attended by known HB_sAg-positive persons
- Hemodialysis patients
- Healthcare workers and others with occupational risk of exposure to blood or blood-contaminated body fluid
- International travelers to areas of high or intermediate HBV endemicity
- Inmates of long-term correctional facilities

Adapted from American Academy of Pediatrics, Report of the Committee on Infectious Diseases, *Red Book*, 25th ed, 2000, 296.

See **Table 6** for recommended Hepatitis B immunization schedule.

Table 6. Recommended Childhood and Adolescent Immunization Schedule United States, 2005

Age ► / Vaccine ▼	Birth	1 mo	2 mo	4 mo	6 mo	12 mo	15 mo	18 mo	24 mo	4-6 y	11-12 y	13-18 y
Hepatitis B[1]	HepB #1	only if mother $HB_sAg(-)$			HepB #3				HepB series			
		HepB #2										
Diphtheria, tetanus, pertussis[2]			DTaP	DTaP	DTaP		DTaP			DTaP	Td	Td
Haemophilus influenzae type b[3]			Hib	Hib	Hib	Hib						
Inactivated poliovirus			IPV	IPV	IPV					IPV		
Measles, mumps, rubella[4]						MMR #1				MMR #2	MMR #2	
Varicella[5]						Varicella			Varicella			
Pneumococcal[6]			PCV	PCV	PCV	PCV			PCV	PPV		
Influenza[7]					Influenza (yearly)				Influenza (yearly)			
Vaccines below this line are for selected populations												
Hepatitis A[8]									Hepatitis A series			

Range of recommended ages | Preadolescent assessment | Catch-up immunization

This schedule indicates the recommended ages for routine administration of currently licensed childhood vaccines, as of December 1, 2004, for children through age 18 years. Any dose not given at the recommended age should be given at any subsequent visit when indicated and feasible. [shaded box] Indicates age groups that warrant special effort to administer those vaccines not given previously. Additional vaccines may be licensed and recommended during the year. Licensed combination vaccines may be used whenever any components of the combination are indicated and the vaccine's other components are not contraindicated. Providers should consult the manufacturers' package inserts for detailed recommendations. Clinically significant adverse events that follow immunization should be reported to the Vaccine Adverse Event Reporting System (VAERS). Guidance about how to obtain and complete a VAERS form can be found on the Internet: http://**www.vaers.org** or by calling **800-822-7967**.

1 **Hepatitis B (HepB) vaccine.** All infants should receive the first dose of hepatitis B vaccine soon after birth and before hospital discharge; the first dose may also be given by age 2 months if the infant's mother is HB_sAg-negative. Only monovalent HepB can be used for the birth dose. Monovalent or combination vaccine containing HepB may be used to complete the series. Four doses of vaccine may be administered when a birth dose is given. The second dose should be given at least 4 weeks after the first dose, except for combination vaccines, which cannot be administered before age 6 weeks. The third dose should be given at least 16 weeks after the first dose and at least 8 weeks after the second dose. The last dose in the vaccination series (third or fourth dose) should not be administered before age 24 weeks.

Infants born to HB_sAg-positive mothers should receive HepB vaccine and 0.5 mL hepatitis B immune globulin (HBIG) within 12 hours of birth at separate sites. The second dose is recommended at age 1-2 months. The last dose in the vaccination series should not be administered before age 24 weeks. These infants should be tested for HB_sAg and anti-HB_s at 9-15 months of age.

Infants born to mothers whose HB_sAg status is unknown should receive the first dose of the HepB vaccine series within 12 hours of birth. Maternal blood should be drawn as soon as possible to determine the mother's HB_sAg status; if the HB_sAg test is positive, the infant should receive HBIG as soon as possible (no later than age 1 week). The second dose is recommended at age 1-2 months. The last dose in the vaccination series should not be administered before age 24 weeks.

2 **Diphtheria, tetanus toxoids, and acellular pertussis (DTaP) vaccine.** The fourth dose of DTaP may be administered as early as age 12 months, provided that 6 months have elapsed since the third dose and the child is unlikely to return at age 15-18 months. The final dose in the series should be given at age ≥4 years. **Tetanus and diphtheria toxoids (Td)** is recommended at age 11-12 years if at least 5 years have elapsed since the last dose of tetanus and diphtheria toxoid-containing vaccine. Subsequent routine Td boosters are recommended every 10 years.

3 ***Haemophilus influenzae* type b (Hib) conjugate vaccine.** Three Hib conjugate vaccines are licensed for infant use. If PRP-OMP (PedvaxHIB® or ComVax® [Merck]) is administered at ages 2 and 4 months, a dose at age 6 months is not required. DTaP/Hib combination products should not be used for primary immunization in infants at ages 2, 4, or 6 months, but can be used as boosters following any Hib vaccine. The final dose in the series should be given at age ≥12 months.

4 **Measles, mumps, and rubella vaccine (MMR).** The second dose of MMR is recommended routinely at age 4-6 years but may be administered during any visit, provided at least 4 weeks have elapsed since the first dose and both doses are administered beginning at or after age 12 months. Those who have not previously received the second dose should complete the schedule by the visit at age 11-12-years.

5 **Varicella vaccine** is recommended at any visit at or after age 12 months for susceptible children (ie, those who lack a reliable history of chickenpox). Susceptible persons age ≥13 years should receive 2 doses, given at least 4 weeks apart.

6 **Pneumococcal vaccine.** The heptavalent **pneumococcal conjugate vaccine (PCV)** is recommended for all children age 2-23 months. It is also recommended for certain children age 24-59 months. The final dose in the series should be given at age ≥12 months. **Pneumococcal polysaccharide vaccine (PPV)** is recommended in addition to PCV for certain high-risk groups. See *MMWR*, 2000, 49(RR-9):1-35.

7 **Influenza vaccine** is recommended annually for children age ≥6 months with certain risk factors (including but not limited to asthma, cardiac disease, sickle cell disease, HIV, and diabetes), healthcare workers, and other persons (including household members) in close contact with persons in groups at high risk (see *MMWR*, 2004, 53(RR-6):1-40), and can be administered to all others wishing to obtain immunity. In addition, healthy children age 6-23 months and close contacts of healthy children age 0-23 months are recommended to receive influenza vaccine, because children in this age group are at substantially increased risk for influenza-related hospitalizations. For healthy persons age 5-49 years, the intranasally administered live, attenuated influenza vaccine (LAIV) is an acceptable alternative to the intramuscular trivalent inactivated influenza vacine (TIV). See *MMWR*, 2004, 53(RR-6):1-40. Children receiving TIV should be administered a dosage appropriate for their age (0.25 mL if 6-35 months or 0.5 mL if ≥3 years). Children age ≤8 years who are receiving influenza vaccine for the first time should receive two doses (separated by at least 4 weeks for TIV and at least 6 weeks for LAIV).

8 **Hepatitis A vaccine** is recommended for children and adolescents in selected states and regions, and for certain high-risk groups; consult your local public health authority. Children and adolescents in these states, regions, and high-risk groups who have not been immunized against hepatitis A can begin the hepatitis A vaccination series during any visit. The two doses in the series should be administered at least 6 months apart. See *MMWR*, 1999, 48(RR-12):1-37

Additional information about vaccines, including precautions and contraindications for vaccination and vaccine shortages is available at http://www.cdc.gov.nip or from the National Immunization Information Hotline, 800-232-2522 (English) or 800-232-0233 (Spanish). Approved by the Advisory Committee on Immunization Practices (http://www.cdc.gov/nip/acip), the American Academy of Pediatrics (http://www.aap.org), and the American Academy of Family Physicians (http://www.aafp.org).

Reference:

"Recommended Childhood and Adolescent Immunization Schedule — United States, 2005," *MMWR* , 2005, 53(51 & 52):Q1-3.

IMMUNIZATION GUIDELINES *(Continued)*

CATCH-UP SCHEDULE FOR CHILDREN AND ADOLESCENTS WHO START LATE OR WHO ARE >1 MONTH BEHIND

Tables 7 and 8 give catch-up schedules and minimum intervals between doses for children who have delayed immunizations. There is no need to restart a vaccine series regardless of the time that has elapsed between doses. Use the chart appropriate for the child's age.

Table 7. Catch-up Schedule for Children Age 4 Months - 6 Years

Dose 1 (Minimum Age)	Minimum Interval Between Doses			
	Dose 1 to Dose 2	**Dose 2 to Dose 3**	**Dose 3 to Dose 4**	**Dose 4 to Dose 5**
DTaP (6 wk)	4 wk	4 wk	6 mo	6 mo[1]
IPV (6 wk)	4 wk	4 wk	4 wk[2]	
HepB[3] (birth)	4 wk	8 wk (and 16 wk after 1st dose)		
MMR (12 mo)	4 wk[4]			
VAR (12 mo)				
Hib[5] (6 wk)	**4 wk:** If 1st dose given at age <12 mo **8 wk (as final dose):** If 1st dose given at age 12-14 mo **No further doses needed:** If 1st dose given at age ≥15 mo	**4 wk[6]:** If current age <12 mo **8 wk (as final dose)[6]:** If current age ≥12 mo and 2nd dose given at age <15 mo **No further doses needed**: If previous dose given at age ≥15 mo	**8 wk (as final dose):** This dose only necessary for children age 12 mo - 5 y who received 3 doses before age 12 mo	
PCV[7] (6 wk)	**4 wk:** If 1st dose given at age <12 mo and current age <24 mo **8 wk (as final dose):** If 1st dose given at age ≥12 mo or current age 24-59 mo **No further doses needed:** For healthy children if 1st dose given at age ≥24 mo	**4 wk**: If current age <12 mo **8 wk (as final dose):** If current age ≥12 mo **No further doses needed**: For healthy children if previous dose given at age ≥24 mo	**8 wk (as final dose):** This dose only necessary for children age 12 mo - 5 y who received 3 doses before age 12 mo	

Table 8. Catch-up Schedule for Children Age 7-18 Years

Minimum Interval Between Doses		
Dose 1 to Dose 2	**Dose 2 to Dose 3**	**Dose 3 to Booster Dose**
Td: 4 wk	Td: 6 mo	Td[8]: **6 mo:** If 1st dose given at age <12 mo and current age <11 y **5 y:** If 1st dose given at age ≥12 mo and 3rd dose given at age <7 y and current age ≥11 y **10 y:** If 3rd dose given at age ≥7 y
IPV[9]: 4 wk	IPV[9]: 4 wk	IPV[2,9]
HepB: 4 wk	HepB: 8 wk (and 16 wk after first dose)	
MMR: 4 wk		
VAR[10]: 4 wk		

Footnotes to Tables 7 and 8

[1]**Diphtheria and tetanus toxoids and acellular pertussis vaccine (DTaP):** The fifth dose is not necessary if the fourth dose was given after the fourth birthday.

[2]**Inactivated polio vaccine (IPV):** For children who received an all-IPV or all-oral poliovirus (OPV) series, a fourth dose is not necessary if third dose was given at age ≥4 years. If both OPV and IPV were given as part of a series, a total of four doses should be given, regardless of the child's current age.

[3]**Hepatitis B vaccine (HepB):** All children and adolescents who have not been immunized against hepatitis B should begin the hepatitis B vaccination series during any visit. Providers should make special efforts to immunize children who were born in, or whose parents were born in, areas of the world where hepatitis B virus infection is moderately or highly endemic.

[4]**Measles, mumps, and rubella vaccine (MMR):** The second dose of MMR is recommended routinely at age 4-6 years, but may be given earlier if desired.

[5]***Haemophilus influenzae* type b (Hib) conjugate vaccine:** Vaccine is not generally recommended for children age ≥5 years.

[6]**Hib:** If current age <12 months and the first 2 doses were PRP-OMP (PedvaxHIB® or Comvax® [Merck]), the third (and final) dose should be given at age 12-15 months and at least 8 weeks after the second dose.

[7]**Pneumococcal conjugate vaccine (PCV):** Vaccine is not generally recommended for children age ≥5 years.

[8]**Tetanus and diphtheria toxoids (Td):** For children age 7-10 years, the interval between the third and booster dose is determined by the age when the first dose was given. For adolescents age 11-18 years, the interval is determined by the age when the third dose was given.

[9]**IPV:** Vaccine is not generally recommended for persons age ≥18 years.

[10]**Varicella (VAR):** Give 2-dose series to all susceptible adolescents age ≥13 years.

Reporting Adverse Reactions

Clinically significant adverse events that follow vaccination should be reported to the Vaccine Adverse Event Reporting System (VAERS). Guidance on completing a VAERS form is available at http://www.vaers.org or call 800-822-7967.

Disease Reporting

Suspected cases of vaccine-preventable diseases should be reported to state or local health departments. Additional information about vaccines, including precautions and contraindications for vaccination and vaccine shortages, is available at http://www.cdc.gov/nip or from the National Immunization Information Hotline, 800-232-2522 (English) or 800-232-0233 (Spanish).

IMMUNIZATION GUIDELINES *(Continued)*

Table 9. Recommended Immunization Schedules for Children Not Immunized in the First Year of Life

Recommended Time/Age	Immunization(s)[1]	Comments
Younger Than 7 Years		
First visit	DTaP, Hib, HBV, MMR	If indicated, tuberculin testing may be done at same visit. If child is ≥5 y of age, Hib is not indicated in most circumstances.
Interval after first visit		
1 mo (4 wk)	DTaP, IPV, HBV, Var[2]	The second dose of IPV may be given if accelerated poliomyelitis immunization is necessary, such as for travelers to areas where polio is endemic.
2 mo	DTaP, Hib, IPV	Second dose of Hib is indicated only if the first dose was received when <15 mo.
≥8 mo	DTaP, HBV, IPV	IPV and HBV are not given if the third doses were given earlier.
Age 4-6 y (at or before school entry)	DTaP, IPV, MMR[3]	DTaP is not necessary if the fourth dose was given after the fourth birthday; IPV is not necessary if the third dose was given after the fourth birthday.
Age 11-12 y	See Table 6	
7-12 Years		
First visit	HBV, MMR, dT, IPV	
Interval after first visit		
2 mo (8 wk)	HBV, MMR,[3] Var,[4] dT, IPV	IPV also may be given 1 mo after the first visit if accelerated poliomyelitis immunization is necessary.
8-14 mo	HBV,[4] dT, IPV	IPV is not given if the third dose was given earlier.
Age 11-12 y	See Table 6	

[1]If all needed vaccines cannot be administered simultaneously, priority should be given to protecting the child against those diseases that pose the greatest immediate risk. In the United States, these diseases for children <2 years usually are measles and *Haemophilus influenzae* type b infection; for children >7 years, they are measles, mumps, and rubella. Before 13 years of age, immunity against hepatitis B and varicella should be ensured. DTaP, HBV, Hib, MMR, and Var can be given simultaneously at separate sites if failure of the patient to return for future immunizations is a concern.

[2]Varicella vaccine can be administered to susceptible children any time after 12 months of age. Unimmunized children who lack a reliable history of varicella should be immunized before their 13th birthday.

[3]Minimal interval between doses of MMR is 1 month (4 weeks).

[4]HBV may be given earlier in a 0-, 2-, and 4-month schedule.

Adapted from American Academy of Pediatrics, Report of the Committee on Infectious Diseases, *Red Book*, 25th ed, 2000.

Table 10. Spacing Live and Killed Antigen Administration Guidelines

Antigen Combinations	Recommended Minimum Interval Between Doses
≥2 killed antigens	None. May be given simultaneously or at any interval between doses. Vaccines associated with systemic reactions (cholera, plague, and parenteral typhoid) should be given on separate occasions.
Killed and live antigens	None. May be given simultaneously or at any interval between doses. (**Exception:** Concurrent administration of cholera and yellow fever vaccines should be avoided. Separate these vaccines by at least 3 weeks.)
≥2 live antigens parenteral	4-week minimum interval if not administered simultaneously. Live oral vaccines (eg, Ty21a typhoid vaccine, oral polio vaccine) can be administered simultaneously or at any interval before or after inactivated or live parenteral vaccines.

Table 11. Passive Immunization Agents — Immune Globulins

Immune Globulin	Dosage		Route
Hepatitis B (H-BIG®)			I.M.
percutaneous inoculation	0.06 mL/kg/dose (within 24 hours) (5 mL max)		
perinatal	0.5 mL/dose (within 12 hours of birth)		
sexual exposure	0.06 mL/kg/dose (within 14 days of contact) (5 mL max)		
Immune globulin (IG)			I.M.[1]
hepatitis A prophylaxis	0.02 mL/kg/dose (as soon as possible or within 2 weeks after exposure) (postexposure prophylaxis)		
<2 y:	0.06 mL/kg/dose (≥3 months or long-term exposure) repeat every 5 months with continuous exposure		
≥2 y:	0.02 mL/kg (3- to 5-month exposure) may be given to travelers whose departure is imminent with hepatitis A vaccine 0.06 mL/kg (long-term exposure) and hepatitis A vaccine		
hepatitis B	0.06 mL/kg/dose (H-BIG® should be used)		
hepatitis C	0.06 mL/kg/dose (percutaneous exposure)		
measles[2]	0.25 mL/kg/dose (max: 15 mL/dose) (within 6 days of exposure) 0.5 mL/kg/dose (max: 15 mL/dose) (immunocompromised children)		
Rabies[3]	20 IU/kg/dose (within 3 days)		
Tetanus (serious, contaminated, wounds; <3 previous tetanus vaccine doses)	250-500 units/dose		I.M.
Varicella-zoster[4] (VZIG)	Within 48 hours but not later than 96 hours after exposure		I.M.[5]
	0-10 kg	125 units = 1 vial	
	10.1-20 kg	250 units = 2 vials	
	20.1-30 kg	375 units = 3 vials	
	30.1-40 kg	500 units = 4 vials	
	>40 kg	625 units = 5 vials	

[1]Deep I.M. in the gluteal region for large doses only. Deltoid muscle or the anterolateral aspect of the thigh are preferred sites for injection. No greater than 5 mL/site in adults or large children; 1-3 mL/site in small children and infants. Max: 20 mL at one time. Pregnant women and infants should receive a thimerosol-free preparation.

[2]IG prophylaxis may not be indicated in a patient who has received IGIV within 3 weeks of exposure.

[3]1/2 of dose used to infiltrate the wound with the remaining 1/2 of dose given I.M. Rabies immune globulin is not recommended in previously HDCV immunized patients.

[4]Infants born to women who develop varicella within 5 days before or 48 hours after delivery should receive 125 units I.M. as a single dose.

[5]No greater than 2.5 mL of VZIG/one injection site. Doses >2.5 mL should be divided and administered at different sites.

IMMUNIZATION GUIDELINES *(Continued)*

Table 12. Suggested Intervals Between Administration of Immune Globulin Preparations for Various Indications and Measles Immunization[1]

Indication	Dose (including mg IgG/kg)	Time Interval (mo) Before Measles or Varicella Vaccination
Tetanus (TIG) prophylaxis	I.M.: 250 units (10 mg IgG/kg)	3
Hepatitis A (IG) prophylaxis		
Contact prophylaxis	I.M.: 0.02 mL/kg (3.3 mg IgG/kg)	3
International travel	I.M.: 0.06 mL/kg (10 mg IgG/kg)	3
Hepatitis B prophylaxis (HBIG)	I.M.: 0.06 mL/kg (10 mg IgG/kg)	3
Rabies immune globulin (RIG)	I.M.: 20 IU/kg (22 mg IgG/kg)	4
Varicella prophylaxis (VZIG)	I.M.: 125 units/10 kg (20-40 mg IgG/kg) (max: 625 units)	5
Measles prophylaxis (IG)		
Standard (ie, nonimmunocompromised contact)	I.M.: 0.25 mL/kg (40 mg IgG/kg)	5
Immunocompromised contact	I.M.: 0.50 mL/kg (80 mg IgG/kg)	6
Blood transfusion		
RBCs, washed	I.V.: 10 mL/kg (negligible IgG/kg)	0
RBCs, adenine-saline added	I.V.: 10 mL/kg (10 mg IgG/kg)	3
Packed RBCs	I.V.: 10 mL/kg (20-60 mg IgG/kg)	5
Whole blood cells	I.V.: 10 mL/kg (80-100 mg IgG/kg)	6
Plasma/platelet products	I.V.: 10 mL/kg (160 mg IgG/kg)	7
Replacement therapy for immune deficiencies	I.V.: 300-400 mg/kg (as IGIV)[2]	8
Immune thrombocytopenic purpura[3]	I.V.: 400 mg/kg (as IGIV) I.V.: 1000 mg/kg (as IGIV)	8 10
Kawasaki disease	I.V.: 2 g/kg (as IGIV)	11
RSV prophylaxis	I.V.: 750 mg/kg (as RSV-IVIG)	9
RSVIG monoclonal antibody (Synagis™)	I.M.: 15 mg/kg	None

[1]This table is not intended for determining the correct indications and dosage for the use of immune globulin preparations. Unvaccinated persons may not be fully protected against measles during the entire suggested time interval, and additional doses of immune globulin and/or measles vaccine may be indicated after measles exposure. The concentration of measles antibody in a particular immune globulin preparation can vary by lot. The rate of antibody clearance after receipt of an immune globulin preparation also can vary. The recommended time intervals are extrapolated from an estimated half-life of 30 days of passively acquired antibody and an observed interference with the immune response to measles vaccine for 5 months after a dose of 80 mg IgG/kg.

[2]Measles vaccination is recommended for most HIV-infected children who do not have evidence of severe immunosuppression, but it is contraindicated for patients who have congenital disorders of the immune system.

[3]Formerly referred to as idiopathic thrombocytopenic purpura.

Modified from *Red Book 2000: Report of the Committee on Infectious Diseases*, 25th ed, Elk Grove Village, IL: American Academy of Pediatrics, 390; Recommendations of the Advisory Committee on Immunization Practices (ACIP) and the American Academy of Family Physicians (AAFP), "General Recommendations on Immunization," *MMWR Morb Mortal Wkly Rep*, 2002, 51(RR-2), 1-36.

Table 13. Recommended for Routine Immunization of HIV-Infected Children — United States

Vaccine	Known HIV Infection: Asymptomatic	Known HIV Infection: Symptomatic
DTaP	Yes	Yes
OPV	No	No
IPV	Yes	Yes
MMR	Yes	Yes[1]
Hib	Yes	Yes
Pneumococcal	Yes	Yes
Influenza[2]	Yes	Yes
Varicella	Consider	Consider
BCG	No	No
Hepatitis A	[3]	[3]
Hepatitis B	Yes	Yes

[1]Severely immunocompromised HIV-infected children should not receive MMR.

[2]Administer influenza vaccine each autumn and repeat annually for HIV-exposed infants ≥6 months of age, HIV-infected children and adolescents, and household contacts of HIV-infected persons.

[3]The immune response in immunocompromised persons, including persons with HIV, may be suboptimal.

RECOMMENDATIONS FOR TRAVELERS

Table 14. Recommended Immunizations for Travelers to Developing Countries[1]

Immunizations	Length of Travel: Brief, <2 wk	Intermediate, 2 wk - 3 mo	Long-term Residential, >3 mo
Review and complete age-appropriate childhood schedule • DTaP; poliovirus vaccine, and *H. influenzae* type b vaccine may be given at 4 wk intervals if necessary to complete the recommended schedule before departure • Measles: 2 additional doses given if younger than 12 mo of age at first dose • Varicella • Hepatitis B[2]	+	+	+
Yellow fever[3]	+	+	+
Hepatitis A[4]	+	+	+
Typhoid fever[4]	±	+	+
Meningococcal disease[5]	±	±	±
Rabies[6]	±	+	+
Japanese encephalitis[3]	±	±	+

[1]+ = recommended; ± = consider.

[2]If insufficient time to complete 6-month primary series, accelerated series can be given.

[3]For endemic regions, see *Health Information for International Travel* in *Red Book*®. For high-risk activities in areas experiencing outbreaks, vaccine is recommended even for brief travel.

[4]Indicated for travelers who will consume food and liquids in areas of poor sanitation.

[5]For endemic regions of Africa, during local epidemics, and travel to Saudi Arabia for the Hajj.

[6]Indicated for person with high risk of animal exposure, and for travelers to endemic countries.

Adapted from "Report of the Committee on Infectious Diseases," *2000 Red Book*®, 25th ed, 78.

IMMUNIZATION GUIDELINES *(Continued)*

Table 15. Recommendations for Pre-exposure Immunoprophylaxis of Hepatitis A Virus Infection for Travelers[1]

Age (y)	Likely Exposure (mo)	Recommended Prophylaxis
<2	<3	IG 0.02 mL/kg[2]
	3-5	IG 0.06 mL/kg[2]
	Long-term	IG 0.06 mL/kg at departure and every 5 mo if exposure to HAV continues[2]
≥2	<3[3]	HAV vaccine[4,5] **or**
	3-5[3]	HAV vaccine[4,5] **or** IG 0.06 mL/kg[2]
	Long-term	HAV vaccine[4,5]

[1] IG = immune globulin; HAV= hepatitis A virus.

[2]IG should be administered deep into a large muscle mass. Ordinarily, no more than 5 mL should be administered in one site in an adult or large child; lesser amounts (maximum 3 mL) should be given to small children and infants.

[3]Vaccine is preferable, but IG is an acceptable alternative.

[4]To ensure protection in travelers whose departure is imminent, IG also may be given.

[5]Dose and schedule of hepatitis A vaccine as recommended according to age.

Adapted from "Report of the Committee on Infectious Diseases," *2000 Red Book®*, 25th ed, 282.

PREVENTION OF MALARIA

Drug[1]	Adult Dosage	Pediatric Dosage
	Chloroquine-Sensitive Areas[2]	
Chloroquine phosphate[3,4]	500 mg (300 mg base), once/week[5]	5 mg/kg base once/week, up to adult dose of 300 mg base[5]
	Chloroquine-Resistant Areas[2]	
Mefloquine[4,6,7]	250 mg once/week[5]	<15 kg: 5 mg/kg[5] 15-19 kg: 1/4 tablet[5] 20-30 kg: 1/2 tablet[5] 31-45 kg: 3/4 tablet[5] >45 kg: 1 tablet[5]
or		
Doxycycline[4,8]	100 mg/d[9]	2 mg/kg/d, up to 100 mg/d[9]
or		
Atovaquone/ proguanil[4,10]	250 mg/100 mg (1 tablet) daily[11]	11-20 kg: 62.5 mg/25 mg[10,11] 21-30 kg: 125 mg/50 mg[10,11] 31-40 kg: 187.5 mg/75 mg[10,11] >40 kg: 250 mg/100 mg[10,11]
Alternative:		
Primaquine[8,12,13]	30 mg base daily	0.5 mg/kg base daily
Chloroquine phosphate[3]	500 mg (300 mg base) once/week[5]	5 mg/kg base once/week, up to adult dose of 300 mg base[5]
plus		
Proguanil[14]	200 mg once/day	<2 y: 50 mg once/day 2-6 y: 100 mg once/day 7-10 y: 150 mg once/day >10 y: 200 mg once/day

[1]No drug regimen guarantees protection against malaria. If fever develops within a year (particularly within the first 2 months) after travel to malarious areas, travelers should be advised to seek medical attention. Insect repellents, insecticide-impregnated bed nets, and proper clothing are important adjuncts for malaria prophylaxis.

[2]Chloroquine-resistant *P. falciparum* occurs in all malarious areas except Central America west of the Panama Canal Zone, Mexico, Haiti, the Dominican Republic, and most of the Middle East (chloroquine resistance has been reported in Yemen, Oman, Saudi Arabia, and Iran).

[3]In pregnancy, chloroquine prophylaxis has been used extensively and safely.

[4]For prevention of attack after departure from areas where *P. vivax* and *P. ovale* are endemic, which includes almost all areas where malaria is found (except Haiti), some experts prescribe in addition primaquine phosphate 26.3 mg (15 mg base)/day or, for children, 0.3 mg base/kg/day during the last 2 weeks of prophylaxis. Others prefer to avoid the toxicity of primaquine and rely on surveillance to detect cases when they occur; particularly when exposure was limited or doubtful.

[5]Beginning 1-2 weeks before travel and continuing weekly for the duration of stay and for 4 weeks after leaving.

[6]In the U.S., a 250 mg tablet of mefloquine contains 228 mg mefloquine base. Outside the U.S., each 275 mg tablet contains 250 mg base.

[7]The pediatric dosage has not been approved by the FDA, and the drug has not been approved for use during pregnancy. However, it has been reported to be safe for prophylactic use during the second or third trimester of pregnancy and possibly during early pregnancy as well (CDC Health Information for International Travel, 2001-2003, 113; BL Smoak, Writer JV, Keep LW, et al, "The Effects of Inadvertent Exposure of Mefloquine Chemoprophylaxis on Pregnancy Outcomes and Infants of US Army Servicewomen," *J Infect Dis*, 1997, 176(3):831-3). Mefloquine is not recommended for patients with cardiac conduction abnormalities. Patients with a history of seizures or psychiatric disorders should avoid mefloquine (*Medical Letter*, 1990, 32:13). Resistance to mefloquine has been reported in some areas, such as Thailand; in these areas, doxycycline should be used for prophylaxis. In children <8 years of age, proguanil plus sulfisoxazole has been used (KN Suh and JS Keystone, *Infect Dis Clin Pract*, 1996, 5:541).

[8]An approved drug, but considered investigational for this condition by the U.S. Food and Drug Administration.

[9]Beginning 1-2 days before travel and continuing for the duration of stay and for 4 weeks after leaving. Use of tetracyclines is contraindicated in pregnancy and in children <8 years of age.

PREVENTION OF MALARIA *(Continued)*

Doxycycline can cause gastrointestinal disturbances, vaginal moniliasis, and photosensitivity reactions.

[10]Atovaquone plus proguanil is available as a fixed-dose combination tablet: adult tablets (250 mg atovaquone/100 mg proguanil, *Malarone*) and pediatric tablets (62.5 mg atovaquone/25 mg proguanil, *Malarone Pediatric*). To enhance absorption, it should be taken within 45 minutes after eating (Looareesuwan S, Chulay JD, Canfield CJ, et al, "Malarone (Atovaquone and Proguanil Hydrochloride): A Review of Its Clinical Development for Treatment of Malaria. Malarone Clinical Trials Study Group," *Am J Trop Med Hyg*, 1999, 60(4):533-41). Although approved for once daily dosing, to decrease nausea and vomiting the dose for treatment is usually divided in two.

[11]Shanks GE et al, *Clin Infect Dis*, 1998, 27:494; Lell B, Luckner D, Ndjave M, et al, "Randomised Placebo-Controlled Study of Atovaquone Plus Proguanil for Malaria Prophylaxis in Children," *Lancet*, 1998, 351(9104):709-13. Beginning 1-2 days before travel and continuing for the duration of stay and for 1 week after leaving. In one study of malaria prophylaxis, atovaquone/proguanil was better tolerated than mefloquine in nonimmune travelers (Overbosch D, Schilthuis H, Bienzle U, et al, "Atovaquone-Proguanil Versus Mefloquine for Malaria Prophylaxis in Nonimmune Travelers: Results From a Randomized, Double-Blind Study," *Clin Infect Dis*, 2001, 33(7):1015-21).

[12]Primaquine phosphate can cause hemolytic anemia, especially in patients whose red cells are deficient in glucose-6-phosphate dehydrogenase. This deficiency is most common in African, Asian, and Mediterranean peoples. Patients should be screened for G6PD deficiency before treatment. Primaquine should not be used during pregnancy.

[13]Several studies have shown that daily primaquine, beginning 1 day before departure and continued until 7 days after leaving the malaria area, provides effective prophylaxis against chloroquine-resistant *P. falciparum* (Baird JK, Lacy MD, Basri H, et al, "Randomized, Parallel Placebo-Controlled Trial of Primaquine for Malaria Prophylaxis in Papua, Indonesia," *Clin Infect Dis*, 2001, 33(12):1990-7). Some studies have shown less efficacy against *P. vivax*. Nausea and abdominal pain can be diminished by taking with food.

[14]Proguanil (Paludrine – Wyeth Ayerst, Canada; AstraZeneca, United Kingdom), which is not available alone in the U.S.A. but is widely available in Canada and Europe, is recommended mainly for use in Africa south of the Sahara. Prophylaxis is recommended during exposure and for 4 weeks afterwards. Proguanil has been used in pregnancy without evidence of toxicity (Phillips-Howard PA and Wood D, "The Safety of Antimalarial Drugs in Pregnancy," *Drug Saf*, 1996, 14(3):131-45).

Adapted from "Report of the Committee on Infectious Diseases," *2003 Red Book®*, 26th ed, 760-1.

CONTRAINDICATIONS AND PRECAUTIONS TO COMMONLY USED VACCINES

Vaccine	Contraindications	Precautions[1]	Vaccines Can Be Administered
General for all vaccines, including diphtheria and tetanus toxoids and acellular pertussis vaccine (DTaP); pediatric diphtheria-tetanus toxoid (DT); adult tetanus-diphtheria toxoid (Td); inactivated poliovirus vaccine (IPV); measles-mumps-rubella vaccine (MMR); *Haemophilus influenzae* type b vaccine (Hib); hepatitis A vaccine; hepatitis B vaccine; varicella vaccine; pneumococcal conjugate vaccine (PCV); influenza vaccine; and pneumococcal polysaccharide vaccine (PPV)	• Serious allergic reaction (eg, anaphylaxis) after a previous vaccine dose • Serious allergic reaction (eg, anaphylaxis) to a vaccine component	• Moderate or severe acute illnesses with or without a fever	• Mild acute illness with or without fever • Mild to moderate local reaction (ie, swelling, redness, soreness); low-grade or moderate fever after previous dose • Lack of previous physical examination in well-appearing person • Current antimicrobial therapy • Convalescent phase of illnesses • Premature birth (hepatitis B vaccine is an exception in certain circumstances)[2] • Recent exposure to an infectious disease • History of penicillin allergy, other nonvaccine allergies, receiving allergen extract immunotherapy • Temperature <40.5°C, fussiness or mild drowsiness after a previous dose of diphtheria toxoid-tetanus toxoid-pertussis vaccine (DTP)/DTaP • Family history of seizures[3] • Family history of sudden infant death syndrome • Family history of an adverse event after DTP or DTaP administration • Stable neurologic conditions (eg, cerebral palsy, well-controlled convulsions, developmental delay)
DTaP	• Severe allergic reaction after a previous dose or to a vaccine component • Encephalopathy (eg, coma, decreased level of consciousness, prolonged seizures) within 7 days of administration of previous dose of DTP or DTaP • Progressive neurologic disorder, including infantile spasms, uncontrolled epilepsy, progressive encephalopathy; defer DTaP until neurologic status clarified and stabilized	• Fever >40.5°C ≤48 hours after vaccination with a previous dose of DTP or DTaP • Collapse or shock-like state (ie, hypotonic hyporesponsive episode) ≤48 hours after receiving a previous dose of DTP/DTaP • Seizure ≤3 days of receiving a previous dose of DTP/DTaP[3] • Persistent, inconsolable crying lasting ≥3 hours, ≤48 hours after receiving a previous dose of DTP/DTaP • Moderate or severe acute illness with or without fever	Same as above

CONTRAINDICATIONS AND PRECAUTIONS TO COMMONLY USED VACCINES *(Continued)*

Vaccine	Contraindications	Precautions[1]	Vaccines Can Be Administered
DT, Td	• Severe allergic reaction after a previous dose or to a vaccine component	• Guillain-Barré syndrome ≤6 weeks after previous dose of tetanus toxoid-containing vaccine • Moderate or severe acute illness with or without fever	Same as above
IPV	• Severe allergic reaction to previous dose or vaccine component	• Pregnancy • Moderate or severe acute illness with or without fever	—
MMR[4]	• Severe allergic reaction after a previous dose or to a vaccine component • Pregnancy • Known severe immunodeficiency (eg, hematologic and solid tumors; congenital immunodeficiency; long-term immunosuppressive therapy,[5] or severely symptomatic human immunodeficiency virus [HIV] infection)	• Recent (≤11 months) receipt of antibody-containing blood product (specific interval depends on product) • History of thrombocytopenia or thrombocytopenic purpura • Moderate or severe acute illness with or without fever	• Positive tuberculin skin test • Simultaneous TB skin testing[6] • Breast-feeding • Pregnancy of recipient's mother or other close or household contact • Recipient is child-bearing-age female • Immunodeficient family member or household contact • Asymptomatic or mildly symptomatic HIV infection • Allergy to eggs
Hib	• Severe allergic reaction after a previous dose or to a vaccine component • Age <6 weeks	• Moderate or severe acute illness with or without fever	—
Hepatitis B	• Severe allergic reaction after a previous dose or to a vaccine component	• Infant weighing <2000 g[2] • Moderate or severe acute illness with or without fever	• Pregnancy • Autoimmune disease (eg, systemic lupus erythematosis or rheumatoid arthritis)
Hepatitis A	• Severe allergic reaction after a previous dose or to a vaccine component	• Pregnancy • Moderate or severe acute illness with or without fever	—
Varicella	• Severe allergic reaction after a previous dose or to a vaccine component • Substantial suppression of cellular immunity • Pregnancy	• Recent (≤11 months) receipt of antibody containing blood product (specific interval depends on product) • Moderate or severe acute illness with or without fever	• Pregnancy of recipient's mother or other close or household contact • Immunodeficient family member or household contact[7] • Asymptomatic or mildly symptomatic HIV infection • Humoral immunodeficiency (eg, agammaglobulinemia)
PCV	• Severe allergic reaction after a previous dose or to a vaccine component	• Moderate or severe acute illness with or without fever	—

Vaccine	Contraindications	Precautions[1]	Vaccines Can Be Administered
Influenza	• Severe allergic reaction to previous dose or vaccine component, including egg protein	• Moderate or severe acute illness with or without fever	• Nonsevere (eg, contact) allergy to latex or thimerosal • Concurrent administration of Coumadin® or aminophylline
PPV	• Severe allergic reaction after a previous dose or to a vaccine component	• Moderate or severe acute illness with or without fever	—

[1]Events or conditions listed as precautions should be reviewed carefully. Benefits and risks of administering a specific vaccine to a person under these circumstances should be considered. If the risk from the vaccine is believed to outweigh the benefit, the vaccine should not be administered. If the benefit of vaccination is believed to outweigh the risk, the vaccine should be administered. Whether and when to administer DTaP to children with proven or suspected underlying neurologic disorders should be decided on a case-by-case basis.

[2]Hepatitis B vaccination should be deferred for infants weighing <2000 g if the mother is documented to be hepatitis B surface antigen (Hb_sAg)-negative at the time of the infant's birth. Vaccination can commence at chronological age 1 month. For infants born to Hb_sAg)-positive women, hepatitis B immunoglobulin and hepatitis B vaccine should be administered at or soon after birth regardless of weight.

[3]Acetaminophen or other appropriate antipyretic can be administered to children with a personal or family history of seizures at the time of DTaP vaccination and every 4-6 hours for 24 hours thereafter to reduce the possibility of postvaccination fever (source: American Academy of Pediatrics, Pickering LK, ed, "Active Immunization," *2000 Red Book*®, Report of the Committee on Infectious Diseases, 25th ed, Elk Grove Village, IL: American Academy of Pediatrics, 2000).

[4]MMR and varicella vaccines can be administered on the same day. If not administered on the same day, these vaccines should be separated by ≥28 days.

[5]Substantially immunosuppressive steroid dose is considered to be ≥2 weeks of daily receipt of 20 mg or 2 mg/kg body weight of prednisone or equivalent.

[6]Measles vaccination can suppress tuberculin reactivity temporarily. Measles-containing vaccine can be administered on the same day as tuberculin skin testing. If testing cannot be performed until after the day of MMR vaccination, the test should be postponed for ≥4 weeks after the vaccination. If an urgent need exists to skin test, do so with the understanding that reactivity might be reduced by the vaccine.

[7]If a vaccine experiences a presumed vaccine-related rash 7-25 days after vaccination, avoid direct contact with immunocompromised persons for the duration of the rash.

Adapted from "Recommendations and Reports," *MMWR Morb Mortal Wkly Rep*, 2002, 51(RR-2):9-10.

SKIN TESTS FOR DELAYED HYPERSENSITIVITY

Skin tests for delayed hypersensitivity are used diagnostically to assess previous infection (ie, PPD, histoplasmin, and coccidioidin) or used to evaluate cellular immune function by testing for anergy (ie, mumps, *Candida*, tetanus toxoid, trichophyton, PPD). Anergy, a defect in cell-mediated immunity, is characterized by a depressed response or lack of response to skin testing with injected antigens. Anergy has been associated with congenital and acquired immunodeficiencies, and malnutrition.

Candida 1:100

Dose = 0.1 mL intradermally (30% of children younger than 18 months of age and 50% older than 18 months of age respond)

Can be used as a control antigen

Histoplasmin 1:100

Dose = 0.1 mL intradermally (yeast derived)

Mumps 40 cfu per mL

Dose = 0.1 mL intradermally (contraindicated in patients allergic to eggs, egg products, or thimerosal)

Purified Protein Derivative 5 TU (PPD[1] Mantoux Tuberculin)

Screening for tuberculosis:

Children who have no risk factors but who reside in high-prevalence regions: skin test at 4-6 years and 11-16 years of age

Children exposed to HIV-infected individuals, homeless, residents of nursing homes, institutionalized adolescents, users of illicit drugs, incarcerated adolescents and migrant farm workers: skin test every 2-3 years

Children at high risk (children infected with HIV, incarcerated adolescents): annual skin testing

Dose = 0.1 mL intradermally

Definition of positive Mantoux skin test (regardless of previous BCG administration):

Reaction ≥5 mm for high-risk group (children in close contact with known or suspected infectious cases of tuberculosis; children suspected to have disease based on clinical and/or roentgenographic evidence; and children with underlying host factors (immunosuppressive conditions, receiving immunosuppressive therapy, and HIV infection).

Reaction ≥10 mm for children <4 years; those with medical diseases who are at increased risk for dissemination or for those at increased risk because of environmental exposure.

Reaction ≥15 mm for children ≥4 years of age including those with no risk factors.

[1]PPD 1 TU (first strength) is only used in individuals suspected of being highly sensitive. PPD 250 TU (second strength) is used only for individuals who fail to respond to a previous injection of 5 TU, or anergic patients in whom TB is suspected.

Tetanus Toxoid 1:5

Dose = 0.1 mL intradermally (29% of children younger than 2 years of age and 78% older than 2 years of age respond if they have received 3 immunizing doses)

Can be used as a control antigen.

Tine Test

Indication: survey and screen for exposure to tuberculosis (grasp forearm firmly; stretch the skin of the volar surface tightly; apply the tines to the selected site; press for at least one second so that a circular halo impression is left on the skin)

General Information

1. Intradermal skin tests should be injected in the flexor surface of the forearm.
2. A pale wheal 6-10 mm in diameter should form over the needle tip as soon as the injection is administered. If no bleb forms, the injection must be repeated.
3. Space skin tests at least 2 inches apart to prevent reactions from overlapping.
4. Read skin tests for diameter of induration and presence of erythema at 24, 48, and 72 hours. Reactions occurring before 24 hours are indicative of an immediate rather than a delayed hypersensitivity reaction.
5. False-negative results may occur in patients with malnutrition, viral infections, febrile illnesses, immunodeficiency disorders, severe disseminated infections, uremia, patients who have received immunosuppressive therapy (steroids, antineoplastic agents), patients who have received a recent live attenuated virus vaccine (MMR, measles).
6. False-positive results may occur in patients sensitive to ingredients in the skin test solution such as thimerosal; cross-sensitivity between similar antigens; or with improper interpretation of skin test.
7. Side effects are pain, blisters, extensive erythema and necrosis at the injection site.

   Emergency equipment and epinephrine should be readily available to treat severe allergic reactions that may occur.

Recommended Interpretation of Skin Test Reactions

Reaction	Local Reaction	
	After Intradermal Injections of Antigens	After Dinitrochlorobenzene
1+	Erythema >10 mm and/or induration >1-5 mm	Erythema and/or induration covering <1/2 area of dosing site
2+	Induration 6-10 mm	Induration covering >1/2 area of dose site
3+	Induration 11-20 mm	Vesiculation and induration at dose site or spontaneous flare at days 7-14 at the site
4+	Induration >20 mm	Bulla or ulceration at dose site or spontaneous flare at days 7-14 at the site

References

American Academy of Pediatrics Committee on Infectious Diseases, "Screening for Tuberculosis in Infants and Children," *Pediatrics*, 1994, 93(1):131-4.

American Academy of Pediatrics Committee on Infectious Diseases, "Update on Tuberculosis Skin Testing of Children," *Pediatrics*, 1996, 97(2):282-4.

NORMAL LABORATORY VALUES FOR CHILDREN

		Normal Values
CHEMISTRY		
Albumin	0-1 y	2.0-4.0 g/dL
	1 y to adult	3.5-5.5 g/dL
Ammonia	Newborns	90-150 mcg/dL
	Children	40-120 mcg/dL
	Adults	18-54 mcg/dL
Amylase	Newborns	0-60 units/L
	Adults	30-110 units/L
Bilirubin, conjugated, direct	Newborns	<1.5 mg/dL
	1 mo to adult	0-0.5 mg/dL
Bilirubin, total	0-3 d	2.0-10.0 mg/dL
	1 mo to adult	0-1.5 mg/dL
Bilirubin, unconjugated, indirect		0.6-10.5 mg/dL
Calcium	Newborns	7.0-12.0 mg/dL
	0-2 y	8.8-11.2 mg/dL
	2 y to adult	9.0-11.0 mg/dL
Calcium, ionized, whole blood		4.4-5.4 mg/dL
Carbon dioxide, total		23-33 mEq/L
Chloride		95-105 mEq/L
Cholesterol	Newborns	45-170 mg/dL
	0-1 y	65-175 mg/dL
	1-20 y	120-230 mg/dL
Creatinine	0-1 y	≤0.6 mg/dL
	1 y to adult	0.5-1.5 mg/dL
Glucose	Newborns	30-90 mg/dL
	0-2 y	60-105 mg/dL
	Children to Adults	70-110 mg/dL
Iron		
	Newborns	110-270 mcg/dL
	Infants	30-70 mcg/dL
	Children	55-120 mcg/dL
	Adults	70-180 mcg/dL
Iron binding	Newborns	59-175 mcg/dL
	Infants	100-400 mcg/dL
	Adults	250-400 mcg/dL
Lactic acid, lactate		2-20 mg/dL
Lead, whole blood		<10 mcg/dL
Lipase		
	Children	20-140 units/L
	Adults	0-190 units/L
Magnesium		1.5-2.5 mEq/L
Osmolality, serum		275-290 mOsm/kg
Osmolality, urine		50-1400 mOsm/kg

		Normal Values
CHEMISTRY		
Phosphorus	Newborns	4.2-9.0 mg/dL
	6 wk to 19 mo	3.8-6.7 mg/dL
	19 mo to 3 y	2.9-5.9 mg/dL
	3-15 y	3.6-5.6 mg/dL
	>15 y	2.5-5.0 mg/dL
Potassium, plasma	Newborns	4.5-7.2 mEq/L
	2 d to 3 mo	4.0-6.2 mEq/L
	3 mo to 1 y	3.7-5.6 mEq/L
	1-16 y	3.5-5.0 mEq/L
Protein, total	0-2 y	4.2-7.4 g/dL
	>2 y	6.0-8.0 g/dL
Sodium		136-145 mEq/L
Triglycerides	Infants	0-171 mg/dL
	Children	20-130 mg/dL
	Adults	30-200 mg/dL
Urea nitrogen, blood	0-2 y	4-15 mg/dL
	2 y to Adult	5-20 mg/dL
Uric acid	Male	3.0-7.0 mg/dL
	Female	2.0-6.0 mg/dL
ENZYMES		
Alanine aminotransferase (ALT) (SGPT)	0-2 mo	8-78 units/L
	>2 mo	8-36 units/L
Alkaline phosphatase (ALKP)	Newborns	60-130 units/L
	0-16 y	85-400 units/L
	>16 y	30-115 units/L
Aspartate aminotransferase (AST) (SGOT)	Infants	18-74 units/L
	Children	15-46 units/L
	Adults	5-35 units/L
Creatine kinase (CK)	Infants	20-200 units/L
	Children	10-90 units/L
	Adult male	0-206 units/L
	Adult female	0-175 units/L
Lactate dehydrogenase (LDH)	Newborns	290-501 units/L
	1 mo to 2 y	110-144 units/L
	>16 y	60-170 units/L

Blood Gases

	Arterial	Capillary	Venous
pH	7.35-7.45	7.35-7.45	7.32-7.42
pCO_2 (mm Hg)	35-45	35-45	38-52
pO_2 (mm Hg)	70-100	60-80	24-48
HCO_3 (mEq/L)	19-25	19-25	19-25
TCO_2 (mEq/L)	19-29	19-29	23-33
O_2 saturation (%)	90-95	90-95	40-70
Base excess (mEq/L)	-5 to +5	-5 to +5	-5 to +5

NORMAL LABORATORY VALUES FOR CHILDREN
(Continued)

Thyroid Function Tests

Test	Age	Value
T_4 (thyroxine)	1-7 d	10.1-20.9 mcg/dL
	8-14 d	9.8-16.6 mcg/dL
	1 mo to 1 y	5.5-16.0 mcg/dL
	>1 y	4.0-12.0 mcg/dL
FTI	1-3 d	9.3-26.6
	1-4 wk	7.6-20.8
	1-4 mo	7.4-17.9
	4-12 mo	5.1-14.5
	1-6 y	5.7-13.3
	>6 y	4.8-14.0
T_3	Newborns	100-470 ng/dL
	1-5 y	100-260 ng/dL
	5-10 y	90-240 ng/dL
	10 y to Adult	70-210 ng/dL
T_3 uptake		35%-45%
TSH	Cord	3-22 micro international units/mL
	1-3 d	<40 micro international units/mL
	3-7 d	<25 micro international units/mL
	>7 d	0-10 micro international units/mL

Hematology Values

Age	Hgb (g/dL)	Hct (%)	RBC (mill/mm^3)	RDW	MCV (fL)	MCH (pg)	MCHC (%)	PLTS (x 10^3/mm^3)
0-3 d	15.0-20.0	45-61	4.0-5.9	<18	95-115	31-37	29-37	250-450
1-2 wk	12.5-18.5	39-57	3.6-5.5	<17	86-110	28-36	28-38	250-450
1-6 mo	10.0-13.0	29-42	3.1-4.3	<16.5	74-96	25-35	30-36	300-700
7 mo to 2 y	10.5-13.0	33-38	3.7-4.9	<16	70-84	23-30	31-37	250-600
2-5 y	11.5-13.0	34-39	3.9-5.0	<15	75-87	24-30	31-37	250-550
5-8 y	11.5-14.5	35-42	4.0-4.9	<15	77-95	25-33	31-37	250-550
13-18 y	12.0-15.2	36-47	4.5-5.1	<14.5	78-96	25-35	31-37	150-450
Adult male	13.5-16.5	41-50	4.5-5.5	<14.5	80-100	26-34	31-37	150-450
Adult female	12.0-15.0	36-44	4.0-4.9	<14.5	80-100	26-34	31-37	150-450

NORMAL LABORATORY VALUES FOR CHILDREN
(Continued)

WBC and Diff

Age	WBC (x 10^3/ mm^3)	Segs	Bands	Lymphs	Monos	Eosinophils	Basophils	Atypical Lymphs	No. of NRBCs
0-3 d	9.0-35.0	32-62	10-18	19-29	5-7	0-2	0-1	0-8	0-2
1-2 wk	5.0-20.0	14-34	6-14	36-45	6-10	0-2	0-1	0-8	0
1-6 mo	6.0-17.5	13-33	4-12	41-71	4-7	0-3	0-1	0-8	0
7 mo to 2 y	6.0-17.0	15-35	5-11	45-76	3-6	0-3	0-1	0-8	0
2-5 y	5.5-15.5	23-45	5-11	35-65	3-6	0-3	0-1	0-8	0
5-8 y	5.0-14.5	32-54	5-11	28-48	3-6	0-3	0-1	0-8	0
13-18 y	4.5-13.0	34-64	5-11	25-45	3-6	0-3	0-1	0-8	0
Adults	4.5-11.0	35-66	5-11	24-44	3-6	0-3	0-1	0-8	0

Segs = segmented neutrophils.

Bands = band neutrophils.

Lymphs = lymphocytes.

Monos = monocytes.

Erythrocyte Sedimentation Rates and Reticulocyte Counts

Sedimentation rate, Westergren	Children	0-20 mm/hour
	Adult male	0-15 mm/hour
	Adult female	0-20 mm/hour
Sedimentation rate, Wintrobe	Children	0-13 mm/hour
	Adult male	0-10 mm/hour
	Adult female	0-15 mm/hour
Reticulocyte count	Newborns	2%-6%
	1-6 mo	0%-2.8%
	Adults	0.5%-1.5%

Cerebrospinal Fluid Values, Normal

Cell count		% PMNs
Preterm mean	9 (0-25.4 WBC/mm^3)	57%
Term mean	8.2 (0-22.4 WBC/mm^3)	61%
>1 mo	0.7	0
Glucose		
Preterm	24-63 mg/dL	mean 50
Term	34-119 mg/dL	mean 52
Children	40-80 mg/dL	
CSF glucose/blood glucose		
Preterm	55-105%	
Term	44-128%	
Children	50%	
Lactic acid dehydrogenase	5-30 units/mL	mean 20 units/mL
Myelin basic protein	<4 ng/mL	
Pressure: Initial LP (mm H_2O)		
Newborns	80-110 (<110)	
Infants/children	<200 (lateral recumbent position)	
Respiratory movements	5-10	
Protein		
Preterm	65-150 mg/dL	mean 115
Term	20-170 mg/dL	mean 90
Children		
Ventricular	5-15 mg/dL	
Cisternal	5-25 mg/dL	
Lumbar	5-40 mg/dL	

APGAR SCORING SYSTEM

Sign	Score 0	1	2
Heart rate	Absent	Under 100 beats per minute	Over 100 beats per minute
Respiratory effort	Absent	Slow (irregular)	Good crying
Muscle tone	Limp	Some flexion of extremities	Active motion
Reflex irritability	No response	Grimace	Cough or sneeze
Color	Blue, pale	Pink body, blue extremities	All pink

From Apgar V, "A Proposal for a New Method of Evaluation of the Newborn Infant," *Anesth Analg*, 1953, 32:260.

FETAL HEART RATE MONITORING

Normal Heart Rates

Fetal heart rate (FHR) 120-160 bpm. Isolated accelerations are normal and considered reassuring. Mild (100-120 bpm) and transient bradycardias may be normal. Normal fetal heart rate tracings show beat-to-beat variability of 5-10 bpm (poor beat-to-beat variability suggests fetal hypoxia).

Abnormal Heart Rates

Bradycardia (FHR <120 bpm): Potential causes include fetal distress, drugs, congenital heart block (associated with maternal SLE, congenital cardiac defects).

Tachycardia (FHR >160 bpm): Potential causes include maternal fever, chorioamnionitis, drugs, fetal dysrhythmias, eg, SVT (with or without fetal CHF).

Decreased Beat-to-Beat Variability

Results from fetal CNS depression. Potential causes include fetal hypoxia, fetal sleep, fetal immaturity, and maternal narcotic/sedative administration.

Fetal Heart Rate Decelerations

Type 1 (early decelerations)

- Seen most commonly in late labor
- Mirror uterine contractions in time of onset, duration, and resolution
- Uniform shape
- Usually associated with good beat-to-beat variability
- Heart rate may dip to 60-80 bpm
- Associated with fetal head compression (increases vagal tone)
- Considered benign, and not representative of fetal hypoxia

Type 2 (late decelerations)

- Deceleration 10-30 seconds after onset of uterine contraction
- Heart rate fails to return to baseline after contraction is completed
- Asymmetrical shape (longer deceleration, shorter acceleration)
- Late decelerations of 10-20 bpm may be significant
- Probably associated with fetal CNS and myocardial depression

Type 3 (variable decelerations)

- Heart rate variations do not correlate with uterine contractions
- Variable shape and duration
- Occur occasionally in many normal labors
- Concerning if severe (HR <60 bpm), prolonged (duration >60 seconds), associated with poor beat-to-beat variability, or combined with late decelerations
- Associated with cord compression (including nuchal cord)

Reference

Manual of Neonatal Care, Joint Program in Neonatology, 1991.

CREATININE CLEARANCE ESTIMATING METHODS IN PATIENTS WITH STABLE RENAL FUNCTION

The following formulas provide an acceptable estimate of the patient's creatinine clearance except when:

a. The patient's serum creatinine is changing rapidly (either up or down).

b. Patients are markedly emaciated.

In these situations (a and b above), certain assumptions have to be made:

a. In patients with rapidly rising serum creatinines (ie, increasing by >0.5-0.7 mg/dL/day), it is best to assume that the patient's creatinine clearance is probably less than 10 mL/minute.

b. In emaciated patients, although their actual creatinine clearance is less than their calculated creatinine clearance (because of decreased creatinine production), it is not possible to predict easily how much less.

Estimation of creatinine clearance using serum creatinine and body length (to be used when an adequate timed specimen cannot be obtained). **Note:** This formula may not provide an accurate estimation of creatinine clearance for infants <6 months of age or for patients with severe starvation or muscle wasting.

$CL_{cr} = K \times L/S_{cr}$

where:

Cl_{cr} = creatinine clearance in mL/minute/1.73 m^2
K = constant of proportionality that is age specific

Age	K
Low birth weight ≤1 y	0.33
Full-term ≤1 y	0.45
2-12 y	0.55
13-21 y female	0.55
13-21 y male	0.70

L = length in cm
S_{Cr} = serum creatinine concentration in mg/dL

Reference

Schwartz GJ, Brion LP, and Spitzer A, "The Use of Plasma Creatinine Concentration for Estimating Glomerular Filtration Rate in Infants, Children and Adolescents," *Ped Clin N Amer*, 1987, 34:571-90.

Children 1-18 years

Method 1: (Traub SL, Johnson CE, *Am J Hosp Pharm*, 1980, 37:195-201)

Equation:

$$Cl_{cr} = \frac{0.48 \times (\text{height})}{S_{cr}}$$

where

Cl_{cr} = creatinine clearance in mL/min/1.73 m^2
S_{cr} = serum creatinine in mg/dL
Height = height in cm

Method 2: See nomogram.

Children 1-18 Years

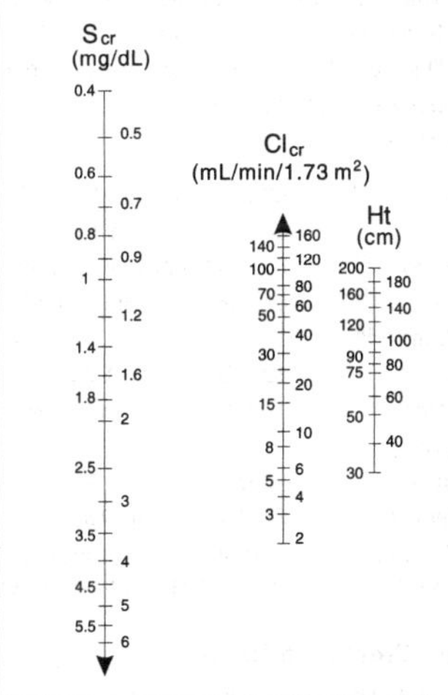

Adults 18 years and older

Method 1: (Cockroft DW and Gault MH, *Nephron*, 1976, 16:31-41)

Estimated creatinine clearance (Cl_{cr}) (mL/min):

$$\text{Male} = \frac{(140 - \text{age})\ \text{IBW (kg)}}{72 \times \text{serum creatinine}}$$

$$\text{Female} = \text{Estimated } Cl_{cr} \text{ male} \times 0.85$$

Note: The use of the patient's ideal body weight (IBW) is recommended for the above formula except when the patient's actual body weight is less than ideal. Use of the IBW is especially important in obese patients. See appendix Growth & Development section for Ideal Body Weight Calculation.

Method 2: (Jelliffe RW, *Ann Intern Med*, 1973, 79:604)

Estimated creatinine clearance (Cl_{cr}) (mL/min/1.73 m²):

$$\text{Male} = \frac{98 - 0.8\ (\text{age} - 20)}{\text{serum creatinine}}$$

$$\text{Female} = \text{Estimated } Cl_{cr} \text{ male} \times 0.90$$

RENAL FUNCTION TESTS

Endogenous creatinine clearance vs age (timed collection)

Creatinine clearance (mL/min/1.73 m^2) = $(Cr_uV/S_{cr}T)$ (1.73/A)

where:

Cr_u	=	Urine creatinine concentration (mg/dL)
V	=	Total urine volume collected during sampling period (mL)
S_{Cr}	=	Serum creatinine concentration (mg/dL)
T	=	Duration of sampling period (min) (24 h = 1440 min)
A	=	Body surface area (m^2)

Age-specific normal values

5-7 d	50.6±5.8 mL/min/1.73 m^2
1-2 mo	64.6±5.8 mL/min/1.73 m^2
5-8 mo	87.7±11.9 mL/min/1.73 m^2
9-12 mo	86.9±8.4 mL/min/1.73 m^2
≥18 mo	
male	124±26 mL/min/1.73 m^2
female	109±13.5 mL/min/1.73 m^2
Adults	
male	105±14 mL/min/1.73 m^2
female	95±18 mL/min/1.73 m^2

Note: In patients with renal failure (creatinine clearance <25 mL/min), creatinine clearance may be elevated over GFR because of tubular secretion of creatinine.

Serum BUN / Serum Creatinine Ratio

Serum BUN (mg/dL):serum creatinine (mg/dL)

Normal BUN:creatinine ratio is 10-15.

BUN:creatinine ratio >20 suggests prerenal azotemia (also seen with high urea-generation states such as GI bleeding).

BUN:creatinine ratio <5 may be seen with disorders affecting urea biosynthesis such as urea cycle enzyme deficiencies and with hepatitis.

Fractional Sodium Excretion

Fractional sodium secretion (FENa) = Na_uS_{cr} /Na_sCr_u x 100%

where:

Na_u	=	Urine sodium (mEq/L)
Na_s	=	Serum sodium (mEq/L)
Cr_u	=	Urine creatinine (mg/dL)
S_{Cr}	=	Serum creatinine (mg/dL)

FENa <1% suggests prerenal failure
FENa >2% suggest intrinsic renal failure
(for newborns, normal FENa is approximately 2.5%)

Note: Disease states associated with a falsely elevated FENa include severe volume depletion (>10%), early acute tubular necrosis and volume depletion in chronic renal disease. Disorders associated with a lowered FENa include acute glomerulonephritis, hemoglobinuric or myoglobinuric renal failure, nonoliguric acute tubular necrosis, and acute urinary tract obstruction. In addition, FENa may be <1% in patients with acute renal failure **and** a second condition predisposing to sodium retention (eg, burns, congestive heart failure, nephrotic syndrome).

Urine Calcium / Urine Creatinine Ratio (spot sample)

Urine calcium (mg/dL): urine creatinine (mg/dL)

Normal values <0.21 (mean values 0.08 males, 0.06 females)

Premature infants show wide variability of calcium:creatinine ratio, and tend to have lower thresholds for calcium loss than older children. Prematures without nephrolithiasis had mean Ca:Cr ratio of 0.75±0.76. Infants with nephrolithiasis had mean Ca:Cr ratio of 1.32±1.03 (Jacinto, et al, *Pediatrics*, vol 81, p 31).

Urine Protein / Urine Creatinine Ratio (spot sample)

P_u/Cr_u	Total Protein Excretion ($mg/m^2/day$)
0.1	80
1	800
10	8000

where:

P_u = Urine protein concentration (mg/dL)

Cr_u = Urine creatinine concentration (mg/dL)

Serum Osmolality

Predicted serum osmolality =

$$2 \times Na\ (mEq/L) + BUN\ (mg/dL) / 2.8 + glucose\ (mg/dL) / 18$$

High Anion Gap (see Toxicology section)

ACID / BASE ASSESSMENT

Henderson-Hasselbalch Equation

$pH = 6.1 + \log (HCO_3^- / (0.03) (pCO_2))$

Alveolar Gas Equation

P_iO_2 = f_iO_2 x (total atmospheric pressure – vapor pressure of H_2O at 37°C)
= f_iO_2 x (760 mm Hg – 47 mm Hg)

PAO_2 = $P_iO_2 - PACO_2 / R$

Alveolar/arterial oxygen gradient = $PAO_2 - PaO_2$

Normal ranges:

Children	15-20 mm Hg
Adults	20-25 mm Hg

Where:

P_iO_2	=	Oxygen partial pressure of inspired gas (mm Hg) (150 mm Hg in room air at sea level)
f_iO_2	=	Fractional pressure of oxygen in inspired gas (0.21 in room air)
PAO_2	=	Alveolar oxygen partial pressure
$PACO_2$	=	Alveolar carbon dioxide partial pressure
PaO_2	=	Arterial oxygen partial pressure
R	=	Respiratory exchange quotient (typically 0.8, increases with high carbohydrate diet, decreases with high fat diet)

Acid / Base Disorders

Acute metabolic acidosis (<12 h duration)

$PaCO_2$ expected = 1.5 (HCO_3^-) + 8±2

or

expected change in pCO = (1-1.5) x change in HCO_3^-

Acute metabolic alkalosis (<12 h duration)

expected change in pCO_2 = (0.5-1) x change in HCO_3^-

Acute respiratory acidosis (<6 h duration)

expected change in HCO_3^- = 0.1 x pCO_2

Acute respiratory acidosis (>6 h duration)

expected change in HCO_3^- = 0.4 x change in pCO_2

Acute respiratory alkalosis (<6 h duration)

expected change in HCO_3^- = 0.2 x change in pCO_2

Acute respiratory alkalosis (>6 h duration)

expected change in HCO_3^- = 0.5 x change in pCO_2

ACUTE DYSTONIC REACTIONS, MANAGEMENT

1. **Confirm that patient has stable airway and adequate respiratory activity.**

2. Administer **one** of the following:

   Diphenhydramine 0.7-1 mg/kg/dose I.V./P.O. q4-6h prn **or**

   Hydroxyzine 0.5-1 mg/kg/dose I.M./P.O. q4-6h prn
   (adult dose: 25-100 mg I.M./P.O. q6h) **or**

   Children >3 years: Benztropine 0.02-0.05 mg/kg/dose or maximum of 1-2 mg I.V./P.O. (avoid use in children <3 years of age except in cases of extreme emergency)

Agents which predispose patients to acute dystonic reactions, such as phenothiazine neuroleptics or antiemetics, often have long therapeutic half-lives. Anticholinergic administration should therefore be continued for 6-24 hours after discontinuation of phenothiazine therapy.

PREPROCEDURE SEDATIVES IN CHILDREN

Purpose: The following table is a guide to aid the clinician in the selection of the most appropriate sedative to sedate a child for a procedure. One must also consider:

- Not all patients require sedation. It is dependent on the procedure and age of the child.
- When sedation is desired, one must consider the time of onset, the duration of action, and the route of administration.
- Each of the following drugs is well absorbed when given by the suggested routes and doses.
- Each drug was assigned an "intensity" based upon the class of drug, dose, and route.[1]
  - Conscious sedation: A medically controlled state of depressed consciousness that retains the patient's ability to independently and continuously maintain a patent airway, respond appropriately to physical stimulation and/or verbal commands. The protective reflexes are maintained.
  - Deep sedation: A medically controlled state of depressed consciousness associated with partial or complete loss of protective reflexes and inability to respond appropriately to physical stimulation and/or verbal commands.
- Those drugs classified as producing deep sedation require more frequent monitoring postprocedure.
- For painful procedures, an analgesic agent needs to be administered.

Sedatives Used to Produce Conscious Sedation

Drug	Route	Dose (mg/kg)	Onset (min)	Duration (h)	Comments
Chloral hydrate	P.O./P.R.	25-100	10-20	4-8	May cause hepatic neoplasms in rats; maximum single dose: infants: 1 g; children: 2 g
Diazepam[2,3] (Valium®)	P.O.	0.2-0.3 90 min prior	60-90	6-8	Maximum oral dose: 10 mg
	I.V.	0.1-0.2	1-3	6-8	Maximum dose I.V.: 5 mg; due to poor absorption and tissue irritation, I.M. route **not** recommended
	P.R.	0.2-0.4	2-10	6-8	May use I.V. solution rectally
"DPT" cocktail[4] (Demerol®, Phenergan®, Thorazine®)	I.M.	Demerol® 1-2, Phenergan® 0.5-1, Thorazine® 0.5-1	30	2-14	May be mixed in single syringe; I.M. only. This combination of agents may have a higher rate of adverse effects compared with alternative sedative/analgesics.

Sedatives Used to Produce Conscious Sedation *(continued)*

Drug	Route	Dose (mg/kg)	Onset (min)	Duration (h)	Comments
Fentanyl	Trans-mucosal	5-15 mcg/kg	5-15	1-2	Maximum trans-mucosal dose: 400 mcg
	I.M.	1-3 mcg/kg	7-15	1-2	
	I.V.	1-3 mcg/kg	Immediate	30-60 min	
Lorazepam[5] (Ativan®)	P.O.	0.05; 90-120 min prior	60	8-12	
	Deep I.M.	0.05; 90-120 min prior	30-60	8-12	
	I.V.	0.05; over 5-10 min	15-30	8-12	
Meperidine (Demerol®)	P.O.	2-4	10-15	2-4	Doses I.M./I.V. >2 mg/kg are considered deep sedation
	I.M.	0.5-2	10-15	2-4	
	I.V.	0.5-2	5	2-3	
Midazolam[6,7] (Versed®)	P.O.	0.2-0.4; 30-45 min prior	20-30	1-2	Maximum oral dose: 15 mg
	Deep I.M.	0.1-0.15; 30-60 min prior	15	1-2	Maximum total dose: 10 mg
	I.V.	**6 mo - 5 y:** 0.05-0.1; **6-12 y:** 0.025-0.05; **>12 y - Adult:** 2.5-5 mg (total dose); give over 10-20 min	1-5	1-2	Maximum concentration: 1 mg/mL; maximum I.M./I.V. dose: 6 mo - 5 y: 6 mg 6 y - Adult: 10 mg
	P.R.	0.3	20-30	1-2	Dilute injection in 5 mL NS; administer rectally
	Intranasal	0.2-0.3	5	30-60 min	Administer nasally: Use a 1 mL needleless syringe into the nares over 15 seconds; use 5 mg/mL concentration; ½ dose may be administered into each nare
Morphine	P.O.	0.2-0.5	20-30	3-5	
	I.M.	0.05-0.2	20-30	3-5	
	I.V.	0.05-0.2	10-15	2-5	

Note: See individual drug monographs for further information.

Sedatives Used to Produce Deep Sedation

Drug	Route	Dose (mg/kg)	Onset (min)	Duration (h)	Comments
Methohexital[8,9] (Brevital®)	I.M.	5-10	5	1-1.5	Maximum concentration for I.M./I.V.: 50 mg/mL; maximum I.M./I.V. dose: 200 mg. Greater incidence of adverse effects with I.V. use.
	I.V.	0.75-2	1	7-10 min	
	P.R.	20-35	5-10	1-1.5	Shorter duration of action than thiopental; rectal given as a 10% solution in sterile water; maximum dose rectal: 500 mg
Pentobarbital	P.O./I.M./P.R.	2-6	10-25	1-4	Maximum I.M./I.V./P.O./P.R. dose: 100 mg
	I.V.	1-3	1	15 min	
Thiopental[10,4] (Pentothal)	I.V.	4-6	0.5-1	5-10 min	
	P.R.	25; immediately prior to procedure	10	1-5	Variable rectal absorption; may use additional 12.5 mg/kg if necessary; maximum rectal dose: 1-1.5 g

Note: See individual drug monographs for further information.

PREPROCEDURE SEDATIVES IN CHILDREN *(Continued)*

Sedatives Used to Produce Dissociative Anesthesia (Monitor as if deep sedation)

Drug	Route	Dose (mg/kg)	Onset (min)	Duration	Comments
Ketamine	P.O.	6-10; 30 min prior	30-45	10-30	Use only under direct supervision of physicians experienced in administering general anesthetics; has analgesic effects; may use injectable product orally diluted in a beverage of the patient's choice
	I.M.	3-7	7	12-25	
	I.V.	0.5-2	1	5-10	

Note: See individual drug monographs for further information.

Footnotes

[1]Committee on Drugs, Section of Anesthesiology, American Academy of Pediatrics, "Guidelines for Monitoring and Management of Pediatric Patient During and After Sedation for Diagnostic and Therapeutic Procedures," *Pediatrics*, 1992, 89:1110-5.

[2]Yager JY and Seshia SS, "Sublingual Lorazepam in Childhood Serial Seizures," *Am J Dis Child*, 1988, 142(9):931-2.

[3]Fell D, Gough MB, Northan AA, et al, "Diazepam Premedication in Children," *Anaesthesia*, 1985, 40:12-7.

[4]Burckart GJ, White III TJ, Siegle RL, et al, "Rectal Thiopental Versus an Intramuscular Cocktail for Sedating Children Before Computer Tomography," *Am J Hosp Pharm*, 1980, 37:222-4.

[5]Burtles R and Astley B, "Lorazepam in Children," *Br J Anaesth*, 1983, 55:275-9.

[6]Roelofse JA, van der Bijl P, Stegmann DH, et al, "Preanesthetic Medication With Rectal Midazolam in Children Undergoing Dental Extractions," *J Oral Maxillofac Surg*, 1990, 48(8):791-7.

[7]Wilton NC, Leigh J, Rosen DR, et al, "Preanesthetic Sedation of Preschool Children Using Intranasal Midazolam," *Anesthesiology*, 1988, 60(6):972-5.

[8]Elman DS and Denson JS, "Preanesthetic Sedation of Children With Intramuscular Methohexital Sodium," *Anesth Analg*, 1965, 44(5):494-8.

[9]Miller JR, Grayson M, and Stoelting VK, "Sedation With Intramuscular Methohexital Sodium," *Am J Ophthalmol*, 1966, 62(1):38-43.

[10]"Drug Evaluations," *AMA*, 1980.

FEBRILE SEIZURES

A febrile seizure is defined as a seizure occurring for no reason other than an elevated temperature. It does not have an infectious or metabolic origin within the CNS (ie, it is not caused by meningitis or encephalitis). Fever is usually >102°F rectally, but the more rapid the rise in temperature, the more likely a febrile seizure may occur. About 4% of children develop febrile seizures at one time of their life, usually occurring between 3 months and 5 years of age with the majority occurring at 6 months to 3 years of age. There are three types of febrile seizures:

1. **Simple** febrile seizures are nonfocal febrile seizures of less than 15 minutes duration. They do not occur in multiples.
2. **Complex** febrile seizures are febrile seizures that are either focal, have a focal component, are longer than 15 minutes in duration, or are multiple febrile seizures that occur within 30 minutes.
3. **Febrile status epilepticus** is a febrile seizure that is a generalized tonic clonic seizure lasting longer than 30 minutes.

Note: Febrile seizures should not be confused with true epileptic seizures associated with fever or "seizure with fever." "Seizure with fever" includes seizures associated with acute neurologic illnesses (ie, meningitis, encephalitis).

Long-term prophylaxis with phenobarbital may reduce the risk of subsequent febrile seizures. The 1980 NIH Consensus paper stated that after the first febrile seizure, long-term prophylaxis should be considered under any of the following:

1. Presence of abnormal neurological development or abnormal neurological exam
2. Febrile seizure was complex in nature:
   - duration >15 minutes
   - focal febrile seizure
   - followed by transient or persistent neurological abnormalities
3. Positive family history of afebrile seizures (epilepsy)

Also consider long-term prophylaxis in certain cases if:

1. the child has multiple febrile seizures
2. the child is <12 months of age

Anticonvulsant prophylaxis is usually continued for 2 years or 1 year after the last seizure, whichever is longer. With the identification of phenobarbital's adverse effects on learning and cognitive function, many physicians will not start long-term phenobarbital prophylaxis after the first febrile seizure unless the patient has more than one of the above risk factors. Most physicians would start long-term prophylaxis if the patient has a second febrile seizure.

Daily administration of phenobarbital and therapeutic phenobarbital serum concentrations ≥15 mcg/mL decrease recurrence rates of febrile seizures. Valproic acid is also effective in preventing recurrences of febrile seizures, but is usually reserved for patients who have significant adverse effects to phenobarbital. The administration of rectal diazepam (as a solution or suppository) at the time of the febrile illness has been shown to be as effective as daily phenobarbital in preventing recurrences of febrile seizures. These rectal dosage forms are just now available in the United States. Some centers in the USA are still using the injectable form of diazepam rectally. The solution for injection is filtered prior to use if drawn from an ampul. A recent study suggests that oral diazepam, 0.33 mg/kg/dose given every 8 hours only when the child has a fever, may reduce the risk of recurrent febrile seizures (see Rosman, et al). (**Note:** A more recent study by Uhari (1995) showed that lower doses of diazepam, 0.2 mg/kg/dose, were not effective.) Carbamazepine and phenytoin are **not** effective in preventing febrile seizures.

FEBRILE SEIZURES *(Continued)*

References

Berg AT, Shinnar S, Hauser WA, et al, "Predictors of Recurrent Febrile Seizures: A Meta-Analytic Review," *J Pediatr*, 1990, 116(3):329-37.

Camfield PR, Camfield CS, Gordon K, et al, "Prevention of Recurrent Febrile Seizures," *J Pediatr*, 1995, 126(6):929-30.

NIH Consensus Statement, "Febrile Seizures: A Consensus of Their Significance, Evaluation and Treatment," *Pediatrics*, 1980, 66(6):1009-12.

Rosman NP, Colton T, Labazzo J, et al, "A Controlled Trial of Diazepam Administration During Febrile Illnesses to Prevent Recurrence of Febrile Seizures," *N Engl J Med*, 1993, 329(2):79-84.

Uhari M, Rantala H, Vainionpää L, et al, "Effect of Acetaminophen and of Low Intermittent Doses of Diazepam on Prevention of Recurrences of Febrile Seizures," *J Pediatr*, 1995, 126(6):991-5.

CAUSES OF NEONATAL SEIZURES

1. Trauma
   a. subdural hematoma
   b. intracortical hemorrhage
   c. cortical vein thrombosis
2. Asphyxia — subependymal hemorrhage
3. Congenital abnormalities (cerebral dysgenesis)
   a. lissencephaly
   b. schizencephaly
4. Hypertension
5. Metabolic
   a. hypocalcemia
      - hypomagnesemia
      - high phosphate load
      - IDM (infants of diabetic mothers)
      - hypoparathyroidism
      - maternal hyperparathyroidism
      - idiopathic
      - DiGeorge's syndrome
   b. hypoglycemia
      - galactosemia
      - IUGR (intrauterine growth retardation)
      - IDM (infants of diabetic mothers)
      - glycogen storage disease
      - idiopathic
      - methylmalonic acidemia
      - propionic acidemia
      - maple syrup urine disease
      - asphyxia
   c. electrolyte imbalance
      - hypernatremia
      - hypomagnesemia
      - hyponatremia
6. Infections
   a. bacterial meningitis
   b. cerebral abscess
   c. herpes encephalitis
   d. Coxsackie meningoencephalitis
   e. cytomegalovirus
   f. toxoplasmosis
   g. syphilis

CAUSES OF NEONATAL SEIZURES *(Continued)*

7. Drug withdrawal
   a. methadone
   b. heroin
   c. barbiturate (short-acting, such as secobarbital and butalbital)
   d. propoxyphene
   e. benzodiazepines (chlordiazepoxide, diazepam)
   f. cocaine
   g. ethanol
   h. codeine
8. Pyridoxine dependency
9. Amino acid disturbances
   a. maple syrup urine disease
   b. urea cycle abnormalities
   c. nonketotic hyperglycinemia
   d. ketotic hyperglycinemia
   e. Leigh disease
   f. isovaleric acidemia
10. Toxins
    a. local anesthetics
    b. isoniazid
    c. lead
    d. indomethacin (from breast feeding)
    e. fentanyl
11. Familial seizures
    a. neurocutaneous syndromes
       - tuberous sclerosis
       - incontinentia pigmenti
    b. genetic syndromes
       - Zellweger's
       - Smith Lemli Opitz
       - neonatal adrenoleukodystrophy
    c. benign familial epilepsy
12. Cerebral hemorrhage
    a. intraventricular
    b. subarachnoid
    c. subdural

Adapted from Painter MJ, Bergman I, and Crumrie P, "Neonatal Seizures," *Pediatr Clin North Am*, 1986, 33:91-107.

ANTIEPILEPTIC DRUGS

Antiepileptic Drugs for Children and Adolescents by Seizure Type and Epilepsy Syndrome

Seizure Type or Epilepsy Syndrome	First Line Therapy	Alternatives
Partial seizures (with or without secondary generalization)	Carbamazepine, oxcarbazepine, or phenytoin	**Second choice:** Gabapentin, lamotrigine, topiramate, or valproate **Third choice:** Tiagabine, zonisamide, phenobarbital, or primidone **Consider:** Benzodiazepine, acetazolamide, vigabatrin, or felbamate
Generalized tonic-clonic seizures	Valproate, carbamazepine, or phenytoin	**Second choice:** Topiramate or lamotrigine **Third choice:** Phenobarbital or primidone **Consider:** Zonisamide
Childhood absence epilepsy		
Before 10 years of age	Ethosuximide (only if no convulsive seizures) or valproate	**Second choice:** Lamotrigine **Third choice:** Methsuximide, acetazolamide, benzodiazepine, topiramate, or zonisamide
After 10 years of age	Valproate	**Second choice:** Lamotrigine **Third choice:** Ethosuximide, methsuximide, acetazolamide, benzodiazepine, topiramate or zonisamide
Juvenile myoclonic epilepsy	Valproate	**Second choice:** Lamotrigine, topiramate, or clonazepam **Third choice:** Phenobarbital, primidone, carbamazepine, or phenytoin **Consider:** Felbamate
Progressive myoclonic epilepsy	Valproate	**Second choice:** Valproate plus clonazepam, or phenobarbital
Lennox-Gastaut and related syndromes	Valproate	**Second choice:** Topiramate, lamotrigine **Third choice:** Ketogenic diet, vagal nerve stimulation, felbamate, benzodiazepine, or phenobarbital **Consider:** Ethosuximide, methsuximide, ACTH or steroids, pyridoxine or vigabatrin
Infantile spasms	ACTH (or steroids), vigabatrin, or valproate	**Second choice:** Topiramate **Third choice:** Lamotrigine, tiagabine, or benzodiazepine **Consider:** Pyridoxine, felbamate, or zonisamide
Benign epilepsy of childhood with centrotemporal spikes	Gabapentin or valproate	**Second choice:** Carbamazepine or phenytoin **Third choice:** Phenobarbital, primidone, or benzodiazepine **Consider:** Lamotrigine or topiramate
Neonatal seizures	Phenobarbital	**Second choice:** Phenytoin **Consider:** Clonazepam, primidone, valproate, or pyridoxine

Adapted from Bourgeois BF, "Antiepileptic Drugs in Pediatric Practice," *Epilepsia*, 1995, 36(Suppl 2):S34-S45 and Bourgeois BF, "New Antiepileptic Drugs in Children: Which Ones for Which Seizures?" *Clin Neuropharmacol*, 2000, 23(3):119-32.

COMA SCALES

Glasgow Coma Scale

Activity	Best Response	Score
Eye opening	Spontaneous	4
	Responds to voice	3
	Responds to pain	2
	No response	1
Verbal response	Oriented and appropriate	5
	Confused / disoriented conversation	4
	Inappropriate words	3
	Nonspecific sounds (incomprehensible)	2
	No response	1
Motor response	Follows commands	6
	Localizes pain	5
	Withdraws to pain	4
	Abnormal flexion (decorticate posturing)	3
	Abnormal extension (decerebrate posturing)	2
	No response	1

Modified Coma Scale for Infants

Activity	Best Response	Score
Eye opening	Spontaneous	4
	Responds to voice	3
	Responds to pain	2
	No response	1
Verbal response	Coos, babbles	5
	Irritable	4
	Cries to pain	3
	Moans to pain	2
	No response	1
Motor response	Normal spontaneous movements	6
	Withdraws to touch	5
	Withdraws to pain	4
	Abnormal flexion (decorticate posturing)	3
	Abnormal extension (decerebrate posturing)	2
	No response	1

Interpretation of Coma Scale Scores
Maximum Score: 15; Minimum Score: 3
(low score indicates greater severity of coma)

Range of Score	Interpretation
3- 8	Coma. Severe brain injury. Immediate action needed. Notify ICU staff STAT. Will require intubation regardless of respiratory status.
9-12	Lethargic. Needs close observation in special care unit. Frequent neuro checks. Notify ICU staff.
13-14	Needs observation
15	Normal

References

James HE, "Neurologic Evaluation and Support in the Child With an Acute Brain Insult," *Pediatr Ann*, 1986, 15(1):16-22.

Jennett B and Teasdale G, "Aspects of Coma After Severe Head Injury," *Lancet*, 1977, 1(8017): 878-81.

ASTHMA

Adapted from National Asthma Education and Prevention Program (NAEPP) Expert Panel Report, "Guidelines for the Diagnosis and Management of Asthma – Update on Selected Topics 2002," NIH Publication No. 02-5075 (www.nhlbi.nih.gov/guidelines/asthma/index.html)

MANAGEMENT OF ASTHMA IN INFANTS, CHILDREN, AND ADULTS

Goals of Asthma Treatment

- Minimal or no chronic symptoms day or night
- Minimal or no exacerbations
- No limitations on activities; no school/work missed
- Minimal use of inhaled short-acting beta$_2$-agonist (<1 time/day, <1 canister/month)
- Minimal or no adverse effects from medications
- Children >5 years of age and adults only: PEF >80% of personal best

Education

- Teach self-management.
- Teach about controlling environmental factors (avoidance of allergens or other factors that contribute to asthma severity).
- Review administration technique and compliance with patient.
- May use a written action plan to help educate.

Stepwise Approach for Managing Infants and Young Children (≤5 Years of Age) With Acute or Chronic Asthma[1]

Symptoms[2]	Long-Term Control (Daily Medications)
STEP 4: Severe Persistent	
Day: Continual Night: Frequent	• **Preferred treatment:** **– High dose inhaled corticosteroid** **AND** **– Long-acting inhaled beta$_2$-agonist** **AND**, if needed – Long-term oral corticosteroids (2 mg/kg/day, generally do not exceed 60 mg/day). (Make repeated attempts to reduce systemic corticosteroids and maintain control with high-dose inhaled corticosteroids.)
STEP 3: Moderate Persistent	
Day: Every day Night: >1 night/week	• **Preferred treatment:** **– Low-dose inhaled corticosteroid** **AND** **Long-acting inhaled beta$_2$-agonist** **OR** **Medium-dose inhaled corticosteroid** • Alternatives: – Low-dose inhaled corticosteroid and either leukotriene receptor antagonist or theophylline
	If needed (especially with recurring severe exacerbations): • **Preferred treatment:** **– Medium-dose inhaled corticosteroid and long-acting inhaled beta$_2$-agonist** • Alternatives: – Medium-dose inhaled corticosteroid and either leukotriene receptor antagonist or theophylline

ASTHMA *(Continued)*

Stepwise Approach for Managing Infants and Young Children (≤5 Years of Age) With Acute or Chronic Asthma[1]

Symptoms[2]	Long-Term Control (Daily Medications)
STEP 2: Mild Persistent	
Day: >2 days/week but <1 time/day Night: >2 nights/month	• **Preferred treatment:** – **Low-dose inhaled corticosteroid (with nebulizer or MDI with holding chamber with or without face mask or DPI)** • Alternatives: Cromolyn (nebulizer is preferred or MDI with holding chamber) **OR** Leukotriene receptor antagonist
STEP 1: Mild Intermittent	
Day: ≤2 days/week Night: ≤2 nights/month	No daily medication needed

[1]Classify severity. The presence of one of the features of severity is sufficient to place a patient in that category. An individual should be assigned to the most severe grade in which any feature occurs. The characteristics noted in this figure are general and may overlap because asthma is highly variable. Furthermore, an individual's classification may change over time.

[2]Patients at any level of severity can have mild, moderate, or severe exacerbations. Some patients with intermittent asthma experience severe and life-threatening exacerbations separated by long periods of normal lung function and no symptoms.

↓ Step Down
Review treatment every 1-6 month; a gradual stepwise reduction in treatment may be possible.

↑ Step Up
If control is not achieved, consider step up. But first: review patient medication technique, adherence, and environmental control (avoidance of allergens or other precipitant factors)

Quick Relief – All Patients

- Bronchodilator as needed for symptoms ≤2 times/week. Intensity of treatment will depend upon severity of exacerbation (see "Management of Asthma Exacerbations"). Either:
  - Preferred treatment: Inhaled short-acting beta$_2$-agonist by nebulizer or face mask and spacer/holding chamber
    or
  - Alternative treatment: Oral beta$_2$-agonist
- With viral respiratory infection:
  - Bronchodilator q4-6h up to 24 hours (longer with physician consult) but, in general, repeat no more than once every 6 weeks.
  - Consider systemic corticosteroid if current exacerbation is severe or patient has history of severe exacerbations.
- Use of short-acting inhaled beta$_2$-agonist on a daily basis, or increasing use, indicates the need to initiate or titrate long-term control therapy.

Notes:

- **The stepwise approach presents guidelines to assist clinical decision making. Asthma is highly variable; clinicians should tailor specific medication plans to the needs and circumstances of individual patients.**
- Gain control as quickly as possible; then decrease treatment to the least medication necessary to maintain control.
- A rescue course of systemic corticosteroid may be needed at any time and step.
- In general, use of short-acting beta$_2$-agonist on a daily basis indicates the need for additional long-term control therapy.

- There are very few studies on asthma therapy for infants.
- Studies comparing medications in children <5 years of age are not available.
- Consultation with an asthma specialist is recommended for moderate or severe persistent asthma. Consider consultation for patient with mild persistent asthma.
- Initiation of long-term control therapy should be considered in infants and young children who have had >3 episodes of wheezing in the past year that lasted >1 day and affected sleep and who have risk factors for asthma.
- Inhaled corticosteroids improve health outcomes for children with mild-moderate persistent asthma. Monitor growth of children taking corticosteroids by any route. If growth appears slowed, weigh the benefits against the risks.
- Antibiotics are not recommended for treatment of acute asthma exacerbations except where there is evidence or suspicion of bacterial infection.

Stepwise Approach for Managing Asthma in Children >5 Years of Age, Adolescents, and Adults: Treatment[1]

Symptoms[2]	Lung Function[3]	Long-Term Control (Daily Medications)
STEP 4: Severe Persistent		
Day: Continual Night: Frequent	PEF/FEV$_1$ ≤60% PEF variability >30%	• **Preferred treatment:** **– High dose inhaled corticosteroid** **AND** **– Long-acting inhaled beta$_2$-agonist** **AND**, if needed – Long-term oral corticosteroids (2 mg/kg/day, generally do not exceed 60 mg/day). (Make repeated attempts to reduce systemic corticosteroids and maintain control with high-dose inhaled corticosteroids.)
STEP 3: Moderate Persistent		
Day: Every day Night: >1 night/week	PEF/FEV$_1$ >60% - <80% PEF variability >30%	• **Preferred treatment:** **– Low-medium dose inhaled corticosteroid** **AND** **– Long-acting inhaled beta$_2$-agonist** • Alternatives: – Increase inhaled corticosteroids within medium-dose range **OR** – Low-medium dose inhaled corticosteroids and either leukotriene receptor antagonist or theophylline
		If needed (especially with recurring severe exacerbations): • **Preferred treatment:** – Increase inhaled corticosteroids within medium-dose range, and add long-acting inhaled beta$_2$-agonist • Alternatives: – Increase inhaled corticosteroids in medium-dose range, and add either leukotriene receptor antagonist or theophylline

ASTHMA *(Continued)*

Stepwise Approach for Managing Asthma in Children >5 Years of Age, Adolescents, and Adults: Treatment[1]

Symptoms[2]	Lung Function[3]	Long-Term Control (Daily Medications)
STEP 2: Mild Persistent		
Day: >2 days/week but <1 time/day Night: >2 nights/month	PEF/FEV$_1$ ≥80% PEF variability 20%-30%	• **Preferred treatment:** – **Low-dose inhaled corticosteroid** • Alternatives: Cromolyn, leukotriene receptor antagonist, nedocromil, or sustained release theophylline (serum concentration 5-15 mcg/mL)
STEP 1: Mild Intermittent		
Day: ≤2 days/week Night: ≤2 nights/month	PEF/FEV$_1$ ≥80% PEF variability <20%	No daily medication needed. A course of systemic corticosteroids is recommended for severe exacerbations.

[1]Classify severity. The presence of one of the features of severity is sufficient to place a patient in that category. An individual should be assigned to the most severe grade in which any feature occurs. The characteristics noted are general and may overlap because asthma is highly variable. Furthermore, an individual's classification may change over time.

[2]Patients at any level of severity can have mild, moderate, or severe exacerbations. Some patients with intermittent asthma experience severe and life-threatening exacerbations separated by long periods of normal lung function and no symptoms.

[3]PEF is % of personal best and FEV$_1$ is % predicted.

↓ Step down
Review treatment every 1-6 months; a gradual stepwise reduction in treatment may be possible.

↑Step up
If control is not maintained, consider step up. First, review patient medication technique, adherence, and environmental control.

Quick Relief – All Patients

- Short-acting bronchodilator: **Inhaled beta$_2$-agonists** as needed for symptoms.
- Intensity of treatment will depend on severity of exacerbation; see "Management of Asthma Exacerbations".
- Use of short-acting inhaled beta$_2$-agonists on a daily basis, or increasing use, indicates the need to initiate or titrate long-term control therapy.

Notes:

- **The stepwise approach presents general guidelines to assist clinical decision making; it is not intended to be a specific prescription. Asthma is highly variable; clinicians should tailor specific medication plans to the needs and circumstances of individual patients.**
- Gain control as quickly as possible; then decrease treatment to the least medication necessary to maintain control.
- A rescue course of systemic corticosteroids may be needed at any time and at any step.
- Some patients with intermittent asthma experience severe and life-threatening exacerbations separated by long periods of normal lung function and no symptoms. This may be especially common with exacerbations provoked by

respiratory infections. A short course of systemic corticosteroids is recommended.

- At each step, patients should control their environment to avoid or control factors that make their asthma worse.
- Antibiotics are not recommended for treatment of acute asthma exacerbations except where there is evidence or suspicion of bacterial infection.
- Consultation with an asthma specialist is recommended for moderate or severe persistent asthma.
- Peak flow monitoring for patients with moderate-severe asthma should be considered.

ASTHMA *(Continued)*

Management of Asthma Exacerbations: Home Treatment[1]

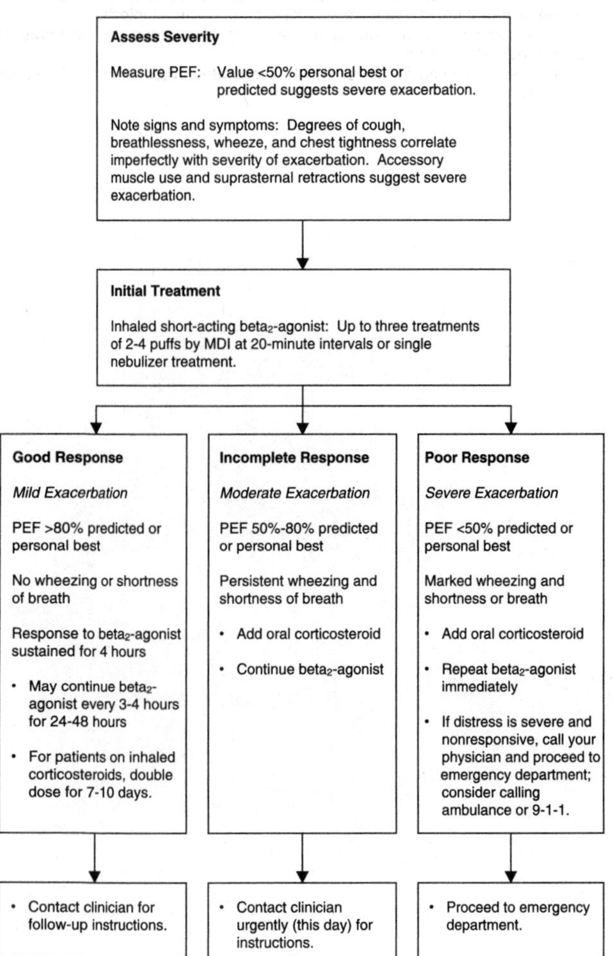

[1]Patients at high risk of asthma-related death should receive immediate clinical attention after initial treatment. Additional therapy may be required.

Management of Asthma Exacerbations: Emergency Department and Hospital-Based Care

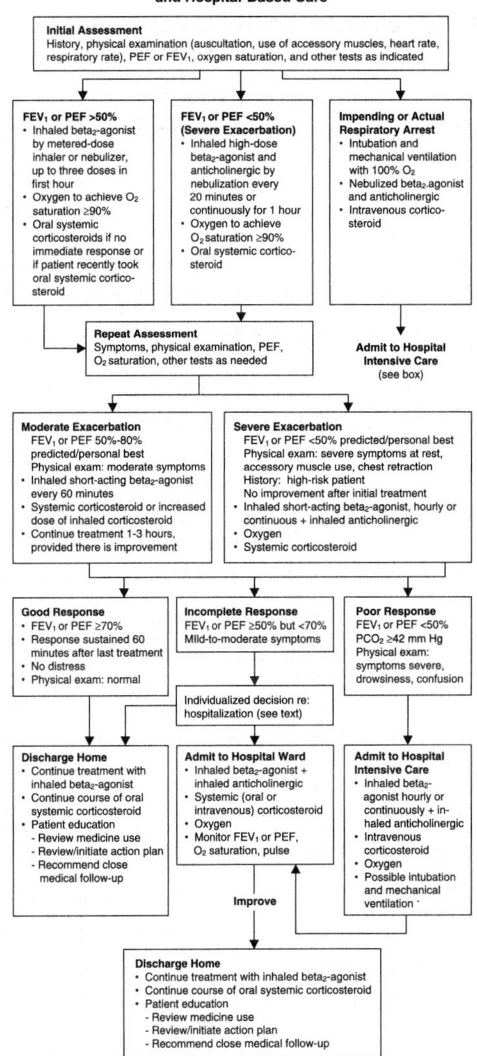

ASTHMA *(Continued)*

ESTIMATED COMPARATIVE DAILY DOSAGES FOR INHALED CORTICOSTEROIDS

Children ≤12 Years

Drug	Low Dose	Medium Dose	High Dose
Beclomethasone dipropionate CFC	84-336 mcg	336-672 mcg	>672 mcg
42 mcg/puff	2-8 puffs	8-16 puffs	>16 puffs
84 mcg/puff	1-4 puffs	4-8 puffs	>8 puffs
Beclomethasone dipropionate HFA	80-160 mcg	160-320 mcg	>320 mcg
40 mcg/puff	2-4 puffs	4-8 puffs	>8 puffs
80 mcg/puff	1-2 puffs	2-4 puffs	>4 puffs
Budesonide DPI	200-400 mcg	400-800 mcg	>800 mcg
200 mcg/inhalation	1-2 inhalations	2-4 inhalations	>4 inhalations
Budesonide inhalation suspension for nebulization	0.5 mg	1 mg	2 mg
Flunisolide	500-750 mcg	1000-1250 mcg	>1250 mcg
250 mcg/puff	2-3 puffs	4-5 puffs	>5 puffs
Fluticasone			
MDI: 44, 110, 220 mcg/puff	88-176 mcg	176-440 mcg	>440 mcg
DPI: 50, 100, 250 mcg/dose	100-200 mcg	200-400 mcg	>400 mcg
Triamcinolone acetonide	400-800 mcg	800-1200 mcg	>1200 mcg
100 mcg/puff	4-8 puffs	8-12 puffs	>12 puffs

Adolescents / Adults

Drug	Low Dose	Medium Dose	High Dose
Beclomethasone dipropionate CFC	168-504 mcg	504-840 mcg	>840 mcg
42 mcg/puff	4-12 puffs	12-20 puffs	>20 puffs
84 mcg/puff	2-6 puffs	6-10 puffs	>10 puffs
Beclomethasone dipropionate HFA	80-240 mcg	240-480 mcg	>480 mcg
40 mcg/puff	2-6 puffs	6-12 puffs	>12 puffs
80 mcg/puff	1-3 puffs	3-6 puffs	>6 puffs
Budesonide DPI	200-600 mcg	600-1200 mcg	>1200 mcg
200 mcg/inhalation	1-3 inhalations	3-6 inhalations	>6 inhalations
Flunisolide	500-1000 mcg	1000-2000 mcg	>2000 mcg
250 mcg/puff	2-4 puffs	4-8 puffs	>8 puffs
Fluticasone			
MDI: 44, 110, 220 mcg/puff	88-264 mcg	264-660 mcg	>660 mcg
DPI: 50, 100, 250 mcg/dose	100-300 mcg	300-600 mcg	>600 mcg
Triamcinolone acetonide	400-1000 mcg	1000-2000 mcg	>2000 mcg
100 mcg/puff	4-10 puffs	10-20 puffs	>20 puffs

Notes:

- **The most important determinant of appropriate dosing is the clinician's judgment of the patient's response to therapy.** The clinician must monitor the patient's response on several clinical parameters and adjust the dose accordingly. The stepwise approach to therapy emphasizes that once control of asthma is achieved, the dose of mediation should be carefully titrated to the minimum dose required to maintain control, thus reducing the potential for adverse effect.
- The reference point for the range in the dosages for children is data on the safety on inhaled corticosteroids in children, which, in general, suggest that the dose ranges are equivalent to beclomethasone dipropionate 200-400 mcg/day (low dose), 400-800 mcg/day (medium dose), and >800 mcg/day (high dose).
- Some dosages may be outside package labeling.
- Metered-dose inhaler (MDI) dosages are expressed as the actuator dose (the amount of drug leaving the actuator and delivered to the patient), which is the labeling required in the United States. This is different from the dosage expressed as the valve dose (the amount of drug leaving the valve, all of which is not available to the patient), which is used in many European countries and in some of the scientific literature. Dry powder inhaler (DPI) doses (eg, Turbuhaler) are expressed as the amount of drug in the inhaler following activation.

ESTIMATED CLINICAL COMPARABILITY OF DOSES FOR INHALED CORTICOSTEROIDS

Data from *in vitro* and in clinical trials suggest that the different inhaled corticosteroid preparations are not equivalent on a per puff or microgram basis. However, it is not entirely clear what implications these differences have for dosing recommendations in clinical practice because there are few data directly comparing the preparations. Relative dosing for clinical comparability is affected by differences in topical potency, clinical effects at different doses, delivery device, and bioavailability. The Expert Panel developed recommended dose ranges for different preparations based on available data and the following assumptions and cautions about estimating relative doses needed to achieve comparable clinical effect.

Relative Topical Potency Using Human Skin Blanching

- The standard test for determining relative topical anti-inflammatory potency is the topical vasoconstriction (MacKenzie skin blanching) test.
- The MacKenzie topical skin blanching test correlates with binding affinities and binding half-lives for human lung corticosteroid receptors (see following table) (Dahlberg, et al, 1984; Hogger and Rohdewald 1994).
- The relationship between relative topical anti-inflammatory effect and clinical comparability in asthma management is not certain. However, recent clinical trials suggest that different *in vitro* measures of anti-inflammatory effect is not certain. However, recent clinical trials suggest that different *in vitro* measures of anti-inflammatory effect correlate with clinical efficacy (Barnes and Pedersen 1993; Johnson 1996; Kamada, et al, 1996; Ebden, et al, 1986; Leblanc, et al, 1994; Gustaffson, et al, 1993; Lundback, et al, 1993; Barnes, et al, 1993; Fabbri, et al, 1993; Langdon and Capsey, 1994; Ayres, et al, 1995; Rafferty, et al, 1985; Bjorkander, et al, 1982, Stiksa, et al, 1982; Willey, et al, 1982.)

ASTHMA *(Continued)*

Medication	Topical Potency (Skin Blanching)[1]	Corticosteroid Receptor Binding Half-Life	Receptor Binding Affinity
Beclomethasone dipropionate (BDP)	600	7.5 hours	13.5
Budesonide (BUD)	980	5.1 hours	9.4
Flunisolide (FLU)	330	3.5 hours	1.8
Fluticasone propionate (FP)	1200	10.5 hours	18.0
Triamcinolone acetonide (TAA)	330	3.9 hours	3.6

[1]Numbers are assigned in reference to dexamethasone, which has a value of "1" in the MacKenzie test.

Relative Doses to Achieve Similar Clinical Effects

- Clinical effects are evaluated by a number of outcome parameters (eg, changes in spirometry, peak flow rates, symptom scores, quick-relief beta$_2$-agonist use, frequency of exacerbations, airway responsiveness).
- The daily dose and duration of treatment may affect these outcome parameters differently (eg, symptoms and peak flow may improve at lower doses and over a shorter treatment time than bronchial reactivity) (van Essen-Zandvliet, et al, 1992; Haahtela, et al, 1991)
- Delivery systems influence comparability. For example, the delivery device for budesonide (Turbuhaler) delivers approximately twice the amount of drug to the airway as the MDI, thus enhancing the clinical effect (Thorsson, et al, 1994; Agertoft and Pedersen, 1993).
- Individual patients may respond differently to different preparations, as noted by clinical experience.
- Clinical trials comparing effects in reducing symptoms and improving peak expiratory flow demonstrate:
  - BDP and BUD achieved comparable effects at similar microgram doses by MDI (Bjorkander, et al, 1982; Ebden, et al, 1986; Rafferty, et al, 1985).
  - BDP achieved effects similar to twice the dose of TAA on a microgram basis.

Reference

National Asthma Education and Prevention Program (NAEPP), Clinical Practice Guidelines, Expert Panel Report 2, "Guidelines for the Diagnosis and Management of Asthma," NIH Publication No. 97-4051, July 1997.

NORMAL RESPIRATORY RATES

Hour After Birth	Average Respiratory Rate	Range
1st hour	60 breaths/minute	20-100
2-6 hours	50 breaths/minute	20-80
>6 hours	30-40 breaths/minute	20-60

Age (years)	Mean RR (breaths/minute)
0-2	25-30
3-9	20-25
10-18	16-20

BLOOD LEVEL SAMPLING TIME GUIDELINES

Drug	Infusion Time	Therapeutic Range	When to Draw Levels
Amikacin sulfate			
I.V.	30 min	Peak: 20-30 mcg/mL	Peak: 30 min after end of 30 min infusion
		Trough: <10 mcg/mL	Trough: Within 30 min before next dose
I.M.			Peak: 1 h after I.M. injection
			Trough: Within 30 min before next dose
Carbamazepine		4-12 mcg/mL	Just before next dose
Chloramphenicol			
I.V.	30 min	Peak: 15-25 mcg/mL	Peak: 90 min after end of 30 min infusion
			Trough: Just before next dose
P.O.			Peak: 2 h post-P.O. dose
Cyclosporine			
I.V./P.O.		BMT 100-200 ng/mL	Just before next dose
		Liver transplant 200-300 ng/mL	
		Renal transplant 100-200 ng/mL	
Digoxin			
I.V./P.O.		Age and disease related: 0.8-2 ng/mL	6 h postdose to just before next dose
Ethosuximide			
P.O.		40-100 mcg/mL	Just before next dose
Flucytosine			
P.O.		25-100 mcg/mL	Peak: 2 h postdose after at least 4 d of therapy
Fosphenytoin (measure phenytoin levels)			
I.V.		Phenytoin: 10-20 mcg/mL	Peak: 2 h after end of an infusion
I.M.			Peak: 4 h after I.M. injection
Gentamicin			
I.V.	30 min	Peak: 4-10 mcg/mL	Peak: 30 min after end of 30 min infusion
		Trough: 0.5-2 mcg/mL	Trough: Within 30 min before next dose
I.M.			Peak: 1 h after I.M. injection
			Trough: Within 30 min before next dose
Phenobarbital		15-40 mcg/mL	Trough: Just before next dose
Phenytoin			
P.O., I.V.		10-20 mcg/mL	Trough: Just before next dose
I.V.			Post-load/Peak: 1 h after end of infusion

Drug	Infusion Time	Therapeutic Range	When to Draw Levels
Theophylline			
I.V. bolus	30 min	10-20 mcg/mL	Peak: 30 min after end of 30 min infusion
Continuous infusion			16-24 h after the start or change in a constant I.V. infusion
P.O. liquid, fast-release tablet (Somophyllin®, Slo-Phyllin® liquid & tablet)			Peak: 1 h postdose Trough: Just before next dose
P.O. slow-release (Theo-Dur®, Slo-Phyllin® GC, Slo-bid®)			Peak: 4 h postdose Trough: Just before next dose
Tobramycin			
I.V.	30 min	Peak: 4-10 mcg/mL	Peak: 30 min after end of 30 min infusion
		Trough: 0.5-2 mcg/mL	Trough: Within 30 min before next dose
I.M.			Peak: 1 h post-I.M. injection
			Trough: Within 30 min before next dose
Trimethoprim			
I.V., dose 20 mg/kg	60 min	Peak: 5-10 mcg/mL	Peak: 30 min after end of 60 min infusion
I.V., dose 8-10 mg/kg		Peak 1-3 mcg/mL	
P.O.			Peak: 1 h postdose
Valproic acid			
P.O.		50-100 mcg/mL	Trough: Just before next dose
Vancomycin	60 min	Peak: 25-40 mcg/mL	Peak: 20-30 min after end of 60 min infusion[1]
		Trough: 5-15 mcg/mL	Trough: Within 30 min before next dose

[1]Some institutions may draw vancomycin peak 1 hour after 1-hour infusion and accept the lower range of therapeutic.

OVERDOSE AND TOXICOLOGY[1]

Drug or Drug Class	Signs / Symptoms	Treatment/Comments
Acetaminophen	Nausea, vomiting, diaphoresis, delirium, fever, coma, vascular collapse, hepatic necrosis, transient azotemia, renal tubular necrosis	Assess severity of ingestion; doses ≥150 mg/kg for children and 7.5 g for adults are thought to be toxic. Obtain serum concentration ≥4 hours postingestion and use acetaminophen nomogram to evaluate need for acetylcysteine. Empty stomach with ipecac (if <1 hour postingestion) or gastric lavage. May administer activated charcoal for one dose, this may decrease absorption of acetylcysteine if given within 1 hour of orally administered acetylcysteine. For unknown ingested quantities and for significant ingestion, give acetylcysteine orally (diluted 1:4 with juice or carbonated beverage); initial: 140 mg/kg then give 70 mg/kg every 4 hours for 17 doses. An I.V. formulation is also available. For I.V. treatment, administer 150 mg/kg (over 15 minutes) followed by 50 mg/kg (over 4 hours), followed by 100 mg/kg (over 16 hours). See acetylcysteine monograph *on page 9999*.
Alpha-adrenergic blocking agents	Hypotension, drowsiness	Induce emesis, give activated charcoal, additional treatment is symptomatic; use I.V. fluids, dopamine, or ephedrine to treat hypotension. Epinephrine may worsen hypotension due to beta effects.
Aminoglycosides	Ototoxicity, nephrotoxicity, neuromuscular toxicity	Hemodialysis or peritoneal dialysis may be useful in patients with decreased renal function.
Anticholinergics, antihistamines	Coma, hallucinations, delirium, tachycardia, dry skin, urinary retention, dilated pupils	For life-threatening arrhythmias or seizures physostigmine may be used.
Anticholinesterase agents	Nausea, vomiting, diarrhea, miosis, CNS depression, excessive salivation, excessive sweating, muscle weakness	Suction oral secretions, decontaminate skin, atropinize patient; atropine dose must be individualized. Infants and children: Initial dose: 0.01-0.02 mg/kg/dose; may need to increase as high as 0.05 mg/kg. Adults: Initial atropine dose: 1 mg; may need to increase to 2-5 mg/dose; pralidoxime (2-PAM) may need to be added for severe intoxications.
Barbiturates	Respiratory depression, circulatory collapse, bradycardia, hypotension, hypothermia, slurred speech, confusion	Repeated oral doses of activated charcoal given every 3-6 hours will increase clearance: Children: 1-2 g/kg/dose; adults: 30-60 g. Assure GI motility, adequate hydration, and renal function. Urinary alkalinization with I.V. sodium bicarbonate will increase renal elimination of longer-acting barbiturates (eg, phenobarbital).

Drug or Drug Class	Signs / Symptoms	Treatment/Comments
Benzodiazepines	Respiratory depression, apnea, hypoactive reflexes, hypotension, slurred speech, unsteady gait, coma	For comatose patient, use gastric lavage with endotracheal tube in place to prevent aspiration; flumazenil, a benzodiazepine antagonist, can be used to reverse the effects of benzodiazepines. See Flumazenil monograph *on page 9999* for dose. Action of flumazenil may be shorter than duration of benzodiazepine; repeat doses as needed. Norepinephrine, phenylephrine, or dopamine may be used to treat hypotension; dialysis is of limited value; support blood pressure and respiration.
Beta-adrenergic blockers	Hypotension, bronchospasm, bradycardia, hyperglycemia, or hypoglycemia	Induce emesis, followed by activated charcoal; treat symptomatically; glucagon, atropine, isoproterenol, or cardiac pacing may be needed to treat bradycardia, conduction defects, or hypotension
Carbamazepine	Dizziness, drowsiness, ataxia, involuntary movements, opisthotonos, seizures, nausea, vomiting, agitation, nystagmus, coma, urinary retention, respiratory depression, tachycardia	Use supportive therapy, general poisoning management as needed; use repeated oral doses of activated charcoal given every 3-6 hours to decrease serum concentrations; children 1-2 g/kg/dose, adults: 30-60 g/dose; charcoal hemoperfusion may be needed; treat hypotension with I.V. fluids, dopamine, or norepinephrine; monitor EKG; diazepam may control convulsions but may exacerbate respiratory depression
Cardiac glycosides	Hyperkalemia may develop rapidly and result in life-threatening cardiac arrhythmias, progressive bradyarrhythmias, 2nd or 3rd degree heart block unresponsive to atropine, ventricular fibrillation, asystole	Obtain serum drug level, induce emesis or perform gastric lavage; give activated charcoal to reduce further absorption; atropine may reverse heart block, phenytoin will improve A-V conduction; digoxin immune Fab (digoxin specific antibody fragments) is used in life-threatening cases, each 38 mg of digoxin immune Fab binds with 0.5 mg of digoxin or digitoxin; see Digoxin Immune Fab monograph *on page 9999* for dosing recommendations
Heparin	Severe hemorrhage	1 mg of protamine sulfate will neutralize approximately 90 units of heparin sodium (bovine) or 115 units of heparin sodium (porcine) or 100 units of heparin calcium (porcine)
Hydantoin derivatives	Nausea, vomiting, nystagmus, slurred speech, ataxia, coma	Gastric lavage or emesis; repeated oral doses of activated charcoal may increase clearance of phenytoin. Children: 1-2 g/kg/dose, adults: 30-60 g/dose activated charcoal every 3-6 hours until nontoxic serum concentration is obtained; assure adequate GI motility, supportive therapy; dialysis may be helpful.

OVERDOSE AND TOXICOLOGY[1] *(Continued)*

Drug or Drug Class	Signs / Symptoms	Treatment/Comments
Iron	Lethargy, nausea, vomiting, green or tarry stools, hypotension, weak rapid pulse, metabolic acidosis, shock, coma, hepatic necrosis, renal failure, local GI erosions	Induce emesis if awake or lavage with saline solution; give deferoxamine mesylate I.V. at 15 mg/kg/hour in cases of severe poisoning (serum Fe >350 mcg/mL) and continue chelation therapy for 24 hours after child is excreting normal color urine; urine output should be maintained at >2 mL/kg/hour to avoid hypovolemic shock
Isoniazid	Nausea, vomiting, blurred vision, CNS depression, intractable seizures, coma, metabolic acidosis	Control seizures with diazepam; if suspected ingestion of >80 mg/kg, give pyridoxine I.V. equal dose to the suspected overdose of isoniazid; lavage after seizure control is reached; force diuresis with I.V. fluids; hemo- or peritoneal dialysis may be beneficial in severe cases
Nonsteroidal anti-inflammatory drugs	Dizziness, abdominal pain, sweating, apnea, nystagmus, cyanosis, hypotension, coma	Induce emesis; give activated charcoal via NG tube; provide symptomatic and supportive care.
Opiates and morphine analogs	Respiratory depression, miosis, hypothermia, bradycardia, circulatory collapse, pulmonary edema, apnea	Establish airway and adequate ventilation; give naloxone 0.1 mg/kg for children up to 5 years of age or 20 kg; for those >5 years or 20 kg give 2 mg naloxone; repeat doses every 2-3 minutes if needed; additional doses may be needed every 20-60 minutes. May need to institute continuous infusion, as duration of action of opiates can be longer than duration of action of naloxone.
Phenothiazines	Deep, unarousable sleep, anticholinergic symptoms, extrapyramidal signs, diaphoresis, rigidity, tachycardia, cardiac dysrhythmias, hypotension, or hypertension	Emesis or gastric lavage; do **not** dialyze; use I.V. benztropine mesylate 0.02-0.05 mg/kg/dose or for adults 1-2 mg/dose slowly over 3-6 minutes for extrapyramidal signs; use loading dose of phenytoin 10-15 mg/kg slow I.V. push for ventricular dysrhythmias; use I.V. fluids and norepinephrine or phenylephrine to treat hypotension; avoid epinephrine which may cause hypotension due to phenothiazine-induced alpha-adrenergic blockade and unopposed epinephrine B_2 action; dantrolene orally 0.5 mg/kg/dose every 12 hours may help with the rigidity

Drug or Drug Class	Signs / Symptoms	Treatment/Comments
Salicylates	Nausea, vomiting, respiratory alkalosis, hyperthermia, dehydration, hyperapnea, tinnitus, headache, dizziness, metabolic acidosis, coma	Induce emesis or gastric lavage immediately; give charcoal with cathartic via NG tube; correct fluid imbalance by giving D_5LR at 10-20 mL/kg/hour for 1-2 hours, more rapid fluid resuscitation may be needed for patients in shock; use sodium bicarbonate to correct metabolic acidosis and enhance renal elimination by alkalinizing the urine; give supplemental potassium after renal function has been determined to be adequate. Monitor electrolytes; obtain serum salicylate level ≥6 hours postingestion; use poisoning nomogram to assess the significance of the ingestion and the need for more aggressive measures.
Tricyclic antidepressants	Agitation, confusion, hallucinations, urinary retention, hypothermia, hypotension, tachycardia, arrhythmias, widened QRS complex, prolonged PR intervals	Maintain normal temperature; correct acidosis with sodium bicarbonate to increase protein binding and decrease free fraction; correction of acidosis may decrease cardiovascular toxicities; avoid disopyramide, procainamide, and quinidine; lidocaine, phenytoin or propranolol may be necessary; reserve physostigmine for refractory life-treating anticholinergic toxicities. For life-threatening arrhythmias or seizures: Children: I.V., slow: Physostigmine 0.01-0.03 mg/kg/dose up to 0.5 mg/dose over 2-3 minutes, repeat in 5 minutes (maximum total dose is 2 mg). Adolescents and adults: 2 mg/dose physostigmine, may repeat 1-2 mg in 20 minutes and give 1-4 mg slow I.V. over 5-10 minutes if signs and symptoms recur.
Warfarin	Internal or external hemorrhage, hematuria	For moderate overdoses, give oral or I.V. phytonadione; for severe hemorrhage, give fresh frozen plasma or whole blood
Xanthine derivatives	Vomiting, abdominal pain, bloody diarrhea, tachycardia, extrasystoles, tachypnea, tonic/clonic seizures	Induce emesis, except in a convulsive patient; give activated charcoal orally; repeated oral doses of activated charcoal may increase clearance; children: 1-2 g/kg/dose, adults: 30-60 g/dose of activated charcoal every 3-6 hours until nontoxic serum concentrations are obtained. Assure adequate GI motility, supportive therapy; charcoal hemoperfusion can also be effective in decreasing serum concentrations.

[1]As for all overdoses and toxic ingestions, provide airway, breathing, and cardiac support; use appropriate general poisoning management and give general supportive therapy when needed (eg, I.V. fluids, blood pressure support, control seizures, etc). Consult more specific toxicology references (eg, Leikin JB and Paloucek FP, *Poisoning & Toxicology Handbook*, Hudson, OH: Lexi-Comp Inc, 1998, and Poisondex®) for further information.

COMMONLY USED ANTIDOTES FOR ACUTE OVERDOSES

While certain drugs may modify symptoms produced by a toxin, only a relatively few toxins have specific antidotes. The purpose of this chart is to identify those drugs, non-medicinal chemicals, plants, snakes, and spiders to which specific antidotes exist. Please refer to the specific monograph for dosing information. This information does not preclude the use of "conventional" therapeutic modalities for the treatment of intoxication (eg, emesis, lavage, charcoal, etc).

Poisoning Agent	Antidote(s)	Indications	Comments
Chemicals, Nonmedicinal			
Arsenic	Dimercaprol (BAL in Oil®)	• Symptomatic arsenic exposure	• Monitor for hypertension, tachycardia, hyperpyrexia, and urticaria • Pretreatment with diphenhydramine may diminish side effects
Calcium oxide	Edetate calcium disodium (EDTA) (Calcium Disodium Versenate®)	• Eye exposure from calcium oxide	• Immediate irrigation with saline followed by an irrigation with 0.01-0.05 M EDTA solution for at least 15 minutes
Carbon monoxide	Oxygen	• Any suspected carbon monoxide intoxication • Hyperbaric oxygen for any patient with signs and symptoms of severe intoxication regardless of the carboxyhemoglobin concentration • Patients with ischemic heart disease, acute ECG changes, anemia, seizure history, or pregnancy should receive hyperbaric oxygen if the carboxy hemoglobin (COHB) >20% or if any acute symptoms are present	
Carbamate insecticides	Atropine	• Symptomatic bradycardia • Myoclonic seizures, severe hallucinations, weakness, arrhythmias, excessive salivation, involuntary urination and defecation	• Caution should be used in patients with narrow-angle glaucoma, cardiovascular disease, or pregnancy • Plasma and/or erythrocyte cholinesterase levels will be depressed from normal
Copper	Penicillamine (Cuprimine®, Depen®)	• Symptomatic copper intoxication	• Little experience with chelation therapy in the setting of acute ingestion

Poisoning Agent	Antidote(s)	Indications	Comments
Cyanide	Amyl nitrite, sodium nitrite, sodium thiosulfate (cyanide antidote kit)	• Begin treatment at the first sign of toxicity if exposure is known or strongly expected	• Do not use methylene blue to reduce elevated methemoglobin levels • Oxygen therapy may be useful when combined with sodium thiosulfate therapy
Ethylene glycol	Ethanol **OR** Fomepizole (Antizol®)	• Ingestion of >0.25 mL/kg ethylene glycol • Ethylene glycol serum level >20 mg/dL • History or strong clinical suspicion of ingestion and at least two of the following criteria: Arterial pH <7.3 Serum bicarbonate <20 mEq/L Osmolality gap >10 mOsm/L Urinary oxalate crystals present	• Goal: Blood ethanol concentration at least 100 mg/dL (22 mmol/L) • Indications for use of fomepizole over ethanol: Ingestion of multiple substances resulting in depressed level of consciousness, altered consciousness, lack of adequate intensive care staffing or laboratory support to monitor ethanol, critically-ill patient with anion gap metabolic acidosis of unknown origin and potential exposure to ethylene glycol, or patients with active hepatic disease • Continue therapy until ethylene glycol level <10 mg/dL • Monitor blood glucose especially in children as ethanol may cause hypoglycemia
Hydrazine	Pyridoxine (vitamin B_6)	• Antidote for seizures and coma	
Hydrofluoric acid (HF)	Calcium gluconate	• Dermal burns (topical treatment with calcium gluconate gel for dermal exposures of HF <20% concentration) •SubQ injections of calcium gluconate for dermal exposures of HF >20% concentration or failure to respond to calcium gluconate gel	• Oral calcium also used as fluoride-binding agent following oral ingestion • Hypocalcemia occurs frequently following oral ingestion and dermal exposure • Topical calcium gels are not available commercially in U.S.; may be compounded; see Extemporaneous Preparations, Calcium Supplements *on page 9999* •Injections of calcium gluconate should not be used in digital area
Hydrogen sulfide	Amyl nitrite **AND** Sodium nitrite	• Severe anoxia, if therapy can be started early – within one hour of exposure	• Do **NOT** use sodium thiosulfate

COMMONLY USED ANTIDOTES FOR ACUTE OVERDOSES *(Continued)*

Poisoning Agent	Antidote(s)	Indications	Comments
Lead	Edetate calcium disodium (EDTA) (Calcium Disodium Versenate®) **with or without** Dimercaprol (BAL in Oil®)	Use both calcium EDTA and BAL: • Symptoms of lead encephalopathy and/or blood lead level >70 mcg/dL • Symptomatic without encephalopathy or asymptomatic with blood lead level >70 mcg/dL Use only EDTA for: • Asymptomatic with blood lead level 45-69 mcg/dL	• Do not confuse or interchange therapy of **calcium** disodium edetate with disodium edetate (Chealamide®, Disotate®, Endrate®) – tetany and possibly fatal hypocalcemia may occur • Calcium EDTA should only be administered after adequate urine flow is established • If urine flow is not established, hemodialysis must accompany calcium EDTA dosing
	Succimer (Chemet®)	• Lead level >45 mcg/dL in patients without encephalopathy or protracted vomiting	• Do not use with calcium disodium edetate or BAL
Manganese	Edetate calcium disodium (EDTA) (Calcium Disodium Versenate®)		• Do not confuse or interchange therapy of **calcium** disodium edetate with disodium edetate (Chealamide®, Disotate®, Endrate®) – tetany and possibly fatal hypocalcemia may occur • Calcium EDTA should only be administered after adequate urine flow is established
Methanol	Ethanol **OR** Fomepizole (Antizol®)	• Anion gap metabolic acidosis associated with a history of methanol ingestion • Methanol blood level >20 mg/dL (6.2 mmoles/L) • Any symptomatic patient with a history of methanol ingestion	• Goal: Ethanol blood level 100-130 mg/dL (22-28 mmoles/L) • Continue therapy until methanol blood level <10 mg/dL • Fomepizole therapy is considered investigational
Organophosphate insecticides	Atropine Pralidoxime (2-PAM, Protopam®)	• Symptomatic bradycardia • Myoclonic seizures, severe hallucinations, weakness, arrhythmias, excessive salivation, involuntary urination and defecation	• Caution should be used in patients with narrow-angle glaucoma, cardiovascular disease, or pregnancy •Most effective when used in initial 24-36 hours after exposure • Plasma and/or erythrocyte cholinesterase levels will be depressed from normal

Poisoning Agent	Antidote(s)	Indications	Comments
Drug / Drug Class			
Acetaminophen	Acetylcysteine (Mucomyst®)	• Serum acetaminophen level >150 mcg/mL at 4 hours postingestion (see Acetaminophen *on page 9999*) • Acute ingestion with dose ≥150 mg/kg (child) or 7.5 g (adolescent/ adult) within 24 hours of presentation if results of plasma levels cannot be obtained within 8-10 hours of ingestion • Unknown quantity ingested and <24 hours have elapsed since the time of ingestion or unable to obtain serum acetaminophen levels within 12 hours of ingestion • Consider repeating an acetaminophen level 4-6 hours after an initial 4-hour level that is under the treatment range if extended release acetaminophen was ingested • Patients presenting >24 hours postacute ingestion who have measurable levels or biochemical evidence of hepatic injury	• Activated charcoal has been shown to adsorb acetylcysteine; therefore, administer activated charcoal before 4-hour acetaminophen level is drawn • If patient vomits within 1 hour of an oral acetylcysteine dose, readminister the dose • I.V. N-acetylcysteine is now available in the U.S. (see acetylcysteine monograph *on page 9999*).
Anticholinergics	Physostigmine (Antilirium®)	• Refractory seizures or arrhythmias unresponsive to conventional therapy • Symptoms should be life-threatening	• Due to potential for producing severe adverse effects, (eg, seizures, bradycardia) routine use of physostigmine is controversial • Atropine should be available to reverse life-threatening cholinergic effects of physostigmine
Baclofen	Physostigmine (Antilirium®)	• Distinguish anticholinergic delirium from other causes of altered mental status	• Long-lasting reversal of anticholinergic signs and symptoms is generally not achieved due to the relatively short duration of action of physostigmine • Atropine should be available to reverse life-threatening cholinergic effects of physostigmine

COMMONLY USED ANTIDOTES FOR ACUTE OVERDOSES *(Continued)*

Poisoning Agent	Antidote(s)	Indications	Comments
Benzodiazepines	Flumazenil (Romazicon®)	• Reverses sedative effects of benzodiazepines	• May precipitate benzodiazepine withdrawal in dependent patients • Not indicated for ethanol, barbiturate, general anesthetic, or narcotic overdose • Mixed drug overdose patients who have ingested drugs that increase the likelihood of seizures (eg, cocaine, lithium, cyclic antidepressants) are at extremely high risk for seizures when flumazenil is used • Action of flumazenil may be shorter than duration of benzodiazepines; repeat doses of flumazenil may be needed • Contraindicated in patients given benzodiazepines for potentially life-threatening conditions (eg, increased intracranial pressure, seizures) and patients with signs of serious cyclic-antidepressant overdosage
Beta-blockers	Isoproterenol (Isuprel®)	• Reversal of bradycardia and hypotension	
	Glucagon	• Reversal of bradycardia unresponsive to isoproterenol	• Glucagon activates adenyl cyclase system at a different site than isoproterenol • Requires liver glycogen stores for hyperglycemic response • I.V. glucose must also be given in treatment of hypoglycemia
Calcium channel blockers	Calcium chloride **OR** Calcium gluconate	• Reversal of cardiovascular effects of calcium channel blockers (calcium antagonists)	• Monitor serum calcium levels • Calcium is most effective in mild to moderate intoxications • May not be effective in correcting symptomatic bradyarrhythmias

Poisoning Agent	Antidote(s)	Indications	Comments
Digitalis glycosides	Digoxin immune Fab (Digibind®)	• Treatment of potentially life-threatening digoxin or digitoxin intoxication in carefully selected patients [serum digoxin level >10 ng/mL or ingestion of >4 mg (child) or >10 mg (adult)] • Life-threatening ventricular arrhythmias secondary to digoxin or digitoxin • Hyperkalemia (K^+ >5 mEq/L) in the setting of digitalis toxicity • Life-threatening cardiac arrhythmias, progressive bradyarrhythmias, second or third degree heart block unresponsive to atropine	• Monitor potassium levels and continuous EKG • Digibind® interferes with the interpretation of serum digoxin/digitoxin levels
Heparin, Enoxaparin, Dalteparin	Protamine	• Severe hemorrhage	• Effect can be immediate and last for 2 hours • Protamine dosage related to anticoagulant dosage and time of anticoagulant administration • Monitor PTT • Monitor for hypotension
Insulin	Dextrose (25%-50%)	• Severe, symptomatic hypoglycemia	• Very hypertonic solutions; dilute with sterile water prior to I.V. administration
Iron	Deferoxamine (Desferal®)	• Serum iron level >350 mcg/mL • Inability to obtain serum iron level within a reasonable time and patient is symptomatic	• Passing of vin rose colored urine indicates free iron was present • Discontinue therapy when urine returns to normal color • Monitor for hypotension during treatment
Isoniazid	Pyridoxine (vitamin B_6)	• Ingestion of >80 mg/kg isoniazid	
Neuromuscular blocking agents, nondepolarizing (eg, pancuronium)	Edrophonium **OR** Neostigmine **OR** Pyridostigmine	• Reversal of neuromuscular blockade	• Atropine should be available to treat acute cholinergic crisis • Not effective for reversal of **depolarizing** neuromuscular blocking agents (eg, succinylcholine)

COMMONLY USED ANTIDOTES FOR ACUTE OVERDOSES *(Continued)*

Poisoning Agent	Antidote(s)	Indications	Comments
Opiates	Naloxone (Narcan®)	• Reversal of symptoms associated with severe toxicity	• May precipitate withdrawal symptoms in patients with physical dependence to opiates • For prolonged intoxication, a continuous infusion may be used
Phenothiazines	Diphenhydramine (Benadryl®) **OR** Benztropine (Cogentin®)	• Reversal of phenothiazine-induced dystonic reactions	
	Sodium bicarbonate	• Reversal of "quinidine-like" cardiovascular effects (eg, prolonged QRS complex) – QRS duration >100 msec – Ventricular dysrhythmias and hypotension	• Goal is arterial pH of 7.45-7.55 and urine pH of 7.5-8 • Attempts at urine alkalinization may be dangerous in patients with renal dysfunction or where sodium and fluid overload may compromise respiratory or cardiac status
Tricyclic antidepressants	Sodium bicarbonate	• Reversal of "quinidine-like" cardiovascular effects (eg, prolonged QRS complex) – QRS duration >100 msec – Ventricular dysrhythmias and hypotension	• Goal is arterial pH of 7.45-7.55 and urine pH of 7.5-8 • Attempts at urine alkalinization may be dangerous in patients with renal dysfunction or where sodium and fluid overload may compromise respiratory or cardiac status
Warfarin	Phytonadione (vitamin K_1)	• Large, acute ingestion • Prothrombin time greater than normal	• Vitamin K is relatively contraindicated in patients with prosthetic heart valves unless toxicity is life-threatening
Zinc	Edetate calcium disodium (EDTA) **and/or** Dimercaprol (BAL in Oil®)	• Symptomatic zinc ingestion	• Few case reports • Monitor zinc levels
Plants			
Foxglove Oleander	Digoxin immune Fab (Digibind®)	• Severely intoxicated patients who fail to respond to conventional therapy • Life-threatening ventricular arrhythmias, progressive bradyarrhythmias, or second- or third degree heart block not responsive to atropine • Hyperkalemia (K^+ >5 mEq/L) in the setting of digitalis toxicity	• Monitor potassium levels and continuous EKG
Mushroom (genus *Gyomitra*)	Pyridoxine (vitamin B_6)		

Poisoning Agent	Antidote(s)	Indications	Comments
Mushrooms containing muscarine (inocybe or clitocybe)	Atropine	•Myoclonic seizures, severe hallucinations, weakness, arrhythmias, excessive salivation, involuntary urination and defecation	•Atropine should only be used when indicated; otherwise use may result in anticholinergic poisoning
Snake Bites			
Coral snakes (Eastern and Texas coral snakes only)	Antivenin *(Micrurus fulvius)*		• Not effective for Arizona or Sonoran coral snakes • Skin testing is recommended • Treatment for hypersensitivity reactions, including anaphylaxis, should be available
Pit vipers (Rattlesnakes, cottonmouths, copperheads)	Antivenin *(Crotalidae)* Polyvalent (equine origin)	• Administration within 4 hours of envenomation is ideal; however, administer within 30 hours in all severe cases of poisoning	• Skin testing is recommended • Treatment for hypersensitivity reactions, including anaphylaxis, should be available
Spiders, Scorpions			
Black widow spider	Antivenin *(Lactrodectus mactans)*	• Severe symptoms including respiratory failure, seizures, or pain and spasms not relieved by calcium, muscle relaxants, or analgesics • Symptomatic pregnant patients • Children <5 years or adults >60 years (at greatest risk for severe toxicity)	• Either dermal or conjunctival sensitivity testing should be done prior to administration of antivenin
Scorpion	Antivenin *(Centruroides)*		• No FDA-approved *Centruroides* antivenin in U.S.; only a *Centruroides exilicauda (sculpturatus)*-specific antivenin is available in Arizona (for intrastate use only)

Leikin JR and Paloucek FP, "Poisoning & Toxicology Compendium," Hudson, OH: Lexi-Comp, Inc, 1998.

Mowry JB, Furbee RB, and Chyka PA, "Poisoning," *Essentials of Critical Care Pharmacology,* 3rd ed, Baltimore, MD: Williams & Wilkens, 1994, 501-29.

Zed PJ and Krenzelok EP, "Treatment of Acetaminophen Overdose,"*Am J Health Syst Pharm,* 1999, 56(11):1081-91.

ANION GAP

Definition: The difference in concentration between unmeasured cation and anion equivalents in serum.

Anion gap = $Na^+ - Cl^- - HCO_3^-$
(The normal anion gap is 10-14 mEq/L.)

Differential diagnosis of increased anion gap

- Organic anions
  - Lactate (sepsis, hypovolemia, large tumor burden)
  - Pyruvate
  - Uremia
  - Ketoacidosis (β-hydroxybutyrate and acetoacetate)
  - Amino acids and their metabolites
  - Other organic acids (eg, formate from methanol, glycolate from ethylene glycol)
- Inorganic anions
  - Hyperphosphatemia
  - Sulfates
  - Nitrates
- Medications and toxins
  - Penicillins and cephalosporins
  - Salicylates (including aspirin)
  - Cyanide
  - Carbon monoxide

Differential diagnosis of decreased anion gap

- Organic cations
  - Hypergammaglobulinemia
- Inorganic cations
  - Hyperkalemia
  - Hypercalcemia
  - Hypermagnesemia
- Medications and toxins
  - Lithium
- Hypoalbuminemia

LABORATORY DETECTION OF DRUGS IN URINE

Agent	Time Detectable in Urine[1]
Alcohol	12-24 h
Amobarbital	2-4 d
Amphetamine	2-4 d
Butalbital	2-4 d
Cannabinoids	
Occasional use	2-7 d
Regular use	30 d
Cocaine (benzoylecgonine)	12-72 h
Codeine	2-4 d
Chlordiazepoxide	30 d
Diazepam	30 d
Ethanol	12-24 h
Heroin (morphine)	2-4 d
Hydromorphone	2-4 d
Marijuana	
Occasional use	2-7 d
Regular use	30 d
Methamphetamine	2-4 d
Methaqualone	2-4 d
Morphine	2-4 d
Pentobarbital	2-4 d
Phencyclidine (PCP)	
Occasional use	2-7 d
Regular use	30 d
Phenobarbital	30 d
Secobarbital	2-4 d

[1]The periods of detection for the various abused drugs listed above should be taken as estimates since the actual figures will vary due to metabolism, user, laboratory, and excretion.

Adapted from Chang JY, "Drug Testing and Interpretation of Results," *Pharmchem Newsletter*, 1989, 17:1.

OSMOLALITY

Definition: The summed concentrations of all osmotically active solute particles.

Predicted serum osmolality =

2 Na^+ (mEq/L) + glucose (mg/dL) / 18 + BUN (mg/dL) / 2.8

The normal range of serum osmolality is 285-295 mOsm/L.

Differential diagnosis of increased serum osmolal gap (increased by >10 mOsm/L)

Medications and toxins

- Alcohols (ethanol, methanol, isopropanol, glycerol, ethylene glycol)
- Mannitol
- Paraldehyde

SALICYLATE INTOXICATION

Serum Salicylate Level and Severity of Intoxication Single Dose Acute Ingestion Nomogram

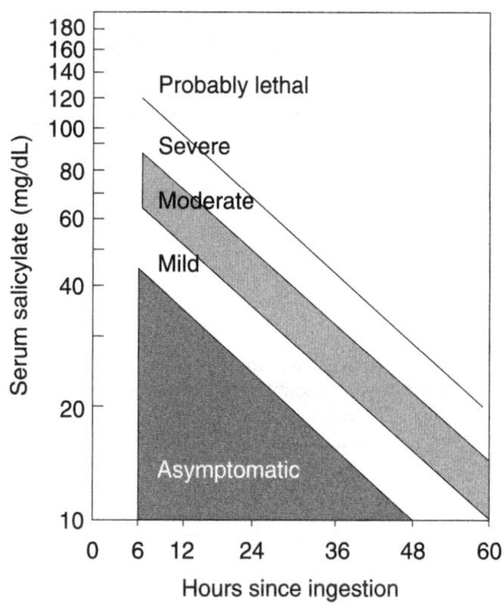

Nomogram relating serum salicylate concentration and expected severity of intoxication at varying intervals following the ingestion of a single dose of salicylate.
From Done AK, "Aspirin Overdosage: Incidence, Diagnosis, and Management," *Pediatrics*, 1978, 62:890-7 with permission.

ACETAMINOPHEN

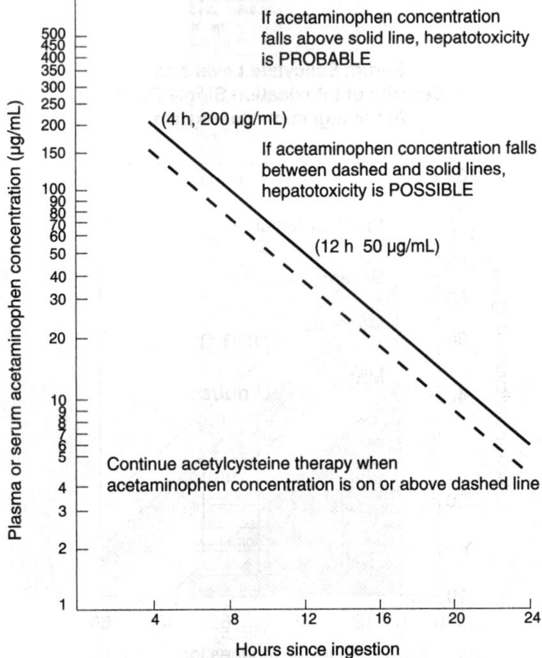

Nomogram relating plasma or serum acetaminophen concentration and probability of hepatotoxicity at varying intervals following ingestion of a single toxic dose of acetaminophen. Modified from Rumack BH, Matthew H, "Acetaminophen Poisoning and Toxicity", Pediatrics, 1975, 55:871-6,
© American Academy of Pediatrics, 1975, and from Rumack BH, et al, "Acetaminophen Overdose", *Arch Intern Med*, 1981, 141:380-5,
© American Medical Association.

MEDICATIONS FOR WHICH A SINGLE DOSE MAY BE FATAL WHEN INGESTED BY A TODDLER

Medication[1]	Minimal Potential Fatal Dose (mg/kg)	Maximal Dose Unit Available (mg)
Antiarrhythmics		
Disopyramide	15	150
Flecainide	25	150
Procainamide	70	1000
Quinidine	15	324
Antimalarials		
Chloroquine	20	500
Hydroxychloroquine	20	200
Quinine	80	650
Antipsychotics		
Chlorpromazine	25	200
Loxapine	30-70	50
Thioridazine	15	200
Calcium channel blockers		
Diltiazem	15	360
Nifedipine	15	90
Verapamil	15	360
Camphor	100	1 g/5 mL
Methyl salicylate	200	1.4 g/mL
Narcotics		
Codeine	7-14	60
Hydrocodone	1.5	60 mg/5 mL
Methadone	1-2	40
Morphine		200
Oral hypoglycemics		
Chlorpropamide	5	25
Glibenclamide	0.1	2.5
Glipizide	0.1	5
Podophyllin 25%	15-20	1.25 g/5 mL
Theophylline	8.4	500
Tricyclic antidepressants		
Amitriptyline	15	100
Desipramine	15	150
Imipramine	15	75

[1]Assumptions: Toddler would weigh 10 kg; the lowest described or estimated fatal dose (adjusted for body weight) was used; the toddler is healthy, with normal drug metabolism.

Adapted from Bar-Oz B, Levichek Z, and Koren G, "Medications That Can Be Fatal for a Toddler With One Tablet or Teaspoonful: A 2004 Update," *Paediatr Drugs*, 2004, 6(2):123-6.

BREAST-FEEDING AND DRUGS

Prior to recommending or prescribing medications to a lactating woman, the following should be considered:

- Is drug therapy necessary?
- Can drug exposure to the infant be minimized? (Using a different route of administration, timing of the dose in relation to breast-feeding, length of therapy, using breast milk stored prior to treatment, etc)
- The infants age and health status (their own ability to metabolize the medication)
- The pharmacokinetics of the drug
- Will the drug interact with a medication the infant is prescribed?
- If medications must be used, pick the safest drug possible.
- In situations where the only drug available may have adverse effects in the nursing infant, consider measuring the infants blood levels.

The tables presented below have been adapted from the American Academy of Pediatrics Committee on Drugs report "Transfer of Drugs and Other Chemicals Into Human Milk," September 2001. It should not be inferred that if a medication is not in the tables it is considered safe for administration to a lactating woman; only that published reports concerning their use were not available at the time the report was published.

Table 1. Cytotoxic Drugs

Cyclophosphamide	Doxorubicin
Cyclosporine	Methotrexate

These are medications thought to interfere with cellular metabolism in the nursing infant. Immune suppression may be possible; effects on growth or carcinogenesis are not known. In addition, doxorubicin is concentrated in human milk; methotrexate is associated with neutropenia in the nursing infant.

Table 2. Drugs of Abuse

Amphetamine	Marijuana
Cocaine	Phencyclidine
Heroin	

Drugs of abuse are not only dangerous to the nursing infant, but also to the mother. Women should be encouraged to avoid their use completely. Effects to the infant reported with amphetamine use in the mother include irritability and poor sleeping; it is also a substance that is concentrated in human milk. Cocaine may cause irritability, vomiting, diarrhea, tremors, or seizures in the infant. Heroin may also cause tremors as well as restlessness, vomiting, and poor feeding.

Nicotine, which was previously on this list, is associated with decreased milk production, decreased weight gain in the infant, and possible increased respiratory illness in the infant. Although there are still questions outstanding regarding smoking and breast-feeding, women should be counseled on the possible effects to their infants and offered aid to smoking cessation if appropriate.

Table 3. Radioactive Compounds That Require Temporary Cessation of Breast-Feeding

Drug	Recommended Time for Cessation of Breast-Feeding
Copper 64 (^{64}Cu)	Radioactivity in milk present at 50 h
Gallium 67 (^{67}Ga)	Radioactivity in milk present for 2 wk
Indium 111 (^{111}In)	Very small amount present at 20 h
Iodine 123 (^{123}I)	Radioactivity in milk present up to 36 h
Iodine 125 (^{125}I)	Radioactivity in milk present for 12 d
Iodine 131 (^{131}I)	Radioactivity in milk present 2-14 d, depending on study
Iodine^{131}	If used for thyroid cancer, high radioactivity may prolong exposure to infant
Radioactive sodium	Radioactivity in milk present 96 h
Technetium-99m (^{99m}Tc), ^{99m}Tc macroaggregates, ^{99m}Tc O4	Radioactivity in milk present 15 h to 3 d

Consider pumping and storing milk prior to study for use during the radioactive period. Pumping should continue after the study to maintain milk production; however, this milk should be discarded until radioactivity is gone. Notify nuclear medicine physician prior to study that the mother is breast-feeding; a short-acting radionuclide may be appropriate. Contact Radiology Department after testing is complete to screen milk samples before resuming feeding.

Table 4a. Psychotropic Drugs Whose Effect on Nursing Infants Is Unknown But May Be of Concern

Antianxiety	Antidepressant	Antipsychotic
Alprazolam	Amitriptyline	Chlorpromazine
Diazepam	Amoxapine	Chlorprothixene
Lorazepam	Bupropion	Clozapine[1]
Midazolam	Clomipramine	Haloperidol
Perphenazine	Desipramine	Mesoridazine
Prazepam[1]	Dothiepin	Trifluoperazine
Quazepam	Doxepin	
Temazepam	Fluoxetine	
	Fluvoxamine	
	Imipramine	
	Nortriptyline	
	Paroxetine	
	Sertraline[1]	
	Trazodone	

[1]Drug is concentrated in human milk.

Psychotropic medications usually appear in the breast milk in low concentrations. Although adverse effects in the infant may be limited to a few case reports, the long half-life of these medications and their metabolites should be considered. In addition, measurable amounts may be found in the infants plasma and also brain tissue. Long-term effects are not known. Colic, irritability, feeding and sleep disorders, and slow weight gain are effects reported with fluoxetine. Chlorpromazine may cause galactorrhea in the mother, while drowsiness and lethargy have been reported in the nursing infant. A decline in developmental scores has been reported with chlorpromazine and haloperidol.

BREAST-FEEDING AND DRUGS *(Continued)*

Table 4b. Additional Drugs Whose Effect on Nursing Infants Is Unknown But May Be of Concern

Drug	Reported Effect in Nursing Infant
Amiodarone	Hypothyroidism
Chloramphenicol	Idiosyncratic bone marrow suppression
Clofazimine	Increase in skin pigmentation; high transfer of mothers dose to infant is possible
Lamotrigine	Therapeutic serum concentrations in infant
Metoclopramide[1]	
Metronidazole	
Tinidazole	

[1]Drug is concentrated in human milk.

No adverse effects to the infant have been reported for metoclopramide; however, it should be recognized that it is a dopaminergic agent. Metronidazole and tinidazole are *in vitro* mutagenic agents. In cases where single dose therapy is appropriate for the mother, breast-feeding may be discontinued for 12-24 hours to allow excretion of the medication.

Table 5. Drugs That Have Been Associated With Significant Effects on Some Nursing Infants and Should Be Given to Nursing Mothers With Caution[1]

Drug	Reported Effect
Acebutolol	Hypotension, bradycardia, tachypnea
5-Aminosalicylic acid	Diarrhea (one case)
Atenolol	Cyanosis, bradycardia
Bromocriptine	Suppresses lactation; may be hazardous to the mother
Aspirin (salicylates)	Metabolic acidosis (one case)
Clemastine	Drowsiness, irritability, refusal to feed, high-pitched cry, neck stiffness (one case)
Ergotamine	Vomiting, diarrhea, convulsions (doses used in migraine medications
Lithium	One-third to one-half therapeutic blood concentration in infants
Phenindone	Anticoagulant: increased prothrombin and partial thromboplastin time in one infant; not used in the United States
Phenobarbital	Sedation; infantile spasms after weaning from milk-containing phenobarbital, methemoglobinemia (one case)
Primidone	Sedation, feeding problems
Sulfasalazine (salicylazosulfapyridine)	Bloody diarrhea (one case)

[1]Blood concentration in the infant may be of clinical importance; measure when possible.

Table 6. Maternal Medication Usually Compatible With Breast-Feeding

Drug	Reported Effect
Acetaminophen	
Acetazolamide	
Acitretin	
Acyclovir[1]	
Alcohol (ethanol)	Large amounts may lead to drowsiness, diaphoresis, deep sleep, weakness, decreased linear growth, and/or abnormal weight gain. Ingestion of 1 g/kg/d decreases mothers milk ejection reflex.
Allopurinol	
Amoxicillin	
Antimony	
Atropine	
Azapropazone (apazone)	
Aztreonam	
B_1 (thiamine)	
B_6 (pyridoxine)	
B_{12}	
Baclofen	
Barbiturate	Refer to Table 5
Bendroflumethiazide	Lactation suppressed
Bishydroxycoumarin (Dicumarol®)	
Bromide	Rash, weakness, absence of cry with maternal intake of 5.4 g/d
Butorphanol	
Caffeine	Irritability and poor sleep may be seen with >2-3 cups/d; excreted slowly
Captopril	
Carbamazepine	
Carbetocin	
Carbimazole	Goiter
Cascara	
Cefadroxil	
Cefazolin	
Cefotaxime	
Cefoxitin	
Cefprozil	
Ceftazidime	
Ceftriaxone	
Chloral hydrate	Sleepiness
Chloroform	
Chloroquine	
Chlorothiazide	
Chlorthalidone	Slow excretion
Cimetidine[1]	

BREAST-FEEDING AND DRUGS *(Continued)*

Table 6. Maternal Medication Usually Compatible With Breast-Feeding *(continued)*

Drug	Reported Effect
Ciprofloxacin	Theoretically, may affect cartilage in weight-bearing joints; pseudomembranous colitis reported in one infant
Cisapride	
Cisplatin	Not found in milk
Clindamycin	
Clogestone	
Codeine	
Colchicine	
Contraceptive pill with estrogen and progesterone	Breast enlargement (rare), decreased milk production and protein count (unconfirmed)
Cycloserine	
D (vitamin)	Infant calcium levels should be monitored if mother receives pharmacologic doses
Danthron	Bowel activity increased
Dapsone	No effects reported, but sulfonamide detected in infants urine
Dexbrompheniramine maleate with d-isoephedrine	Crying, poor sleeping patterns, irritability
Diatrizoate	
Digoxin	
Diltiazem	
Dipyrone	
Disopyramide	
Domperidone	
Dyphylline[1]	
Enalapril	
Erythromycin[1]	
Estradiol	Withdrawal, vaginal bleeding
Ethambutol	
Ethanol	See alcohol
Ethosuximide	No effects reported, but detected in infants urine
Fentanyl	
Fexofenadine	
Flecainide	
Fleroxacin	In one report, a single 400 mg dose was administered to the mother and breast milk not given to infant for 48 hours
Fluconazole	
Flufenamic acid	
Fluorescein	
Folic acid	
Gadopentetic (Gadolinium)	
Gentamicin	
Gold salts	

Table 6. Maternal Medication Usually Compatible With Breast-Feeding *(continued)*

Drug	Reported Effect
Halothane	
Hydralazine	
Hydrochlorothiazide	
Hydroxychloroquine[1]	
Ibuprofen	
Indomethacin	Seizure (one case)
Iodides	May affect thyroid activity; see Iodine
Iodine	Goiter
Iodine (povidone-iodine/ vaginal douche)	Increased iodine levels in breast milk; iodine odor on infants skin
Iohexol	
Iopanoic acid	
Isoniazid	Metabolite secreted in breast milk; no hepatotoxicity reported in infant
Interferon alfa	
Ivermectin	
K_1 (vitamin)	
Kanamycin	
Ketoconazole	
Ketorolac	
Labetalol	
Levonorgestrel	
Levothyroxine	
Lidocaine	
Loperamide	
Loratadine	
Magnesium sulfate	
Medroxyprogesterone	
Mefenamic acid	
Meperidine	
Methadone	
Methimazole (active metabolite of carbimazole)	
Methyldopa	
Methprylon	Drowsiness
Metoprolol[1]	
Metrizamide	
Metrizoate	
Mexiletine	
Minoxidil	
Morphine	No effects reported but found in infants serum
Moxalactam	
Nadolol[1]	
Nalidixic acid	Hemolysis reported in infant with glucose-g-phosphate dehydrogenase deficiency
Naproxen	

BREAST-FEEDING AND DRUGS *(Continued)*

Table 6. Maternal Medication Usually Compatible With Breast-Feeding *(continued)*

Drug	Reported Effect
Nefopam	
Nifedipine	
Nitrofurantoin	Hemolysis reported in infant with G6PD deficiency
Norethynodrel	
Norsteroids	
Noscapine	
Ofloxacin	Theoretically, may affect cartilage in weight-bearing joints
Oxprenolol	
Phenylbutazone	
Phenytoin	
Piroxicam	
Prednisolone	
Prednisone	
Procainamide	
Progesterone	
Propoxyphene	
Propranolol	
Propylthiouracil	
Pseudoephedrine[1]	
Pyridostigmine	
Pyrimethamine	
Quinidine	
Quinine	
Riboflavin	
Rifampin	
Scopolamine	
Secobarbital	
Senna	
Sotalol	
Spironolactone	
Streptomycin	
Sulbactam	
Sulfapyridine	Use with caution in infants with G6PD deficiency and in ill, stressed, or premature infants
Sulfisoxazole	Use with caution in infants with G6PD deficiency and in ill, stressed, or premature infants
Sumatriptan	
Suprofen	
Terbutaline	
Terfenadine	
Tetracycline	Negligible absorption by infant; potential to stain infants unerupted teeth
Theophylline	Irritability

Table 6. Maternal Medication Usually Compatible With Breast-Feeding *(continued)*

Drug	Reported Effect
Thiopental	
Thiouracil	
Ticarcillin	
Timolol	
Tolbutamide	Jaundice is possible
Tolmetin	
Trimethoprim and sulfamethoxazole	
Triprolidine	
Valproic acid	
Verapamil	
Vitamin (see individual entries, eg, B_1, B_6, B_{12}, D, K)	
Warfarin	
Zolpidem	

[1]Drug is concentrated in human milk.

Table 7. Selected Food and Environmental Agents

Agent	Effect Related to Breast-Feeding
Aspartame	Use with caution if mother or infant has phenylketonuria
Chocolate	Irritability or increased bowel activity observed in infant when >16 oz/d consumed by mother
Fava beans	Hemolysis reported in infant with G6PD deficiency
Hexachlorobenzene	Skin rash, diarrhea, vomiting, dark urine, neurotoxicity, death
Hexachlorophene	No effects reported; however, possibility of milk contamination following nipple washing
Lead	Neurotoxicity possible
Mercury, methylmercury	Possible effects on neurodevelopment
Silicone breast implants	Breast-feeding not contraindicated
Vegetarian diet	B_{12} deficiency

References

American Academy of Pediatrics Committee on Drugs, "Transfer of Drugs and Other Chemicals Into Human Milk," *Pediatrics*, 2001, 108(3): 776-89.

2000 Red Book: Report of the Committee on Infectious Diseases, 25th ed, Elk Grove Village, IL: American Academy of Pediatrics, 2000, 98-104.

COMPATIBILITY OF MEDICATIONS MIXED IN A SYRINGE

	Atropine	Chlorpromazine	Codeine	Diphenhydramine	Droperidol	Fentanyl	Glycopyrrolate	Hydroxyzine	Meperidine	Metoclopramide	Midazolam	Morphine	Pentazocine	Pentobarbital†	Prochlorperazine	Promazine	Promethazine	Trimethobenzamide
Atropine		C	•	C	C	C	C	C	C	C	C	C	C	C	C	C	C	•
Chlorpromazine	C		•	C	C	C	C	C	C	C	C	C	C	X	C	C	C	•
Codeine	•	•		•	•	•	C	C	•	•	•	•	•	X	•	•	•	•
Diphenhydramine	C	C	•		C	C	C	C	C	C	C	C	C	X	C	C	C	•
Droperidol	C	C	•	C		C	C	C	C	C	C	C	C	X	C	C	C	•
Fentanyl	C	C	•	C	C		C	C	C	C	C	C	C	X	C	C	C	•
Glycopyrrolate	C	C	C	C	C	C		C	C	•	C	C	X	X	C	C	C	C
Hydroxyzine	C	C	C	C	C	C	C		C	C	C	C	C	X	C	C	C	•
Meperidine	C	C	•	C	C	C	C	C		C	C	X	C	X	C	C	C	•
Metoclopramide	C	C	•	C	C	C	•	C	C		C	C	C	•	C	C	C	•
Midazolam	C	C	•	C	C	C	C	C	C	C		C	•	X	X	C	C	C
Morphine	C	C	•	C	C	C	C	C	C	C	C		C	X	C*	C	C	•
Pentazocine	C	C	•	C	C	C	C	C	C	C	•	C		X	C	C	C	C
Pentobarbital†	C	X	X	X	X	X	X	X	X	•	X	X	X		X	X	X	•
Prochlorperazine	C	C	•	C	C	C	C	C	C	C	X	C*	C	X		C	C	•
Promazine	C	C	•	C	C	C	C	C	C	C	C	C	C	X	C		C	•
Promethazine	C	C	•	C	C	C	C	C	C	C	C	C	C	X	C	C		•
Trimethobenzamide	•	•	•	•	•	•	C	•	•	•	C	•	C	•	•	•	•	

C = physically compatible if used within 15 minutes after mixing in a syringe.
X = incompatible.
• = no documented information.
C* = potential incompatibility produced by certain manufacturers.
† = compatibility profile is characteristic of most barbiturate salts, such as phenobarbital and secobarbital.

The following combinations have been found to be compatible:

atropine / meperidine / promethazine
atropine / meperidine / hydroxyzine
meperidine / promethazine / chlorpromazine

The following drugs should not be mixed with any other drugs in the same syringe:

diazepam, chlordiazepoxide

References

Forman JK and Sourney PF, "Visual Compatibility of Midazolam Hydrochloride With Common Preoperative Injectable Medications," *Am J Hosp Pharm*, 1987, 44(10):2298-9.

King JC, "Guide to Parenteral Admixtures," St Louis, MO: Cutter Laboratories, 1986.

Parker WA, *Hosp Pharm*, 1984, 19:475-8.

Trissel LA, "Handbook on Injectable Drugs," 5th ed, Bethesda, MD: American Society of Health-System Pharmacists, Inc, 1988.

Stevenson JG and Patriarca C, "Incompatibility of Morphine Sulfate and Prochlorperazine Edisylate in Syringes," *Am J Hosp Pharm*, 1985, 42:2651.

CONTROLLED SUBSTANCES

Note: These are federal classifications. Your individual state may place a substance into a more restricted category. When this occurs, the more restricted category applies. Consult your state law.

Schedule I = C-I

The drugs and other substances in this schedule have no legal medical uses except research. They have a **high** potential for abuse. They include opiates, opium derivatives, and hallucinogens.

Schedule II = C-II

The drugs and other substances in this schedule have legal medical uses and a **high** abuse potential which may lead to severe dependence. They include former "Class A" narcotics, amphetamines, barbiturates, and other drugs.

Schedule III = C-III

The drugs and other substances in this schedule have legal medical uses and a **lesser** degree of abuse potential which may lead to **moderate** dependence. They include former "Class B" narcotics and other drugs.

Schedule IV = C-IV

The drugs and other substances in this schedule have legal medical uses and **low** abuse potential which may lead to **moderate** dependence. They include barbiturates, benzodiazepines, propoxyphenes, and other drugs.

Schedule V = C-V

The drugs and other substances in this schedule have legal medical uses and **low** abuse potential which may lead to **moderate** dependence. They include narcotic cough preparations, diarrhea preparations, and other drugs.

FEVER DUE TO DRUGS

Most Common

Atropine	Cephalosporins	Procainamide
Amphotericin B	Interferon	Quinidine
Asparaginase	Methyldopa	Salicylates (high doses)
Barbiturates	Penicillins	Streptomycin
Bleomycin	Phenytoin	Sulfonamides

Less Common

Allopurinol	Hydralazine	Nitrofurantoin
Antihistamines	Hydroxyurea	Pentazocine
Azathioprine	Imipenem	Procarbazine
Carbamazepine	Iodides	Propylthiouracil
Cimetidine	Isoniazid	Rifampin
Cisplatin	Mercaptopurine	Streptokinase
Colistimethate	Metoclopramide	Triamterene
Diazoxide	Nifedipine	Vancomycin
Folic acid	NSAIDs	

References

Cunha BA, "Antibiotic Side Effects," *Med Clin North Am*, 2001, 85(1):149-85.

Mackowiak PA and LeMaistre CF, "Drug Fever: A Critical Appraisal of Conventional Concepts. An Analysis of 51 Episodes in Two Dallas Hospitals and 97 Episodes Reported in the English Literature," *Ann Intern Med*, 1987, 106(5):728-33.

Tabor PA, "Drug-Induced Fever," Table 2, "Drugs Implicated in Causing a Fever," *Drug Intell Clin Pharm*, 1986, 20(6):416.

DISCOLORATION OF FECES DUE TO DRUGS

Black
Acetazolamide
Alcohols
Alkalies
Aluminum hydroxide
Aminophylline
Aminosalicylic acid
Amphetamine
Amphotericin
Antacids
Anticoagulants
Aspirin
Betamethasone
Bismuth
Charcoal
Chloramphenicol
Chlorpropamide
Clindamycin
Corticosteroids
Cortisone
Cyclophosphamide
Cytarabine
Dicumarol
Digitalis
Ethacrynic acid
Ferrous salts
Floxuridine
Fluorides
Fluorouracil
Halothane
Heparin
Hydralazine
Hydrocortisone
Ibuprofen
Indomethacin
Iodine drugs
Iron salts
Levarterenol
Levodopa
Manganese
Melphalan
Methylprednisolone
Methotrexate
Methylene blue
Oxyphenbutazone
Paraldehyde
Phenacetin
Phenolphthalein
Phenylbutazone
Phenylephrine
Phosphorous
Potassium salts
Prednisolone
Procarbazine
Pyrvinium
Reserpine
Salicylates
Sulfonamides
Tetracycline
Theophylline
Thiotepa
Triamcinolone
Warfarin

Blue
Chloramphenicol
Methylene blue

Dark Brown
Dexamethasone

Gray
Colchicine

Green
Indomethacin
Iron
Medroxyprogesterone

Greenish Gray
Oral antibiotics
Oxyphenbutazone
Phenylbutazone

Light Brown
Anticoagulants

Orange-Red
Phenazopyridine
Rifampin

Pink
Anticoagulants
Aspirin
Heparin
Oxyphenbutazone
Phenylbutazone
Salicylates

Red
Anticoagulants
Aspirin
Heparin
Oxyphenbutazone
Phenolphthalein
Phenylbutazone
Pyrvinium
Salicylates
Tetracycline syrup

Red-Brown
Oxyphenbutazone
Phenylbutazone
Rifampin

Tarry
Ergot preparations
Ibuprofen
Salicylates
Warfarin

White/Speckling
Aluminum hydroxide
Antibiotics (oral)
Indocyanine green

Yellow
Senna

Yellow-Green
Senna

Adapted from Drugdex® — Drug Consults, Micromedex, Vol 62, Denver, CO: Rocky Mountain Drug Consultation Center, 1998.

DISCOLORATION OF URINE DUE TO DRUGS

Black
Cascara
Cotrimoxazole
Ferrous salts
Iron dextran
Levodopa
Methocarbamol
Methyldopa
Naphthalene
Pamaquine
Phenacetin
Phenols
Quinine
Sulfonamides

Blue
Anthraquinone
DeWitt's pills
Indigo blue
Indigo carmine
Methocarbamol
Methylene blue
Mitoxantrone
Nitrofurans
Resorcinol
Triamterene

Blue-Green
Amitriptyline
Anthraquinone
DeWitt's pills
Doan's® pills
Indigo blue
Indigo carmine
Magnesium salicylate
Methylene blue
Resorcinol

Brown
Anthraquinone dyes
Cascara
Chloroquine
Hydroquinone
Levodopa
Methocarbamol
Methyldopa
Methocarbamol
Metronidazole
Nitrofurans
Nitrofurantoin
Pamaquine
Phenacetin
Phenols
Primaquine
Quinine
Rifabutin
Rifampin
Senna
Sodium diatrizoate
Sulfonamides

Brown-Black
Isosorbide mono- or dinitrate
Methyldopa
Metronidazole
Nitrates
Nitrofurans
Phenacetin
Povidone iodine
Quinine
Senna

Dark
p-Aminosalicylic acid
Cascara
Levodopa
Metronidazole
Nitrites
Phenacetin
Phenol
Primaquine
Quinine
Resorcinol
Riboflavin
Senna

Green
Amitriptyline
Anthraquinone
DeWitt's pills
Indigo blue
Indigo carmine
Indomethacin
Methocarbamol
Methylene blue
Nitrofurans
Phenols
Propofol
Resorcinol
Suprofen

Green-Yellow
DeWitt's pills
Methylene blue

Milky
Phosphates

Orange
Chlorzoxazone
Dihydroergotamine mesylate
Heparin sodium
Phenazopyridine
Phenindione
Rifabutin
Rifampin
Sulfasalazine
Warfarin

Orange-Red-Brown
Chlorzoxazone
Doxidan
Phenazopyridine
Rifampin
Warfarin

Orange-Yellow
Fluorescein sodium
Rifampin
Sulfasalazine

Pink
Aminopyrine
Anthraquinone dyes
Aspirin
Cascara
Danthron
Deferoxamine
Merbromin
Methyldopa
Phenazopyridone
Phenolphthalein
Phenothiazines
Phenytoin
Salicylates
Senna

Purple
Phenolphthalein

Red
Anthraquinone
Cascara
Chlorpromazine
Daunorubicin
Deferoxamine
Dihydroergotamine mesylate
Dimethyl sulfoxide
DMSO
Doxorubicin
Heparin
Ibuprofen
Methyldopa
Oxyphenbutazone
Phenacetin
Phenazopyridine
Phenolphthalein
Phenothiazines
Phensuximide
Phenylbutazone
Phenytoin
Rifampin
Senna

Red-Brown
Cascara
Deferoxamine
Methyldopa
Oxyphenbutazone
Pamaquine
Phenacetin
Phenazopyridine
Phenolphthalein
Phenothiazines
Phenylbutazone
Phenytoin
Quinine
Senna

Red-Purple
Chlorzoxazone
Ibuprofen
Phenacetin
Senna

Rust
Cascara
Chloroquine
Metronidazole
Nitrofurantoin
Pamaquine
Phenacetin
Quinacrine
Riboflavin
Senna
Sulfonamides

Yellow
Nitrofurantoin
Phenacetin
Quinacrine
Riboflavin
Sulfasalazine

Yellow-Brown
Aminosalicylate acid
Bismuth
Cascara
Chloroquine
DeWitt's pills
Methylene blue
Metronidazole
Nitrofurantoin
Pamaquine
Primaquine
Quinacrine
Senna
Sulfonamides

Yellow-Pink
Cascara
Senna

Adapted from Drugdex® — Drug Consults, Micromedex, Vol 62, Denver, CO: Rocky Mountain Drug Consultation Center, 1998.

DRUGS IN PREGNANCY

Medications Known to Be Teratogens

- Alcohol
- Androgens
- Anticonvulsants
- Antineoplastics
- Cocaine
- Diethylstilbestrol
- Etretinate
- Iodides (including radioactive iodine)
- Isotretinoin
- Lithium
- Live vaccines
- Methimazole
- Penicillamine
- Tetracyclines
- Warfarin

Medications Suspected to Be Teratogens

- ACE inhibitors
- Benzodiazepines
- Estrogens
- Oral hypoglycemic drugs
- Progestogens
- Quinolones

Medications With No Known Teratogenic Effects[1]

- Acetaminophen
- Cephalosporins
- Corticosteroids
- Docusate sodium
- Erythromycin
- Multiple vitamins
- Narcotic analgesics
- Penicillins
- Phenothiazines
- Thyroid hormones
- Tricyclic antidepressants

[1]No drug is absolutely without risk during pregnancy. These drugs appear to have a minimal risk when used judiciously in usual doses under the supervision of a medical professional.

Medications With Nonteratogenic Adverse Effects in Pregnancy

- Antithyroid drugs
- Aminoglycosides
- Aspirin
- Barbiturates (chronic use)
- Benzodiazepines
- Beta-blockers
- Caffeine
- Chloramphenicol
- Cocaine
- Diuretics
- Isoniazid
- Narcotic analgesics (chronic use)
- Nicotine
- Nonsteroidal anti-inflammatory agents
- Oral hypoglycemic agents
- Propylthiouracil
- Sulfonamides

Adapted from DiPiro JT, Talbert RL, Hayes PE, et al, "Therapeutic Considerations During Pregnancy and Lactation," *Pharmacotherapy: A Pathophysiologic Approach*, 4th ed, Stamford, CT: Appleton & Lange, 1999.

MILLIEQUIVALENT FOR SELECTED IONS

Approximate Milliequivalents — Weights of Selected Ions

Salt	mEq/g Salt	mg Salt/mEq
Calcium carbonate ($CaCO_3$)	20	50
Calcium chloride ($CaCl_2 \bullet 2H_2O$)	14	73
Calcium gluconate (Ca gluconate$_2 \bullet 1H_2O$)	4	224
Calcium lactate (Ca lactate$_2 \bullet 5H_2O$)	6	154
Magnesium sulfate ($MgSO_4$)	16	60
Magnesium sulfate ($MgSO_4 \bullet 7H_2O$)	8	123
Potassium acetate (K acetate)	10	98
Potassium chloride (KCl)	13	75
Potassium citrate (K_3 citrate$\bullet 1H_2O$)	9	108
Potassium iodide (KI)	6	166
Sodium bicarbonate ($NaHCO_3$)	12	84
Sodium chloride (NaCl)	17	58
Sodium citrate (Na_3 citrate$\bullet 2H_2O$)	10	98
Sodium iodide (NaI)	7	150
Sodium lactate (Na lactate)	9	112
Zinc sulfate ($ZnSO_4 \bullet 7H_2O$)	7	144

Valences and Approximate Weights of Selected Ions

Substance	Electrolyte	Valence	Ionic Wt
Calcium	Ca^{++}	2	40
Chloride	Cl^-	1	35.5
Magnesium	Mg^{++}	2	24
Phosphate	PO_4^{3-}	3	95[1]
	HPO_4^{2-}	2	96
	$H_2PO_4^-$	1	97
Potassium	K^+	1	39
Sodium	Na^+	1	23
Sulfate	SO_4^{2-}	2	96[1]

[1]The atomic weight of phosphorus is 31, and of sulfur is 32.

PEDIATRIC MEDICATION ADMINISTRATION

Adapted from *Giving Your Child Medicine – Ways to Ensure Your Child Receives the Correct Dose of Medicine*, patient booklet, Lexi-Comp, Inc, 2002.

General Advice

Administering medicine to a sick child can be extremely challenging for parents and caregivers. Dosages are calculated by taking the child's age and/or weight into consideration. Infants and young children require very small doses of medicines, thus making accurate measurement very important.

Special measuring devices are available to accurately and easily provide the prescribed dosage. Measuring out a dose with common household utensils can lead to unacceptable inaccuracies. Improper measurement can also cause increased side effects, and over- or under-dosing.

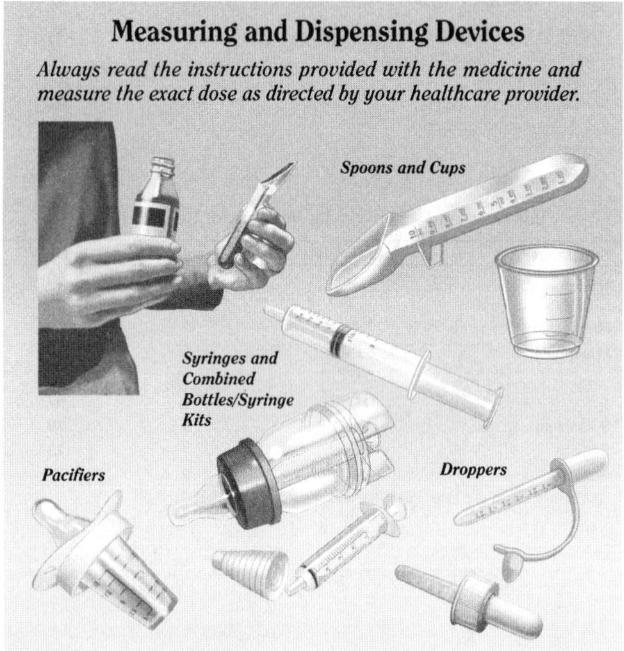

Liquids

Use either an oral syringe, a medicine dropper, a medicine spoon, or a medicine cup (only for older children) when giving your child oral liquids. You can purchase any of these at a local pharmacy if not provided with your child's medicine. There are specialized pacifiers and bottles designed as medicine delivery aids for children <2 years of age.

- If the medicine can be given on an empty stomach, give right before a feeding.
- Hold an infant in the normal feeding position, or put in a highchair or car seat.

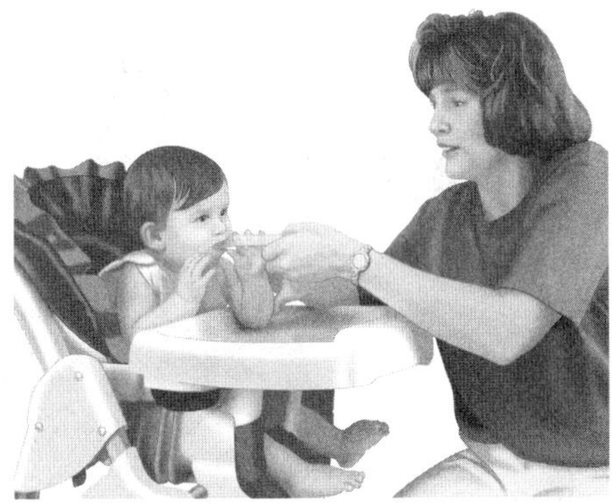

If the child refuses to take the medicine because of bad taste, check with a pharmacist to see if the medicine can be mixed with fruit juice, milk, or another liquid. Pharmacists may be able to flavor the medicine to disguise the taste. You may use a popsicle to partially numb the mouth, give the medicine, and then use the popsicle again to help improve taste.

- Prepare the medicine. Open the infant's mouth by gently squeezing his/her cheeks or by using your finger to pull out a corner of the infant's mouth.
- Slowly squirt the medicine into the side of the infant's mouth. Do not squirt it to the back of the throat because this can cause choking or gagging.
- Gently stroke the infant under the chin to encourage swallowing while still holding the cheeks together.
- Alternatively, pour medicine into a small cup and dip your little finger in it. Let the infant suck it off your finger.
- Young children may want to be in control of taking the medicine by guiding the dropper or spoon into their mouth.
- Rinse measuring device with warm water after each use.

Droppers or cups which come with specific medicines should not be used to administer other medicine.

PEDIATRIC MEDICATION ADMINISTRATION *(Continued)*

Eye Drops and Ointments

- Wash your hands before and after use.
- Hold container between hands to bring eye drops or ointment to room temperature before using.
- Clean child's eye of secretions and old medicine if necessary.
- Gently wipe the eye with a damp gauze or cotton pad.
- Tilt child's head back and to the side of the affected eye.
- Do not touch the container tip to eye, lid, or other skin.

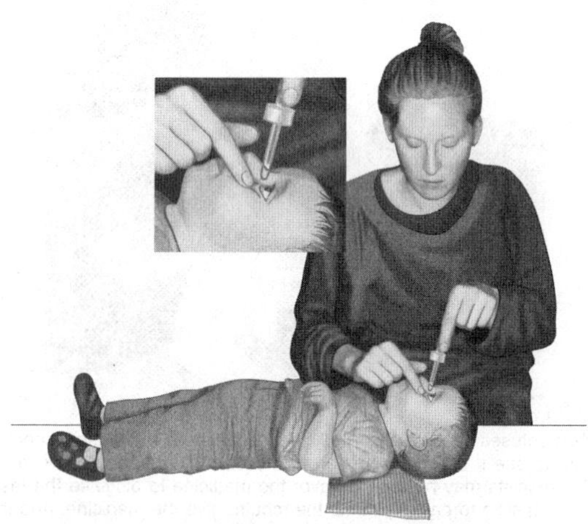

Drops

- If the drops are a suspension, shake the bottle well.
- Gently press the skin under the lower eyelid and pull the lower eyelid away from the eye slightly until you can see a small pouch.
- Insert 1 drop. Wait 1 minute between drops if more than one eye medicine is prescribed.
- After using medicine, ask the child to keep eyes closed. Apply light pressure to the inside corner of the eye.
- Do this for 3-5 minutes. This keeps the medicine in the eye.

Ointment

- If you are using an ointment, gently pull down the lower lid and squeeze in the prescribed amount.
- Release the lower eyelid and instruct the child to keep eyes closed for 1-2 minutes. This will put the medicine in contact with the eye.

Ear Drops

- Wash your hands before and after use.
- Warm the medicine by holding the bottle between your hands.
- If the drops are a suspension, shake the bottle well.
- For children <3 years of age, pull the outer ear outward and downward.
- For children ≥3 years of age, pull the outer ear outward and upward.
- Instill prescribed number of drops in affected ear without touching dropper to ear.
- Have child stay on side for 2 minutes or insert cotton plug into ear.
- Repeat procedure in other ear if necessary.

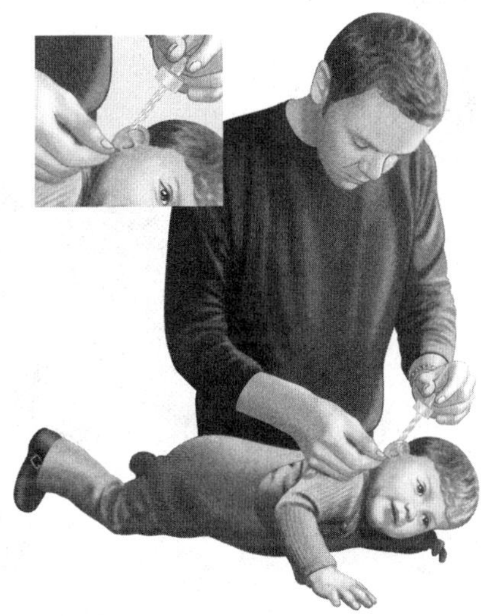

Topical Creams and Ointments

If no specific directions have been given, follow these general guidelines:

- For use on skin only. Keep out of mouth, nose, and eyes (may burn).
- Wash your hands before and after use.
- Clean affected area and dry well before use.
- Apply a thin layer of medicine to the affected skin and rub in gently. Some medicines can be poured or squeezed onto a gauze pad, cotton swab, or cotton ball to apply.
- Do not put coverings (bandages, dressings) over the area unless told to do so by a healthcare provider.

PEDIATRIC MEDICATION ADMINISTRATION *(Continued)*

Nose Drops

- Wash your hands before and after use.
- Warm the medicine by holding the bottle between your hands.
- If the drops are a suspension, shake the bottle well.
- Try to clear mucus out of nose. For infants and small children, you can use a nasal aspirator (bulb syringe) or gently twirl a moist cotton swab inside each nostril.

  Do not reach too far into the nostril with the swab or bulb syringe.

  For older children, have the child blow nose.
- Infants can be cradled in your arms in a lying position with head tilted back slightly.

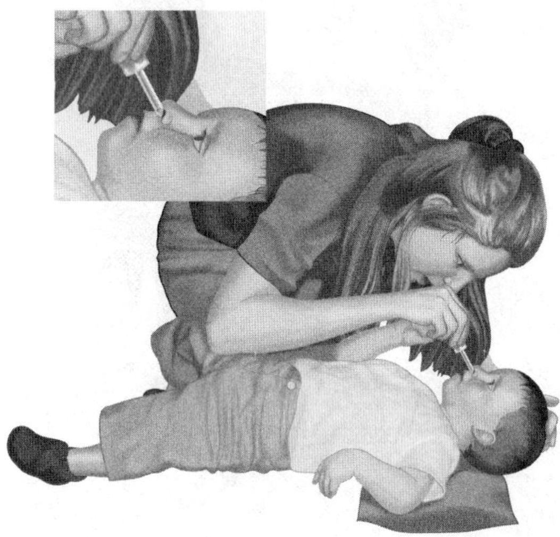

- Young children should lie on their back with a small pillow between their shoulders.
- Have them tilt head back over top of pillow. Older children can sit up with the head tilted back.
- Tell older children they may be able to taste the medicine.
- Draw the correct amount of medicine into the dropper, insert the dropper slightly into the nostril, and squeeze the medicine in without touching dropper to the nose.
- Repeat procedure in other nostril if necessary.
- Keep the child's head tilted back for 2 minutes.
- If child coughs, sit him/her upright.

Rectal Suppositories

- Wash your hands before and after use.
- If appropriate, store suppository in refrigerator or run it under cold water with the wrapper still on to make it firm enough to place in rectum. Ask pharmacist if you are able to safely store medicine in a refrigerator.
- Infants should be facedown across your knees. An older child can lie on his/her side with knees drawn to chest.
- Remove the wrapper.
- Moisten suppository with water or place a small amount of petroleum jelly on the tip.
- Consider use of a disposable glove.
- Gently insert the smooth, rounded end of the suppository into the rectum and up beyond the sphincter ($^1/_2$ to 1 inch beyond the sphincter). Use your pinky finger for children <3 years of age and your index finger for those ≥3 years.
- If the suppository is inserted far enough, it should stay in place. If it comes out, reinsert it slightly farther than before.
- Hold the buttocks together for a couple of minutes to prevent the child from expelling the suppository.
- Have child remain in the same position for about 20 minutes, if possible. If not, have him/her sit or lie down without going to the bathroom.

If in doubt...

Speak to your healthcare provider or your pharmacist about any concerns you have regarding the medicine prescribed for your child.

IF YOUR CHILD HAS A REACTION TO ANY MEDICINE, GET HELP IMMEDIATELY.

Do's and Don'ts

DO wash your child's hands immediately if medicine gets on them.

DO use distractions such as toys, songs, stories, or rhymes to keep your child busy while trying to give medicine.

DO get another adult to help hold the infant while you give the medicine, or use a car seat to hold the infant or child still.

DO try a different form of the medicine. A child might prefer a chewable tablet or a form that can be sprinkled on food.

DO teach your child about the illness and why he/she has to take medicine. Your healthcare provider or librarian may have books about children who are sick or need to take medicine.

DO help your child gain some control by letting him/her make age-appropriate decisions about care.

DO use prescription as directed, even if your child is feeling better.

DO store medicine out of the reach of children and pets.

DO NOT measure medicine for an infant with a medicine cup (use an oral syringe, a medicine dropper, or a medicine spoon).

DO NOT use a teaspoon or tablespoon from your silverware to measure medicine for your child.

SEROTONIN SYNDROME

Diagnostic Criteria for Serotonin Syndrome

- Recent addition or dosage increase of any agent increasing serotonin activity or availability (usually within 1 day)
- Absence of abused substances, metabolic infectious etiology, or withdrawal
- No recent addition or dosage increase of a neuroleptic agent prior to onset of signs and symptoms
- Presence of three or more of the following: (% incidence)

Agitation (34%)
Abdominal pain (4%)
Ataxia/incoordination (40%)
Diaphoresis (45%)
Diarrhea (8%)
Hyperpyrexia (45%)
Hypertension/hypotension (35%)
Hyperthermia
Hyperreflexia (52%)
Mental status change – cognitive behavioral changes:
  Anxiety (15%)
  Euphoria/hypomania (21%)
  Confusion (51%)
  Agitation (34%)
  Disorientation
  Coma/unresponsiveness (29%)
Muscle rigidity (51%)
Mydriasis
Myoclonus (58%)
Nausea (23%)
Nystagmus (15%)
Restlessness/hyperactivity (48%)
Salivation (2%)
Seizures (12%)
Shivering (26%)
Sinus tachycardia (36%)
Tachypnea (26%)
Tremor (43%)
Unreactive pupils (20%)

Drugs (as Single Causative Agent) Which Can Induce Serotonin Syndrome

Specific serotonin reuptake inhibitors (SSRI)
MDMA (Ecstasy)
Clomipramine

Drug Combinations Which Can Induce Serotonin Syndrome[1]

Alprazolam – Clomipramine
Amphetamines – MAO inhibitors
Amphetamines – SSRIs (Citalopram, Fluoxetine, Fluvoxamine, Paroxetine, Sertraline)
Amphetamines – Tricyclic antidepressants
Amitriptyline – Dihydroergotamine
Amitriptyline – Lithium – Trazodone
Amitriptyline – Sertraline
Anorexiants – MAO inhibitors
Bromocriptine – Levodopa/Carbidopa
Buspirone – Nefazodone
Buspirone – SSRIs (Citalopram, Fluoxetine, Fluvoxamine, Paroxetine, Sertraline)
Buspirone – Trazodone
Buspirone – Tricyclic antidepressants
Carbamazepine – Fluoxetine
Citalopram – Moclobemide
Clomipramine – Alprazolam
Clomipramine – Clorgiline
Clomipramine – Lithium
Clomipramine – MAO inhibitors
Clomipramine – Moclobemide
Clomipramine – S-adenosylmethionine
Clomipramine – Tranylcypromine
Clorgiline – Clomipramine
Dextromethorphan – MAO inhibitors
Dextromethorphan – SSRIs (Citalopram, Fluoxetine, Fluvoxamine, Paroxetine, Sertraline)
Dextropropoxyphene – Phenelzine – Trazodone
Dihydroergotamine – Amitriptyline
Dihydroergotamine – Paroxetine

Dihydroergotamine – SSRIs (Citalopram, Fluoxetine, Fluvoxamine, Paroxetine, Sertraline)
Dihydroergotamine – Tricyclic antidepressants
Fentanyl – SSRIs (Citalopram, Fluoxetine, Fluvoxamine, Paroxetine, Sertraline)
Fluoxetine – Carbamazepine
Fluoxetine – Remoxipride
Fluoxetine – Tryptophan
Levodopa/Carbidopa – Bromocriptine
Linezolid - SSRIs (Citalopram, Fluoxetine, Fluvoxamine, Paroxetine, Sertraline)
Linezolid – Tramadol
Linezolid – Tricyclic antidepressants
Lithium – Amitriptyline – Trazodone
Lithium – Clomipramine
Lithium – SSRIs (Citalopram, Fluoxetine, Fluvoxamine, Paroxetine, Sertraline)
Lithium – Tricyclic antidepressants
Lithium – Venlafaxine
Lysergic acid diethylamide (LSD) – SSRIs (Citalopram, Fluoxetine, Fluvoxamine, Paroxetine, Sertraline)
Metoclopramide – Sertraline
Metoclopramide – Venlafaxine
MAO inhibitors – Amphetamines
MAO inhibitors – Anorexiants
MAO inhibitors – Clomipramine
MAO inhibitors – Dextromethorphan
MAO inhibitors – Meperidine
MAO inhibitors – Nefazodone
MAO inhibitors – Serotonin agonists
MAO inhibitors – S-adenosylmethionine
MAO inhibitors – SSRIs (Citalopram, Fluoxetine, Fluvoxamine, Paroxetine, Sertraline)
MAO inhibitors – St John's Wort
MAO inhibitors – Tramadol
MAO inhibitors – Trazodone
MAO inhibitors – Tricyclic antidepressants
MAO inhibitors – Tryptophan
MAO inhibitors – Venlafaxine
Meperidine – MAO inhibitors
Meperidine – Moclobemide
Meperidine – Nefazodone
Meperidine – SSRIs (Citalopram, Fluoxetine, Fluvoxamine, Paroxetine, Sertraline)
Moclobemide – Citalopram
Moclobemide – Clomipramine
Moclobemide – Meperidine
Moclobemide – Pethidine
Moclobemide – SSRIs (Citalopram, Fluoxetine, Fluvoxamine, Paroxetine, Sertraline)
Moclobemide – Tricyclic antidepressants
Nefazodone – Buspirone
Nefazodone – MAO inhibitors
Nefazodone – Meperidine
Nefazodone – Serotonin agonists
Nefazodone – SSRIs (Citalopram, Fluoxetine, Fluvoxamine, Paroxetine, Sertraline)
Nefazodone – Trazodone
Nefazodone – Tramadol
Nefazodone – Valproic Acid
Nortriptyline – Trazodone
Paroxetine – Dihydroergotamine
Paroxetine – Trazodone
Pethidine – Moclobemide
Phenelzine – Trazodone – Dextropropoxyphene
Remoxipride – Fluoxetine
S-adenosylmethionine – Clomipramine
S-adenosylmethionine – MAO inhibitors
S-adenosylmethionine – SSRIs (Citalopram, Fluoxetine, Fluvoxamine, Paroxetine, Sertraline)
S-adenosylmethionine – Tricyclic antidepressants
Selegiline (high-dose) – SSRIs (Citalopram, Fluoxetine, Fluvoxamine, Paroxetine, Sertraline)
Selegiline (high-dose) – Tricyclic antidepressants
Selegiline (high-dose) – Venlafaxine
Serotonin agonists (Sumatriptan, others) – MAO inhibitors
Serotonin agonists (Sumatriptan, others) – Nefazodone
Serotonin agonists (Sumatriptan, others) – SSRIs (Citalopram, Fluoxetine, Fluvoxamine, Paroxetine, Sertraline)
Serotonin agonists (Sumatriptan, others) – TCAs
Serotonin agonists (Sumatriptan, others) – Tramadol
Sertraline – Amitriptyline
Sibutramine – SSRIs (Citalopram, Fluoxetine, Fluvoxamine, Paroxetine, Sertraline)

SEROTONIN SYNDROME *(Continued)*

SSRIs – Amphetamines
SSRIs – Buspirone
SSRIs – Dextromethorphan
SSRIs – Dihydroergotamine
SSRIs – Fentanyl
SSRIs – Linezolid
SSRIs – Lithium
SSRIs – Lysergic acid diethylamide (LSD)
SSRIs – MAO inhibitors
SSRIs – Meperidine
SSRIs – Moclobemide
SSRIs – Nefazodone
SSRIs – S-adenosylmethionine
SSRIs – Selegiline (high-dose)
SSRIs – Serotonin agonists
SSRIs – Sibutramine
SSRIs – St John's Wort
SSRIs – Tramadol
SSRIs – Trazodone
SSRIs – Tricyclic antidepressants
SSRIs – Tryptophan
St John's Wort – MAO inhibitors
St John's Wort – SSRIs (Citalopram, Fluoxetine, Fluvoxamine, Paroxetine, Sertraline)
St John's Wort – Tricyclic antidepressants
Sympathomimetics – Tricyclic antidepressants
Tramadol – Linezolid
Tramadol – MAO inhibitors
Tramadol – Nefazodone
Tramadol – Serotonin agonists
Tramadol – SSRIs (Citalopram, Fluoxetine, Fluvoxamine, Paroxetine, Sertraline)
Tramadol – TCAs
Tranylcypromine – Clomipramine
Trazodone – Buspirone
Trazodone – Lithium – Amitriptyline
Trazodone – MAO inhibitors
Trazodone – Nefazodone
Trazodone – Nortriptyline
Trazodone – Paroxetine
Trazodone – SSRIs (Citalopram, Fluoxetine, Fluvoxamine, Paroxetine, Sertraline) (theoretical)
Tricyclic antidepressants – Amphetamines
Tricyclic antidepressants – Buspirone
Tricyclic antidepressants – Dihydroergotamine
Tricyclic antidepressants – Linezolid
Tricyclic antidepressants – Lithium
Tricyclic antidepressants – MAO inhibitors
Tricyclic antidepressants – Moclobemide
Tricyclic antidepressants – S-adenosylmethionine
Tricyclic antidepressants – Serotonin agonists
Tricyclic antidepressants – SSRIs (Citalopram, Fluoxetine, Fluvoxamine, Paroxetine, Sertraline)
Tricyclic antidepressants – St John's Wort
Tricyclic antidepressants – Sympathomimetics
Tricyclic antidepressants – Tramadol
Tryptophan – Fluoxetine
Tryptophan – MAO inhibitors
Tryptophan – SSRIs (Citalopram, Fluoxetine, Fluvoxamine, Paroxetine, Sertraline)
Valproic acid – Nefazodone
Venlafaxine – Lithium
Venlafaxine – MAO inhibitors
Venlafaxine – Selegiline (high-dose)

[1]When administered within 2 weeks of each other.

Guidelines for Treatment of Serotonin Syndrome

Therapy is primarily supportive with intravenous crystalloid solutions utilized for hypotension and cooling blankets for mild hyperthermia. Norepinephrine is the preferred vasopressor. Chlorpromazine or dantrolene sodium may have a role in controlling fevers, although there is no proven benefit. Benzodiazepines are the first-line treatment in controlling rigors and thus, limiting fever and rhabdomyolysis, whilo clonazepam may be specifically useful in treating myoclonus. Endotracheal intubation and paralysis may be required to treat refractory muscular contractions. Tachycardia or tremor can be treated with beta-blocking agents; although due to its blockade of 5-HTIA receptors, the syndrome may worsen. Serotonin blockers such as diphenhydramine, cyproheptadine, or chlorpromazine have been used with variable efficacy. Methysergide and nitroglycerin (I.V. infusion with lorazepam) also has been utilized with variable efficacy in case reports. It appears that cyproheptadine is most consistently beneficial.

Recovery seen within 1 day in 70% of cases; mortality rate is about 11%.

References

Gardner DM and Lynd LD, "Sumatriptan Contraindications and the Serotonin Syndrome," *Ann Pharmacother*, 1998, 32(1):33-8

Gitlin MJ, "Venlafaxine, Monoamine Oxidase Inhibitors, and the Serotonin Syndrome," *J Clin Psychopharmacol*, 1997, 17:66-7.

Heisler MA, Guidery JR, and Arnecke B, "Serotonin Syndrome Induced by Administration of Venlafaxine and Phenelzine," *Ann Pharmacother*, 1996, 30:84.

Hodgman MJ, Martin TG, and Krenzelok EP, "Serotonin Syndrome Due to Venlafaxine and Maintenance Tranylcypromine Therapy," *Hum Exp Toxicol*, 1997, 16:14-7.

John L, Perreault MM, Tao T, et al, "Serotonin Syndrome Associated With Nefazodone and Paroxetine," *Ann Emerg Med*, 1997, 29:287-9.

LoCurto MJ, "The Serotonin Syndrome," *Emerg Clin North Am*, 1997, 15(3):665-75.

Martin TG, "Serotonin Syndrome," *Ann Emerg Med*, 1996, 28:520-6.

Mills K, "Serotonin Toxicity: A Comprehensive Review for Emergency Medicine," *Top Emerg Med*, 1993, 15:54-73.

Mills KC, "Serotonin Syndrome: A Clinical Update," *Crit Care Clin*, 1997, 13(4):763-83.

Nisijima K, Shimizu M, Abe T, et al, "A Case of Serotonin Syndrome Induced by Concomitant Treatment With Low-Dose Trazodone, and Amitriptyline and Lithium," *Int Clin Psychopharmacol*, 1996, 11:289-90.

Sobanski T, Bagli M, Laux G, et al, "Serotonin Syndrome After Lithium Add-On Medication to Paroxetine," *Pharmacopsychiatry*, 1997, 30:106-7.

Sporer, "The Serotonin Syndrome: Implicated Drugs, Pathophysiology and Management," *Drug Safety*, 1995, 13(2):94-104.

Sternbach H, "The Serotonin Syndrome," *Am J Psychiatry*, 1991, 146:705-7.

Van Berkum MM, Thiel J, Leikin JB, et al, "A Fatality Due to Serotonin Syndrome," *Medical Update for Psychiatrists*, 1997, 2:55-7.

SODIUM CONTENT OF SELECTED MEDICINALS

Name and Dosage Unit[1]	Sodium	
	mg	mEq
Antibiotics		
Amikacin sulfate, 1 g	29.9	1.3
Aminosalicylate sodium, 1 g	109	4.7
Ampicillin, suspension, 250 mg/5 mL, 5 mL	10	0.4
Ampicillin sodium, 1 g	66.7	3
Carbenicillin disodium, 382 mg (tablet)	23	1
Cefazolin sodium, 1 g	47	2
Cefotaxime sodium, 1 g	50.6	2.2
Cefoxitin sodium, 1 g	53	2.3
Ceftriaxone sodium, 1 g	60	2.6
Cefuroxime, 1 g	54.2	2.4
Chloramphenicol sodium succinate, 1 g	51.8	2.3
Dicloxacillin, 250 mg (capsule)	13	0.6
Erythromycin ethyl succinate, suspension 200 mg/5 mL	29	1.3
Erythromycin Base Filmtab®, 250 mg	70	3
Metronidazole, 500 mg I.V.	322	14
Nafcillin sodium, 1 g	66.7	2.9
Nitrofurantoin, suspension, 25 mg/5 mL	7	0.3
Penicillin G potassium, 1,000,000 units I.V.	7.6	0.3
Penicillin G sodium, 1,000,000 units I.V.	46	2
Penicillin V potassium, suspension, 250 mg/5 mL	38	1.7
Piperacillin sodium, 1 g	42.6	1.8
Ticarcillin disodium, 1 g	119.6	5.2
Antacids, Liquid (content per 5 mL)		
ALternaGEL®	2	0.1
Gaviscon®	13	0.57
Maalox®	1.3	0.06
Tums E-X™	<4.8	<0.2
Sodium Content of Miscellaneous Medicinals		
Acetazolamide sodium, 500 mg	47.2	2.05
Chlorothiazide sodium, 500 mg	57.5	2
Cisplatin, 10 mg	35.4	1.54
Edetate calcium disodium, 1 g	122	5.3
Fleet® Enema, 4.5 oz	5000[2]	218
Fleet® Phospho®-Soda, 20 mL	2217	96.4
Hydrocortisone sodium succinate, 1 g	47.5	2.07
Hypaque® M 75%, injection, 20 mL	200	8.7
Hypaque® M 90%, injection, 20 mL	220	9.6
Metamucil® Instant Mix (orange)	6	0.27

Name and Dosage Unit[1]	Sodium	
	mg	mEq
Methotrexate sodium, 100 mg vial	20	0.86
Methotrexate sodium, 100 mg vial (low sodium)	15	0.65
Naproxen sodium, 250 mg (tablet)	23	1
Neutra-Phos®, capsule and 75 mL reconstituted solution	164	7.13
Pentobarbital sodium, 50 mg/mL	5	0.2
Phenobarbital sodium, 65 mg, 1 mL vial	6	0.3
Phenytoin sodium, 1 g	88	3.8
Promethazine expectorant, 5 mL	53	2.3
Shohl's solution modified, 1 mL	23	1
Sodium ascorbate, 500 mg acid equivalent	65.3	2.84
Sodium bicarbonate, 50 mL 8.4%	1150	50
Sodium nitroprusside, 50 mg	7.8	0.34
Sodium polystyrene sulfonate, 1 g	94.3[3]	4.1
Thiopental sodium, 1 g	86.8	3.8
Valproate sodium, 250 mg/5 mL, 5 mL	23	1

[1]Product formulations and hence sodium content are subject to change by the manufacturer.

[2]Average systemic absorption 250-300 mg.

[3]Total sodium content. Only about 33% is liberated in clinical use.

SUGAR-FREE LIQUID PHARMACEUTICALS

The following sugar-free liquid preparations are listed by therapeutic category and alphabetically within each category. Please note that product formulations are subject to change by the manufacturer. Some of these products may contain sorbitol, alcohol, xylitol, or other sweeteners which may be partially metabolized to provide calories.

Analgesics

Acetaminophen Elixir (various)
APAP/APAP Plus
Febrol® and Febrol® EX
Mapap® Drops
Methadone Hydrochloride Intensol
Paregoric USP (Abbott)
Silapap®
Tylenol® Drops

Antacids / Antiflatulents

Alcalak®
Aldroxicon®
Aluminum Hydroxide Suspension
Citrocarbonate® Granules
Gaviscon® Liquid
Maalox® Plus Suspension
Maalox® Suspension
Maalox® Therapeutic Concentrate
Magnesia and Alumina Oral Suspension USP (Abbott, Phillips Roxane)
Milk of Bismuth
Milk of Magnesia USP
Mylanta® Liquid
Mylicon® Drops
Pepto-Bismol® Liquid and Tablets
Riopan Plus®
Riopan® Suspension

Antiasthmatics

Alupent® Syrup
Elixophyllin® Elixir
Lufyllin® Elixir
Organidin® NR

Antidepressants

Celexa™ Solution
Prozac® Solution
Sinequan® Oral Concentrate

Antidiarrheals

Corrective Mixture With Paregoric
Diotame®
Kaolin Mixture With Pectin NF (Abbott)
Kaolin-Pectin Suspension (Phillips Roxane)
Konsyl® Powder
Lomanate®
Lomotil® Liquid
Paregoric USP (various)

Parepectolin® (various)
Pepto-Bismol®
St Joseph® Antidiarrheal

Antiepileptics

Mysoline® Suspension

Antihistamine-Decongestants

Bromphen® Elixir
Dimetapp® Elixir
Isoclor® Liquid and Capsules
Naldecon® Pediatric Drops and Syrup
Naldecon® Syrup
Phenergan® Syrup
Rondec® DM Drops
S-T® Forte® Liquid
Tavist® Syrup
Vistaril® Oral Suspension
Zyrtec® Syrup

Anti-infectives

Augmentin® Suspension
Furadantin® Oral Suspension
NegGram® Suspension
Sulfamethoxazole and Trimethoprim Suspension (Biocraft, Beecham, Burroughs Wellcome)
Vibramycin® Syrup
Zovirax® Suspension

Corticosteroids

Decadron® Elixir
Dexamethasone Solution (Roxane)
Dexamethasone Intensol Solution
Pediapred® Oral Liquid
Prelone® Syrup

Cough Medicines

Chlorgest-HD®
Codiclear® DH Syrup
Codimal® DM
Contac Jr® Liquid
Dimetane®-DC Cough Syrup
Dimetane®-DX Cough Syrup
Entuss® Expectorant Liquid
Histafed® Pediatric Liquid
Hycomine® Syrup and Pediatric Syrup
Medicon® D
Medi-Synal®
Naldecon-DX® Pediatric Drops and Syrup
Naldecon-DX® Adult Liquid
Non-Drowsy Comtrex®
Organidin® NR
Potassium Iodide Solution (various)
Robitussin-CF® Liquid
Robitussin® Night Relief Liquid
Rondec®-DM Drops
Rondec®-DM Syrup
Ryna® Liquid
Ryna-C® Liquid

SUGAR-FREE LIQUID PHARMACEUTICALS *(Continued)*

Ryna-CX® Liquid
Scot-Tussin® DM Syrup
Scot-Tussin® Expectorant
Scot-Tussin® DM Cough Chasers
Silexin® Cough Syrup
Sudodrin®/Sudodrin® Forte®
Terpin® Hydrate With Codeine Elixir (various)
Tolu-Sed® Cough Syrup
Tolu-Sed® DM
Tricodene® Liquid
Tussirex® Sugar-Free

Dental Preparations and Fluoride Preparations

Cepacol® Mouthwash
Cepastat® Mouthwash and Gargle
Chloraseptic® Mouthwash and Gargle
Fluorigard® Mouthrinse
Fluorinse®
Flura-Drops®
Flura-Loz®
Flura® Tablets
Gel-Kam®
Karigel®
Karigel® N
Luride® Drops
Luride® SF Lozi-Tabs
Luride® 0.25 and 0.5 Lozi-Tabs
Luride® Lozi-Tabs
Pediaflor® Drops
Phos-Flur® Rinse/Supplement
Point-Two® Mouthrinse
Prevident® Disclosing Drops
Thera-Flur® Gel and Drops

Diagnostic Agents

Gastrografin®

Dietary Substitutes

Co-Salt®

Iron Preparations / Blood Modifiers

Amicar® Syrup
Geritol® Complete Tablets
Geritonic™ Liquid
Hemo-Vite® Liquid
Iberet® Liquid
Iberet®-500 Liquid
Niferex®
Nu-Iron® Elixir
Vita-Plus H® Half Strength, Sugar-Free
Vita-Plus H®, Sugar-Free

Laxatives

Aromatic Cascara Fluidextract USP
Castor Oil
Castor Oil (flavored)
Castor Oil USP

Colace®, Liquid
Emulsoil®
Fiberall® Powder
Hydrocil® Instant Powder
Hypaque® Oral Powder
Kondremul®
Kondremul® With Cascara
Kondremul® With Phenolphthalein
Konsyl® Powder
Liqui-Doss®
Magnesium Citrate Solution NF
Metamucil® Instant Mix (lemon-lime or orange)
Metamucil® SF Powder
Milk of Magnesia
Milk of Magnesia/Cascara Suspension
Milk of Magnesia/Mineral Oil Emulsion (various)
Mineral Oil (various)
Neoloid® Liquid
NuLYTELY®
Sodium Phosphate & Biphosphate Oral Solution USP (Phillips Roxane)

Potassium Products

Cena-K® Solution
K-G® Elixir
Kaochlor-Eff® Tablets for Solution
Kaochlor® S-F Solution
Kaon® Elixir (grape and lemon-lime flavor)
Kaon-Cl® 20% Liquid
Kay Ciel® Elixir
Kay Ciel® Powder
Klor-Con®/25 Powder
Klor-Con® EF Tablets
Klor-Con® Liquid 20%
Klor-Con® Powder
Potassium Chloride Oral Solution USP 5%, 10%, and 20% (various)
Potassium Gluconate Elixir NF
Rum-K® Solution
Tri-K® Liquid

Sedatives-Tranquilizers-Antipsychotics

Butabarbital Sodium Elixir
Butisol Sodium® Elixir
Haldol® Concentrate
Loxitane® C Drops
Mellaril® Concentrate
Serentil® Concentrate
Thorazine® Concentrate

Vitamin Preparations-Nutritionals

Aquasol A® Drops
Bugs Bunny™ Chewable Tablets
Bugs Bunny™ Plus Iron Chewable Tablets
Bugs Bunny™ With Extra C Chewable Tablets
Bugs Bunny™ Plus Minerals Chewable Tablets
Calciferol™ Drops
Caltrate® 600 Tablets
Cod Liver Oil (various)
DHT™ Intensol Solution (Roxane)

SUGAR-FREE LIQUID PHARMACEUTICALS *(Continued)*

Drisdol® in Propylene Glycol
Flintstones™ Complete Chewable Tablets
Flintstones™ With Extra C Chewable Tablets
Flintstones™ Plus Iron Chewable Tablets
Oyst-Cal® 500 Tablets
Pediaflor®
PMS® Relief
Poly-Vi-Flor® Drops
Poly-Vi-Flor®/Iron Drops
Poly-Vi-Sol® Drops
Poly-Vi-Sol®/Iron Drops
Posture® Tablets
Spiderman™ Children's Chewable Vitamin Tablets
Spiderman™ Children's Plus Iron Tablets
Theragran® Jr Children's Chewable Tablets
Tri-Vi-Flor® Drops
Tri-Vi-Sol® Drops
Tri-Vi-Sol®/Iron Drops
Vi-Daylin® ADC Drops
Vi-Daylin® ADC/Fluoride Drops
Vi-Daylin® ADC Plus Iron Drops
Vi-Daylin® Drops
Vi-Daylin®/Fluoride Drops
Vi-Daylin® Plus Iron Drops
Vitalize®

Miscellaneous

Altace™ Capsules
Bicitra® Solution
Colestid® Granules
Digoxin® Elixir (Roxane)
Lipomul®
Lithium Citrate Syrup
Nicorette® Chewing Gum
Polycitra®-K Solution
Polycitra®-LC Solution
Tagamet® Liquid

References

Hill EM, Flaitz CM, and Frost GR, "Sweetener Content of Common Pediatric Oral Liquid Medications," *Am J Hosp Pharm*, 1988, 45:135-42.

Kumar A, Rawlings RD, and Beaman DC, "The Mystery Ingredients: Sweeteners, Flavorings, Dyes, and Preservatives in Analgesic/Antipyretic, Antihistamine/Decongestant, Cough and Cold, Antidiarrheal, and Liquid Theophylline Preparations," *Pediatrics*, 1993, 91:927-33.

"Sugar Free Products," *Drug Topics Red Book*, 1992, 17-8.

CARBOHYDRATE CONTENT OF MEDICATIONS

Description (Brand Name)	Dosage Unit	Grams Carbohydrate per Dosage Unit
Analgesics / Antipyretics		
Acetaminophen extended release caplets (Tylenol®)	650 mg	<0.03
Acetaminophen extra strength caplets (Tylenol®)	500 mg	<0.05
Acetaminophen extra strength gel caps (Tylenol®)	500 mg	<0.05
Acetaminophen infant drops (grape and cherry) (Tylenol®)	0.8 mL	<0.71
Acetaminophen liquid suspension cherry) (Tylenol®)	160 mg/5 mL	<5
Acetaminophen regular strength caplets (Tylenol®)	325 mg	<0.04
Acetaminophen elixir (Tylenol®)	160 mg/5 mL	<1.6
Acetaminophen extra strength liquid (Tylenol®)	1000 mg/30 mL	<5.7
Acetaminophen junior strength swallowable caplets (Tylenol®)	160 mg	<0.4
Acetaminophen grape flavored suspension (Tylenol®)	160 mg/5 mL	<4.8
Acetaminophen elixir with codeine (Tylenol® With Codeine) *0.35 g ethyl alcohol/5 mL	120 mg/5 mL	3
Acetaminophen with codeine tablets (Tylenol® With Codeine)	All strengths	0.05
Acetaminophen chewable tablets (Tylenol®)	80 mg	0.25
Effervescent flavored antacid and pain reliever (Alka-Selzer®)	325 mg	0.01
Ibuprofen tablets (Advil®)	200 mg	0.23
Ibuprofen drops (Motrin®)	40 mg/mL	<0.41
Ibuprofen suspension (Motrin®)	100 mg/5 mL	<0.63
Ibuprofen chewable tablets (Motrin®)	50 mg	<0.28
Ibuprofen chewable tablets (Motrin®)	100 mg	<0.54
Antibiotics		
Amoxicillin pediatric drops (Amoxil®)	50 mg/mL	1.6
Amoxicillin oral suspension (Amoxil®)	125 mg/5 mL	1.7
Amoxicillin oral suspension (Amoxil®)	250 mg/5 mL	1.85
Amoxicillin chewable tablets (Amoxil®)	125 mg	0.05
Amoxicillin chewable tablets (Amoxil®)	250 mg	0.34

CARBOHYDRATE CONTENT OF MEDICATIONS *(Continued)*

Description (Brand Name)	Dosage Unit	Grams Carbohydrate per Dosage Unit
Amoxicillin capsules (Amoxil®)	250 mg	0
Amoxicillin capsules (Amoxil®)	500 mg	0
Amoxicillin oral suspension (Trimox®)	125 mg/5 mL	3.3
Amoxicillin oral suspension (Trimox®)	250 mg/5 mL	3.3
Amoxicillin capsules (Trimox®)	250 mg	0
Amoxicillin capsules (Trimox®)	500 mg	0
Amoxicillin/clavulanate potassium oral suspension (Augmentin®)	125 mg/5 mL	0.52
Amoxicillin/clavulanate potassium oral suspension (Augmentin®)	200 mg/5 mL	0.06
Amoxicillin/clavulanate potassium oral suspension (Augmentin®)	250 mg/5 mL	0.6
Amoxicillin/clavulanate potassium oral suspension (Augmentin®)	400 mg/5 mL	0.06
Amoxicillin/clavulanate potassium chewable tablets (Augmentin®)	125 mg	0.08
Amoxicillin/clavulanate potassium chewable tablets (Augmentin®)	250 mg	0.34
Amoxicillin/clavulanate potassium chewable tablets (Augmentin®)	400 mg	0.36
Amoxicillin/clavulanate potassium tablets (Augmentin®)	250 mg	0.02
Amoxicillin/clavulanate potassium tablets (Augmentin®)	500 mg	0.02
Amoxicillin/clavulanate potassium tablets (Augmentin®)	875 mg	0.03
Ampicillin oral suspension (Omnipen®)	125 mg/5 mL	4
Ampicillin oral suspension (Omnipen®)	250 mg/5 mL	4
Azithromycin oral suspension (Zithromax®)	100 mg/5 mL	3.86
Azithromycin tablets (Zithromax®)	250 mg	0.06
Cefaclor oral suspension (Ceclor®)	125 mg/5 mL	2.95
Cefaclor oral suspension (Ceclor®)	187 mg/5 mL	2.83
Cefaclor oral suspension (Ceclor®)	250 mg/5 mL	2.83
Cefaclor oral suspension (Ceclor®)	375 mg/5 mL	2.6
Cefaclor pulvules (Ceclor®)	250 mg	0.04
Cefaclor pulvules (Ceclor®)	500 mg	0.07
Cefadroxil oral suspension (Duricef®)	250 mg/5 mL	3
Cefadroxil oral suspension (Duricef®)	125 mg/5 mL	3.1
Cefadroxil capsules (Duricef®)	500 mg	0.13

Description (Brand Name)	Dosage Unit	Grams Carbohydrate per Dosage Unit
Cefadroxil film-coated tablets (Duricef®)	1 g	0.13
Cefixime oral suspension (Suprax®)	100 mg/5 mL	2.7
Cefixime tablets (Suprax®)	200 mg	0.06
Cefixime tablets (Suprax®)	400 mg	0.12
Cefpodoxime proxetil oral suspension (Vantin®)	50 mg/5 mL	3
Cefpodoxime proxetil oral suspension (Vantin®)	100 mg/5 mL	3.05
Cefpodoxime proxetil tablets (Vantin®)	100 mg	0.04
Cefpodoxime proxetil tablets (Vantin®)	200 mg	0.08
Cefprozil oral suspension (Cefzil®)	125 mg/5 mL	2
Cefprozil oral suspension (Cefzil®)	250 mg/5 mL	1.9
Cefprozil tablets (Cefzil®)	250 mg	0.02
Cefprozil tablets (Cefzil®)	500 mg	0.03
Cefuroxime axetil suspension (Ceftin®)	125 mg/5 mL	3.23
Cefuroxime axetil tablets (Ceftin®)	125 mg	0
Cefuroxime axetil tablets (Ceftin®)	250 mg	0
Cefuroxime axetil tablets (Ceftin®)	500 mg	0
Cephalexin oral suspension (Keflex®)	125 mg/5 mL	3.13
Cephalexin oral suspension (Keflex®)	250 mg/5 mL	3.03
Cephalexin pulvules (Keflex®)	250 mg	0.13
Cephalexin pulvules (Keflex®)	500 mg	0.13
Ciprofloxacin tablets (Cipro®)	250 mg	0.04
Ciprofloxacin tablets (Cipro®)	500 mg	0.07
Ciprofloxacin tablets (Cipro®)	750 mg	0.11
Ciprofloxacin oral suspension (Cipro®)	250 mg/5 mL	1.4
Ciprofloxacin oral suspension (Cipro®)	500 mg/5 mL	1.3
Clarithromycin suspension (Biaxin®)	125 mg/5 mL	3
Clarithromycin suspension (Biaxin®)	250 mg/5 mL	2.3
Clarithromycin tablets (Biaxin®)	250 mg	0.07
Clarithromycin tablets (Biaxin®)	500 mg	0
Erythromycin base tablets (Ery-Tab®)	333 mg	0
Erythromycin base tablets (Ery-Tab®)	500 mg	0
Erythromycin estolate oral suspension (Ilosone®)	125 mg/5 mL	1.85
Erythromycin estolate oral suspension (Ilosone®)	250 mg/5 mL	1.8

CARBOHYDRATE CONTENT OF MEDICATIONS *(Continued)*

Description (Brand Name)	Dosage Unit	Grams Carbohydrate per Dosage Unit
Erythromycin estolate pulvules (Ilosone®)	250 mg	0
Erythromycin estolate tablets (Ilosone®)	500 mg	0.11
Erythromycin ethylsuccinate drops (EryPed®)	10 mg/2.5 mL	1.5
Erythromycin ethylsuccinate chewable tablets (EryPed®)	200 mg	1.44
Erythromycin ethylsuccinate suspension (E.E.S.®)	200 mg/5 mL	3.5
Erythromycin ethylsuccinate suspension (E.E.S.®)	400 mg/5 mL	3.5
Erythromycin ethylsuccinate granules (E.E.S.®)	200 mg/5 mL	1.5
Erythromycin ethylsuccinate filmtabs (E.E.S.®)	400 mg	0.2
Erythromycin ethyl + sulfisoxazole acetyl suspension (Pediazole®)	200 mg/5 mL	1.9
Erythromycin ethyl + sulfisoxazole acetyl suspension (Pediazole®)	600 mg/5 mL	1.9
Loracarbef oral suspension (Lorabid®)	100 mg/5 mL	3.15
Loracarbef oral suspension (Lorabid®)	200 mg/5 mL	3.03
Loracarbef pulvules (Lorabid®)	200 mg	0.22
Loracarbef pulvules (Lorabid®)	400 mg	0.11
Nitrofurantoin oral suspension (Furadantin®)	25 mg/5 mL	0.7
Penicillin V potassium oral suspension	125 mg/5 mL	2.53
Penicillin V potassium oral suspension	250 mg/5 mL	3.28
Penicillin V potassium tablets	250 mg	0.09
Penicillin V potassium tablets	500 mg	0
Trimethoprim (TMP) and sulfamethoxazole (SMX) suspension (Septra®)	40 mg TMP/200 mg SMX/5 mL	2.35
Trimethoprim (TMP) and sulfamethoxazole (SMX) grape suspension (Septra®)	40 mg TMP/200 mg SMX/5 mL	2.35
Trimethoprim (TMP) and sulfamethoxazole (SMX) tablets (Septra®)	80 mg TMP/400 mg SMX/5 mL	0

Description (Brand Name)	Dosage Unit	Grams Carbohydrate per Dosage Unit
Trimethoprim (TMP) and sulfamethoxazole (SMX) double strength tablets (Septra®)	160 mg TMP/800 mg SMX/5 mL	0
Antiepileptic Drugs		
Carbamazepine suspension (Tegretol®)	100 mg/5 mL	2.65
Carbamazepine chewable tablets (Tegretol®)	100 mg	0.28
Carbamazepine tablets (Tegretol®)	200 mg	0.06
Clonazepam tablets (Klonopin®)	0.5 mg	0.14
Clonazepam tablets (Klonopin®)	1 mg	0.14
Clonazepam tablets (Klonopin®)	2 mg	0.14
Ethosuximide syrup (Zarontin®)	250 mg/5 mL	3.63
Ethosuximide capsules (Zarontin®)	250 mg	0.13
Felbamate solution (Felbatol®)	600 mg/5 mL	1.5
Felbamate tablets (Felbatol®)	400 mg	0.13
Felbamate tablets (Felbatol®)	600 mg	0.19
Gabapentin tablets (Neurontin®)	100 mg	0.03
Gabapentin tablets (Neurontin®)	300 mg	0.07
Gabapentin tablets (Neurontin®)	400 mg	0.1
Lamotrigine tablets (Lamictal®)	25 mg	0.03
Lamotrigine tablets (Lamictal®)	100 mg	0.11
Lamotrigine tablets (Lamictal®)	150 mg	0.16
Lamotrigine tablets (Lamictal®)	200 mg	0.14
Lamotrigine chewable/dispersible tablets (Lamictal®)	5 mg	0
Lamotrigine chewable/dispersible tablets (Lamictal®)	25 mg	0
Phenobarbital elixir *0.71 g ethyl alcohol/5 mL	20 mg/5 mL	3.4
Phenobarbital tablets	15 mg	0.06
Phenobarbital tablets	30 mg	0.07
Phenobarbital tablets	60 mg	0.1
Phenytoin suspension (Dilantin®)	125 mg/5 mL	1.39
Phenytoin infatabs (Dilantin®)	50 mg	0.48
Phenytoin kapseal (Dilantin®)	30 mg	0.15
Phenytoin kapseal (Dilantin®)	100 mg	0.11
Primidone oral suspension (Mysoline®)	250 mg/5 mL	0
Primidone tablets (Mysoline®)	50 mg	0.03
Primidone tablets (Mysoline®)	250 mg	0.03
Sodium divalproex sprinkle capsules (Depakote®)	125 mg	0.05

CARBOHYDRATE CONTENT OF MEDICATIONS *(Continued)*

Description (Brand Name)	Dosage Unit	Grams Carbohydrate per Dosage Unit
Sodium divalproex tablets (Depakote®)	125 mg	0.03
Sodium divalproex tablets (Depakote®)	250 mg	0.05
Sodium divalproex tablets (Depakote®)	500 mg	0.1
Tiagabine tablets (Gabitril®)	4 mg	0.05
Tiagabine tablets (Gabitril®)	12 mg	0.14
Tiagabine tablets (Gabitril®)	16 mg	0.19
Tiagabine tablets (Gabitril®)	20 mg	0.23
Topiramate tablets (Topamax®)	25 mg	0.04
Topiramate tablets (Topamax®)	100 mg	0.17
Topiramate tablets (Topamax®)	200 mg	0.09
Valproic acid syrup (Depakene®)	250 mg/5 mL	4.5
Valproic acid capsules (Depakene®)	250 mg	0
Antifungals		
Fluconazole oral suspension (Diflucan®)	10 mg/mL	2.88
Fluconazole oral suspension (Diflucan®)	40 mg/mL	2.73
Fluconazole tablets (Diflucan®)	50 mg and 100 mg	0
Nystatin oral suspension	100,000 units/mL	0.61
Nystatin oral suspension (Mycostatin®)	100,000 units/mL	0.60
Nystatin tablets (Mycostatin®)	500,000 units	0.11
Antihistamines		
Cetirizine syrup (Zyrtec®)	5 mg/5 mL	3
Cetirizine tablets (Zyrtec®)	5 mg	0.08
Cetirizine tablets (Zyrtec®)	10 mg	0.16
Diphenhydramine elixir (Benadryl®)	5 mL	1.5
Hydroxyzine syrup (Atarax®)	10 mg/5 mL	5.88
Hydroxyzine tablets (Atarax®)	10 mg	0.04
Hydroxyzine tablets (Atarax®)	25 mg	0.05
Hydroxyzine tablets (Atarax®)	50 mg	0.07
Hydroxyzine tablets (Atarax®)	100 mg	0.1
Hydroxyzine suspension (Vistaril®)	25 mg/5 mL	5.83
Hydroxyzine capsules (Vistaril®)	25 mg	0.03
Hydroxyzine capsules (Vistaril®)	50 mg	0.07
Hydroxyzine capsules (Vistaril®)	100 mg	0.11

Description (Brand Name)	Dosage Unit	Grams Carbohydrate per Dosage Unit
Antinausea Medications		
Dimenhydrinate chewable tablets (Dramamine®)	50 mg	<0.5
Meclizine tablets (Dramamine II®)	25 mg	<0.25
Antivirals		
Acyclovir suspension (Zovirax®) *1.75 g of sorbitol	200 mg/5 mL	0
Acyclovir tablets (Zovirax®)	400 mg	0.02
Acyclovir capsules (Zovirax®)	200 mg	0.21
Zidovudine syrup (Retrovir®)	50 mg/5 mL	2.15
Zidovudine tablets (Retrovir®)	300 mg	0.02
Zidovudine capsules (Retrovir®)	100 mg	0.09
Cough and Cold Preparations		
Brompheniramine pseudoephedrine tablets (Dristan® Allergy)	4 mg 60 mg	0
Chlorpheniramine phenylpropanolamine chewable tablets (Allerest® Children's)	1 mg 9.4 mg	0.25
Chlorpheniramine phenylpropanolamine dextromethorphan aspirin effervescent tablets (Alka-Selzer Plus® Cold and Cough)	2 mg 10 mg 20 mg 325 mg	0.01
Chlorpheniramine phenylephrine dextromethorphan syrup	4 mg/5 mL 10 mg/5 mL 15 mg/5 mL	3.6
Dextromethorphan guaifenesin syrup (Robitussin® DM) *2.24 g sorbitol/5 mL	10 mg/5 mL 100 mg/5 mL	0
Dextromethorphan pseudoephedrine syrup (Robitussin® Pediatric Cough and Cold)	7.5 mg/5 mL 15 mg/5 mL	1.35
Triprolidine pseudoephedrine syrup (Actifed®)	1.25 mg/5 mL 30 mg/5 mL	5
Decongestant / Nasal Preparations		
Oxymetazoline nasal spray	0.05%	0
Phenylephrine (Neo-Synephrine® Pediatric Formula Nasal Drops)	0.125%	0
Xylometazoline (Otrivin® Pediatric Nasal Drops)	0.05%	0
Fluoride		
Sodium fluoride (Luride® Drops (peach flavor)	0.5 mg/mL (fluoride ion)	0.7

CARBOHYDRATE CONTENT OF MEDICATIONS *(Continued)*

Description (Brand Name)	Dosage Unit	Grams Carbohydrate per Dosage Unit
Laxatives		
Docusate sodium sorbitol glycerin capsules (Correctol® Extra Gentle Stool Softener)	100 mg	0.13
Docusate sodium liquigels (Surfak®)	240 mg	0.37
Docusate sodium syrup	20 mg/5 mL	1.4
Glycerin suppositories	82.5% glycerin/1.35 g	1.11
Magnesium hydroxide in purified water and mineral oil	300 mg/5 mL	0
Magnesium hydroxide (Phillips'® MOM Mint)	40 mEq elem mg/15 mL	0
Mono and dibesic sodium phosphate enema (Fleets®)	Enema	0
Senna children's syrup (Senokot® Children's)	5 mL	3.3
Senna syrup (Senokot®)	5 mL	3.3
Senna granules (Senokot®)	Teaspoonful	2
Senna tablets (Senokot®)	Tablet	0.03
Senna tablets (Senokot-S®)	Tablet	0.05
Senna tablets (SenokotXTRA®)	Tablet	0.08
Multiple Vitamin and Mineral Supplements		
Multiple vitamin and mineral supplement (Bugs Bunny Complete)	Chewable tablet (sugar free)	0.37
Multiple vitamin and mineral supplement (Bugs Bunny Plus Iron)	Chewable tablet	0.47
Multiple vitamin and mineral supplement (Bugs Bunny With Extra C)	Chewable tablet	0.32
Multiple vitamin and mineral supplement (Centrum® Advanced Formula Liquid)	15 mL	6.25
Multiple vitamin and mineral supplement (Centrum® Advanced Formula Tablets)	Tablet	0.25
Multiple vitamin and mineral supplement (Centrum® Kids Rugrats™ Extra Calcium)	Chewable tablet	<0.5
Multiple vitamin and mineral supplement (Centrum® Kids Rugrats™ Extra C)	Chewable tablet	<0.5
Multiple vitamin and mineral supplement (Centrum® Kids Rugrats™ Complete)	Chewable tablet	<0.5

Description (Brand Name)	Dosage Unit	Grams Carbohydrate per Dosage Unit
Multiple vitamin and mineral supplement (Flinstones® Plus Extra C)	Chewable tablet	<0.6
Multiple vitamin and mineral supplement (Flinstones® Plus Iron)	Chewable tablet	0.65
Multiple vitamin and mineral supplement (Flinstones® Plus Calcium)	Chewable tablet	0.11
Multiple vitamin and mineral supplement (Flinstones® Original)	Chewable tablet	0.70
Multiple vitamin and mineral supplement (Flinstones® Complete)	Chewable tablet (sugar free)	0.37
Multiple vitamin and mineral supplement (Unicap®)	Tablet	0.25
Multiple vitamin and mineral supplement (Unicap®)	Capsule	0.25
Calcium Containing Vitamin Products		
Calcium carbonate capsules (Calci-Mix®)	1250 mg	0
Calcium carbonate tablets (Caltrate® 600)	1500 mg	0.25
Calcium citrate capsules (Citracal®)	2,376 mg	0
Calcium carbonate tablets	640 mg	0.05
Calcium carbonate, iron, vitamin D tablets (Caltrate® 600 + Iron and Vitamin D)	1500 mg	0.25
Calcium carbonate gelcap (Liqui-Cal®)	600 mg	0.16
Calcium carbonate suspension	1250 mg/5 mL	1.75
Calcium citrate + magnesium gelcap	Gelcap	0.15
Calcium citrate, vitamin D, vitamin A tablets (Nutravescent®)	250 mg	0.07
Calcium, elemental (Calcet®)	Tablet	0.07
Calcium-iron multivitamin (Calcet® Plus)	Tablet	0.07
Calcium citrate (Citracal®)	950 mg	0
Iron-Containing Vitamin Products		
Ferrous fumarate (Ferro-Sequels®)	Capsule	0.5
Ferrous sulfate drops (Fer-In-Sol®)	75 mg/0.6 mL	0.7
Ferrous sulfate syrup (Fer-In-Sol®)	90 mg/5 mL	6.25
Iron, vitamin B, vitamin D drops (Poly-Vi-Sol® With Iron)	10 mg/mL	0.63
Iron, vitamins A, D, E, C drops (Vi-Daylin® + Iron Drops)	20 mg/mL	0.75
Iron, vitamins A, D, E, C liquid (Vi-Daylin® Liquid With Iron)	10 mg/5 mL	5

CARBOHYDRATE CONTENT OF MEDICATIONS *(Continued)*

Description (Brand Name)	Dosage Unit	Grams Carbohydrate per Dosage Unit
Iron, vitamins A, D, E, C, folic acid chewable tablets (Vi-Daylin® Chewable With Iron)	12 mg 0.3 mg	0.43
Miscellaneous		
Aminocaproic acid syrup (Amicar®)	250 mg/mL	0.26
Calcium carbonate tablets (Mylanta® Children's Chewables)	400 mg	0.93
Calcium carbonate suspension (Mylanta® Children's Suspension)	400 mg/5 mL	1.5
Calcium carbonate tablets (Tums® Regular)	500 mg	0.75
Calcium carbonate tablets (Tums® 500)	1250 mg	1.9
Calcium carbonate extra strength tablets (Tums® E-X)	750 mg	1.1
Calcium carbonate ultra tablets (Tums® Ultra)	1000 mg	1.5
Calcium carbonate sugar free extra strength tablets (Tums® Extra Strength Sugar Free)	750 mg	0.5
Carnitine solution (Carnitor®)	1 g/10 mL	0.48
Chloral hydrate	500 mg/5 mL	3
Chlorothiazide suspension (Diuril®) *0.025 ethyl alcohol/5 mL	250 mg/5 mL	2
Cimetidine tablets (Tagamet®)	200 mg	0.01
Cimetidine tablets (Tagamet®)	300 mg	0.01
Cimetidine tablets (Tagamet®)	400 mg	0.01
Cimetidine tablets (Tagamet®)	800 mg	0.02
Cimetidine liquid (Tagamet®) *0.5 ethyl alcohol/5 mL	300 mg/5 mL	2.8
Citalopram solution (Celexa™)	10 mg/5 mL	2.5
Clindamycin solution (Cleocin®)	75 mg/5 mL	1.89
Clonidine tablets (Catapres®)	0.1 mg	0.12
Clonidine tablets (Catapres®)	0.2 mg	0.11
Clonidine tablets (Catapres®)	0.3 mg	0.16
Cyclosporine oral suspension (Neoral®)	100 mg/mL	0
Cyclosporine capsules (Neoral®)	25 mg	0.01
Cyclosporine capsules (Neoral®)	100 mg	0.04
Cyclosporine oral suspension (Sandimmune®) *0.12 ethyl alcohol/mL	100 mg/mL	0

Description (Brand Name)	Dosage Unit	Grams Carbohydrate per Dosage Unit
Cyclosporine capsules (Sandimmune®)	25 mg	0
Cyclosporine capsules (Sandimmune®)	50 mg	0.01
Cyclosporine capsules (Sandimmune®)	100 mg	0
Dexamethasone oral solution (Dexamethasone Intensol®) *0.3 ethyl alcohol/mL	0.5 mg/5 mL 1 mg/mL	1.7 0
Diazepam oral solution	5 mg/5 mL	1
Digoxin pediatric elixir (Lanoxin®) *0.1 ethyl alcohol/mL	0.05 mg/mL	0.3
Digoxin tablets (Lanoxin®)	0.25 mg	0.10
Digoxin tablets (Lanoxin®)	0.125 mg	0.09
Famotidine oral suspension (Pepcid®)	40 mg/5 mL	1.19
Famotidine tablets (Pepcid®)	20 mg	0.09
Famotidine tablets (Pepcid®)	40 mg	0.08
Fluoxetine liquid (Prozac®)	20 mg/5 mL	1
Fluoxetine capsules (Prozac®)	10 mg	0.22
Fluoxetine capsules (Prozac®)	20 mg	0.21
Furosemide tablets (Lasix®)	20 mg	0.06
Furosemide tablets (Lasix®)	40 mg	0.11
Furosemide tablets (Lasix®)	80 mg	0.22
Furosemide elixir (Lasix®)	10 mg/mL	0.8
Glycopyrrolate tablets (Robinul®)	1 mg	0.1
Glycopyrrolate tablets (Robinul®)	2 mg	0.18
Loperamide (Imodium® A-D) *0.26 ethyl alcohol/5 mL	1 mg/5 mL	4.13
Megaldrate, simethicone suspension (Riopan Plus®)	5 mL	0.37
Magnesium hydroxide, aluminum hydroxide, simethicone (Mylanta®)	Tablet – regular strength	0.49
Magnesium hydroxide, aluminum hydroxide, simethicone (Mylanta®)	Tablet – double strength	0.83
Magnesium carbonate, calcium carbonate (Mylanta®)	Gel capsule	0
Magnesium hydroxide, aluminum hydroxide, simethicone (different flavors available) (Mylanta®)	Liquid – regular strength, 5 mL	0.67
Magnesium hydroxide, aluminum hydroxide, simethicone (Mylanta®)	Liquid – double strength, 5 mL	0.67
Mesalamine capsules (Pentasa®)	250 mg	0.23
Metoclopramide syrup (Reglan®)	5 mg/5 mL	1.75

CARBOHYDRATE CONTENT OF MEDICATIONS *(Continued)*

Description (Brand Name)	Dosage Unit	Grams Carbohydrate per Dosage Unit
Metoclopramide tablets (Reglan®)	5 mg	0.11
Metoclopramide tablets (Reglan®)	10 mg	0.10
Nifedipine capsules (Procardia®)	10 mg	0.10
Nifedipine capsules (Procardia®)	20 mg	0.12
Potassium chloride (Rum-K®)	10 mEq/5 mL	2.26
Potassium chloride 10% *0.25 ethyl alcohol/5 mL	6.67 mEq/5 mL	0.25
Potassium chloride (Kaochlor® SF) *0.25 ethyl alcohol/5 mL	6.67 mEq/5 mL	0
Potassium citrate/sodium citrate (Polycitra®)		0
Prednisolone syrup (Prelone®)	5 mg/5 mL	2.01
Prednisolone syrup (Prelone®)	15 mg/5 mL	3.55
Prednisolone oral solution (Pediapred®)	5 mg/5 mL	1.53
Prednisone oral solution *0.25 ethyl alcohol/5 mL	5 mg/5 mL	1.8
Ranitidine syrup (Zantac®)	150 mg/10 mL	1
Ranitidine efferdose granules (Zantac®)	150 mg/packet	0
Ranitidine efferdose tablets (Zantac®)	150 mg	0
Ranitidine tablets (Zantac®)	All strengths	0
Simethicone drops (Mylicon®)	40 mg/0.6 mL	<0.071
Theophylline elixir (Elixophyllin®) *0.86 ethyl alcohol/5 mL	26.67 mg/5 mL	0.31
Vitamin D drops (Drisdol®)	8000 units/mL	0
Vitamin E drops (Aquasol E®)	15 units/0.3 mL	0.06

References

Adapted from Feldstein TJ, "Carbohydrate and Alcohol Content of 200 Oral Liquid Medications for Use in Patients Receiving Ketogenic Diets," *Pediatrics*, 1996, 97:506-11.

Adapted from McGhee B and Katyal N, "Avoid Unnecessary Drug-Related Carbohydrates for Patients Consuming the Ketogenic Diet," *J Am Diet Assoc*, 2001, 101(1):87-101.

ORAL MEDICATIONS THAT SHOULD NOT BE CRUSHED OR ALTERED

There are a variety of reasons for crushing tablets or capsule contents prior to administering to the patient. Patients may have nasogastric tubes which do not permit the administration of tablets or capsules; an oral solution for a particular medication may not be available from the manufacturer or readily prepared by pharmacy; patients may have difficulty swallowing capsules or tablets; or mixing of powdered medication with food or drink may make the drug more palatable.

Generally, medications which should not be crushed fall into one of the following categories.

- **Extended-Release Products**. The formulation of some tablets is specialized as to allow the medication within it to be slowly released into the body. This is sometimes accomplished by centering the drug within the core of the tablet, with a subsequent shedding of multiple layers around the core. Wax melts in the GI tract. Slow-K® is an example of this. Capsules may contain beads which have multiple layers which are slowly dissolved with time.

  Common Abbreviations for Extended-Release Products

CD	Controlled dose
CR	Controlled release
CRT	Controlled-release tablet
LA	Long-acting
SR	Sustained release
TR	Timed release
TD	Time delay
SA	Sustained action
XL	Extended release
XR	Extended release

- **Medications Which Are Irritating to the Stomach**. Tablets which are irritating to the stomach may be enteric-coated which delays release of the drug until the time when it reaches the small intestine. Enteric-coated aspirin is an example of this.
- **Foul-Tasting Medication**. Some drugs are quite unpleasant to taste so the manufacturer coats the tablet in a sugar coating to increase its palatability. By crushing the tablet, this sugar coating is lost and the patient tastes the unpleasant tasting medication.
- **Sublingual Medication**. Medication intended for use under the tongue should not be crushed. While it appears to be obvious, it is not always easy to determine if a medication is to be used sublingually. Sublingual medications should indicate on the package that they are intended for sublingual use.
- **Effervescent Tablets**. These are tablets which, when dropped into a liquid, quickly dissolve to yield a solution. Many effervescent tablets, when crushed, lose their ability to quickly dissolve.

Recommendations

1. It is not advisable to crush certain medications.
2. Consult individual monographs prior to crushing capsule or tablet.
3. If crushing a tablet or capsule is contraindicated, consult with your pharmacist to determine whether an oral solution exists or can be compounded.

ORAL MEDICATIONS THAT SHOULD NOT BE CRUSHED OR ALTERED *(Continued)*

Drug Product	Dosage Form	Dosage Reasons / Comments
Accuhist®	Tablet	Slow release[8]
Accutane®	Capsule	Mucous membrane irritant
Aciphex™	Tablet	Slow release
Adalat® CC	Tablet	Slow release
Adderall XR™	Capsule	Slow release[1]
Advicor®	Tablet	Slow release
Afeditab™ CR	Tablet	Slow release
Aggrenox®	Capsule	Slow release **Note:** Capsule may be opened; contents include an aspirin tablet that may be chewed and dipyridamole pellets that may be sprinkled on applesauce
Alavert™ Allergy Sinus 12 Hour	Tablet	Slow release
Allegra-D®	Tablet	Slow release
Altocor™	Tablet	Slow release
Arthritis Bayer® Time Release	Capsule	Slow release
Arthrotec®	Tablet	Enteric-coated
A.S.A.® Enseals®	Tablet	Enteric-coated
Asacol®	Tablet	Slow release
Ascriptin® A/D	Tablet	Enteric-coated
Ascriptin® Extra Strength	Tablet	Enteric-coated
Augmentin XR™	Tablet	Slow release[2, 8]
Avinza™	Capsule	Slow release[1] (not pudding)
Avodart™	Capsule	Teratogenic potential[9]
Azulfidine® EN-tabs®	Tablet	Enteric-coated
Bayer® Aspirin EC	Caplet	Enteric-coated
Bayer® Aspirin, Low Adult 81 mg	Tablet	Enteric-coated
Bayer® Aspirin, Regular Strength 325 mg	Caplet	Enteric-coated
Biaxin® XL	Tablet	Slow release
Biltricide®	Tablet	Taste[8]
Bisacodyl	Tablet	Enteric-coated[3]
Bontril® Slow-Release	Capsule	Slow release
Calan® SR	Tablet	Slow release[8]
Carbatrol®	Capsule	Slow release[1]
Cardene® SR	Capsule	Slow release
Cardizem®	Tablet	Slow release
Cardizem® CD	Capsule	Slow release[1]
Cardizem® LA	Tablet	Slow release
Cardizem® SR	Capsule	Slow release[1]
Carter's Little Pills®	Tablet	Enteric-coated
Cartia® XT	Capsule	Slow release
Ceclor® CD	Tablet	Slow release
Ceftin®	Tablet	Taste[8] **Note:** Use suspension for children
CellCept®	Capsule, tablet	Teratogenic potential[9]

Drug Product	Dosage Form	Dosage Reasons / Comments
Charcoal Plus®	Tablet	Enteric-coated
Chloral Hydrate	Capsule	**Note:** Product is in liquid form within a special capsule[2]
Chlor-Trimeton® 12-Hour	Tablet	Slow release[2]
Cipro™	Tablet	Taste[5]
Cipro® XR	Tablet	Slow release
Claritin-D® 12-Hour	Tablet	Slow release
Claritin-D® 24-Hour	Tablet	Slow release
Colace®	Capsule	Taste[5]
Colestid®	Tablet	Slow release
Comhist® LA	Capsule	Slow release[1]
Commit™	Lozenge	**Note:** Integrity compromised by chewing or crushing
Compazine® Spansule®	Capsule	Slow release[2]
Concerta®	Tablet	Slow release
Contac® 12-Hour	Tablet	Slow release
Cotazym-S®	Capsule	Enteric-coated[1]
Covera-HS™	Tablet	Slow release
Creon® 5, 10, 20	Capsule	Slow release[1]
Crixivan®	Capsule	Taste **Note:** Capsule may be opened and mixed with fruit puree (eg, banana)
Cytovene®	Capsule	Skin irritant
Cytoxan®	Tablet	**Note:** Drug may be crushed, but maker recommends using injection
Dallergy®	Capsule	Slow release
Dallergy-JR®	Capsule	Slow release
Deconamine® SR	Capsule	Slow release[2]
Defen L.A.®	Tablet	Slow release[8]
Depakene®	Capsule	Slow release mucous membrane irritant[2]
Depakote®	Tablet	Slow release
Depakote® ER	Tablet	Slow release
Desoxyn®	Tablet	Slow release
Desyrel®	Tablet	Taste[5]
Detrol® LA	Capsule	Slow release
Dexedrine® Spansule®	Capsule	Slow release
Diamox® Sequels®	Capsule	Slow release
Dilacor® XR	Capsule	Slow release
Dilatrate-SR®	Capsule	Slow release
Diltia XT®	Capsule	Slow release
Ditropan® XL	Tablet	Slow release
Dolobid®	Tablet	Irritant
Donnatal® Extentab®	Tablet	Slow release[2]
Drisdol®	Capsule	Liquid filled[4]
Drixoral®	Tablet	Slow release[2]
Drixoral® Plus	Tablet	Slow release
Drixoral® Sinus	Tablet	Slow release

ORAL MEDICATIONS THAT SHOULD NOT BE CRUSHED OR ALTERED *(Continued)*

Drug Product	Dosage Form	Dosage Reasons / Comments
Dulcolax®	Capsule	Liquid-filled
Dulcolax®	Tablet	Enteric-coated[3]
Duratuss® G	Tablet	Slow release[9]
Duratuss® GP	Tablet	Slow release[8]
Dynabac®	Tablet	Enteric-coated
DynaCirc® CR	Tablet	Slow release
Easprin®	Tablet	Enteric-coated
EC-Naprosyn®	Tablet	Enteric-coated
Ecotrin® Adult Low Strength	Tablet	Enteric-coated
Ecotrin® Maximum Strength	Tablet	Enteric-coated
Ecotrin® Regular Strength	Tablet	Enteric-coated
E.E.S.® 400	Tablet	Enteric-coated[2]
Effexor® XR	Capsule	Slow release
Efidac/24® Pseudoephedrine	Tablet	Slow release
Efidac® 24	Tablet	Slow release
E-Mycin®	Tablet	Enteric-coated
Entex® LA	Capsule	Slow release[2]
Entex® PSE	Capsule	Slow release
Entocort™ EC	Capsule	Enteric-coated[1]
Ergomar®	Tablet	Sublingual form[7]
Eryc®	Capsule	Enteric-coated[1]
Ery-Tab®	Tablet	Enteric-coated
Erythrocin Stearate	Tablet	Enteric-coated
Erythromycin Base	Tablet	Enteric-coated
Eskalith CR®	Tablet	Slow release
Evista®	Tablet	Taste; teratogenic potential[9]
Extendryl JR	Capsule	Slow release
Extendryl SR	Capsule	Slow release[2]
Feldene®	Capsule	Mucous membrane irritant
Feosol®	Tablet	Enteric-coated[2]
Feratab®	Tablet	Enteric-coated[2]
Fergon®	Tablet	Enteric-coated
Fero-Grad 500®	Tablet	Slow release
Ferro-Sequels®	Tablet	Slow release
Flagyl ER®	Tablet	Slow release
Flomax®	Capsule	Enteric-coated[1]
Fosamax®	Tablet	Mucous membrane irritant
Fumatinic®	Capsule	Slow release
Geocillin®	Tablet	Taste
Gleevec®	Tablet	Taste[8] **Note:** May be dissolved in mineral oil or apple juice
Glucophage® XR	Tablet	Slow release
Glucotrol® XL	Tablet	Slow release
Gris-PEG®	Tablet	**Note:** Crushing may result in precipitation of larger particles.

Drug Product	Dosage Form	Dosage Reasons / Comments
Guaifed®	Capsule	Slow release
Guaifed®-PD	Capsule	Slow release
Guaifenex® DM	Tablet	Slow release[8]
Guaifenex® LA	Tablet	Slow release[8]
Guaifenex® PSE	Tablet	Slow release[8]
Guaimax-D®	Tablet	Slow release
Hista-Vent® DA	Tablet	Slow release[8]
Humibid® DM	Tablet	Slow release
Humibid® LA	Tablet	Slow release
Iberet® Filmtab	Tablet	Slow release[2]
Iberet®-500	Tablet	Slow release[2]
Iberet-Folic-500®	Tablet	Slow release
ICAPS® Time Release	Tablet	Slow release
Imdur™	Tablet	Slow release[8]
Inderal® LA	Capsule	Slow release
Inderide® LA	Capsule	Slow release
Indocin® SR	Capsule	Slow release[1,2]
InnoPran XL™	Capsule	Slow release
Ionamin®	Capsule	Slow release
Isoptin® SR	Tablet	Slow release
Isordil® Sublingual	Tablet	Sublingual form[7]
Isosorbide Dinitrate Sublingual	Tablet	Sublingual form[7]
Isosorbide SR	Tablet	Slow release
K+ 8®	Tablet	Slow release[2]
K+ 10®	Tablet	Slow release[2]
Kadian®	Capsule	Slow release[1] **Note:** Do not give via N/G tubes
Kaon-Cl®	Tablet	Slow release[2]
K-Dur®	Tablet	Slow release
Klor-Con®	Tablet	Slow release[2]
Klor-Con® M	Tablet	Slow release[2]
Klotrix®	Tablet	Slow release[2]
K-Lyte®	Tablet	Effervescent tablet[6]
K-Lyte/Cl®	Tablet	Effervescent tablet[6]
K-Lyte DS®	Tablet	Effervescent tablet[6]
K-Tab®	Tablet	Slow release[2]
Lescol® XL	Tablet	Slow release
Levbid®	Tablet	Slow release[8]
Levsinex® Timecaps®	Capsule	Slow release
Lexxel®	Tablet	Slow release
Lipram 4500	Capsule	Enteric-coated[1]
Lipram-CR	Capsule	Enteric-coated[1]
Lipram-PN	Capsule	Enteric-coated[1]
Lipram-UL	Capsule	Enteric-coated[1]
Lipram (all products)	Capsule	Slow release[1]
Liquibid-PD	Tablet	Slow release[8]
Lithobid®	Tablet	Slow release
Lodine® XL	Tablet	Slow release
Lodrane® LD	Capsule	Slow release[1]

ORAL MEDICATIONS THAT SHOULD NOT BE CRUSHED OR ALTERED *(Continued)*

Drug Product	Dosage Form	Dosage Reasons / Comments
Mag-Tab® SR	Tablet	Slow release
Maxifed®	Tablet	Slow release
Maxifed® DM	Tablet	Slow release
Maxifed-G®	Tablet	Slow release
Mestinon® Timespan®	Tablet	Slow release[2]
Metadate® CD	Capsule	Slow release[1]
Metadate™ ER	Tablet	Slow release
Methylin™ ER	Tablet	Slow release
Micro-K®	Capsule	Slow release
Motrin®	Tablet	Taste[5]
MS Contin®	Tablet	Slow release[2]
Mucinex®	Tablet	Slow release
Myfortic®	Tablet	Slow release
Naprelan®	Tablet	Slow release
Nasatab® LA	Tablet	Slow release[8]
Nexium®	Capsule	Slow release[1]
Niaspan®	Tablet	Slow release
Nicotinic Acid	Capsule, tablet	Slow release
Nifediac™ CC	Tablet	Slow release
Nitrostat®	Tablet	Sublingual route[7]
Norflex™	Tablet	Slow release
Norpace® CR	Capsule	Slow release form within a special capsule
Oramorph SR®	Tablet	Slow release[2]
Oruvail®	Capsule	Slow release
OxyContin®	Tablet	Slow release
Palgic®-D	Tablet	Slow release[8]
Pancrease®	Capsule	Enteric-coated[1]
Pancrease® MT	Capsule	Enteric-coated[1]
Pancrecarb MS®	Capsule	Enteric-coated[1]
PanMist®-DM	Tablet	Slow release[8]
PanMist®-Jr	Tablet	Slow release[8]
PanMist®-LA	Tablet	Slow release[8]
Pannaz®	Tablet	Slow release[8]
Papaverine Sustained Action	Capsule	Slow release
Paxil CR™	Tablet	Slow release
Pentasa®	Capsule	Slow release
Perdiem® Fiber Therapy	Granules	Wax coated
PhenaVent™ D	Tablet	Slow release
Plendil®	Tablet	Slow release
Prelu-2®	Capsule	Slow release
Prevacid®	Capsule	Slow release
Prevacid®	Suspension	Slow release **Note:** Contains enteric-coated granules
Prilosec®	Capsule	Slow release

Drug Product	Dosage Form	Dosage Reasons / Comments
Procainamide HCl SR	Tablet	Slow release
Procanbid®	Tablet	Slow release
Procardia®	Capsule	Delays absorption[2, 5]
Procardia XL®	Tablet	Slow release **Note:** AUC is unaffected.
Profen II®	Tablet	Slow release[8]
Profen II DM®	Tablet	Slow release[8]
Profen Forte™ DM	Tablet	Slow release
Pronestyl®-SR	Tablet	Slow release
Propecia®	Tablet	**Note:** Women who are, or may become, pregnant, should not handle crushed or broken tablets
Proscar®	Tablet	**Note:** Women who are, or may become, pregnant, should not handle crushed or broken tablets
Protonix®	Tablet	Slow release
Quibron-T/SR®	Tablet	Slow release[2]
Rescon-Jr	Tablet	Slow release
Respa-DM®	Tablet	Slow release[8]
Respaire®-120 SR	Capsule	Slow release
Ritalin-SR®	Tablet	Slow release
Rondec-TR®	Tablet	Slow release[2]
Rythmol® SR	Capsule	Slow release
Sinemet® CR	Tablet	Slow release
SINUvent® PE	Tablet	Slow release[8]
Slo-Niacin®	Tablet	Slow release[8]
Slow-Mag®	Tablet	Slow release
Somnote™	Capsule	Liquid filled
Sudafed® 12-Hour	Capsule	Slow release[2]
Sular®	Tablet	Slow release
Symax SR	Tablet	Slow release
Taztia XT™	Capsule	Slow release
Tegretol®-XR	Tablet	Slow release
Temodar®	Capsule	**Note:** If capsules are accidentally opened or damaged, rigorous precautions should be taken to avoid inhalation or contact of contents with the skin or mucous membranes[9]
Tessalon®	Capsule	Slow release
Theo-24®	Tablet	Slow release[2]
Theochron®	Tablet	Slow release
Tiazac®	Capsule	Slow release
Topamax®	Capsule	Taste[1]
Topamax®	Tablet	Taste
Touro™ CC	Tablet	Slow release
Touro EX®	Tablet	Slow release
Touro LA®	Tablet	Slow release
Trental®	Tablet	Slow release

ORAL MEDICATIONS THAT SHOULD NOT BE CRUSHED OR ALTERED *(Continued)*

Drug Product	Dosage Form	Dosage Reasons / Comments
TripTone®	Tablet	Slow release
Tylenol® Arthritis Pain	Tablet	Slow release
Tylenol® 8 Hour	Tablet	Slow release
Ultrase®	Capsule	Enteric-coated[1]
Ultrase® MT	Capsule	Enteric-coated[1]
Uniphyl®	Tablet	Slow release
Urocit®-K	Tablet	Wax-coated
Verelan®	Capsule	Slow release[1]
Videx® EC	Capsule	Slow release
Voltaren®-XR	Tablet	Slow release
VoSpire ER™	Tablet	Slow release
Wellbutrin SR®	Tablet	Slow release
Wellbutrin XL™	Tablet	Slow release
Xanax XR®	Tablet	Slow release
Z-Cof LA	Tablet	Slow release[8]
Zephrex LA®	Tablet	Slow release
ZORprin®	Tablet	Slow release
Zyban®	Tablet	Slow release

[1]Capsule may be opened and the contents taken without crushing or chewing; soft food such as applesauce or pudding may facilitate administration; contents may generally be administered via nasogastric tube using an appropriate fluid, provided entire contents are washed down the tube.

[2]Liquid dosage forms of the product are available; however, dose, frequency of administration, and manufacturers may differ from that of the solid dosage form.

[3]Antacids and/or milk may prematurely dissolve the coating of the tablet.

[4]Capsule may be opened and the liquid contents removed for administration.

[5]The taste of this product in a liquid form would likely be unacceptable to the patient; administration via nasogastric tube should be acceptable.

[6]Effervescent tablets must be dissolved in the amount of diluent recommended by the manufacturer.

[7]Tablets are made to disintegrate under the tongue.

[8]Tablet is scored and may be broken in half without affecting release characteristics.

[9]Skin contact may enhance tumor production; avoid direct contact.

Adapted from Mitchell JF, "Oral Dosage Forms That Should Not Be Crushed-2004," available at: www.hospitalpharmacyjournal.com.

NOTES

NOTES

NOTES

NOTES

NOTES

NOTES

NOTES

NOTES

NOTES

Products offered by LEXI-COMP

DRUG INFORMATION HANDBOOK FOR ADVANCED PRACTICE NURSING

by Beatrice B. Turkoski, RN, PhD; Brenda R. Lance, RN, MSN; and Mark F. Bonfiglio, PharmD Foreword by: Margaret A. Fitzgerald, MS, RN, CS-FNP

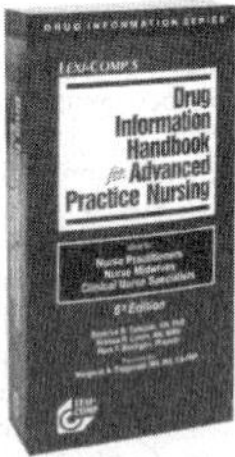

Designed specifically to meet the needs of nurse practitioners, clinical nurse specialists, nurse midwives, and graduate nursing students. The handbook is a unique resource for detailed, accurate information, which is vital to support the advanced practice nurse's role in patient drug therapy management. Over 4750 U.S., Canadian, and Mexican medications are covered in the 1000 monographs. Drug data is presented in an easy-to-use, alphabetically-organized format covering up to 46 key points of information (including dosing for pediatrics, adults, and geriatrics). Appendix contains over 230 pages of valuable comparison tables and additional information. Also included are two indexes, Pharmacologic Category and Controlled Substance, which facilitate comparison between agents.

DRUG INFORMATION HANDBOOK FOR NURSING

by Beatrice B. Turkoski, RN, PhD; Brenda R. Lance, RN, MSN; and Mark F. Bonfiglio, PharmD

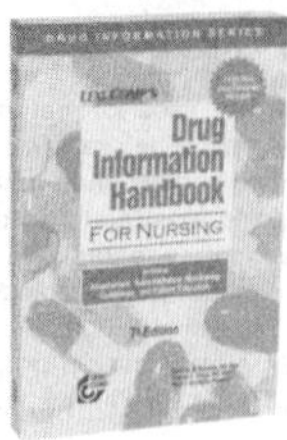

Completely updated and better than ever! We have taken user feedback and created what we believe to be the easiest to use and most complete source of drug information available for nurses. This book is a new size and format for quicker reference with a larger font for easier reading. Registered professional nurses and upper-division nursing students involved with assisting in medication therapy management will find this handbook provides quick access to drug data in a concise, easy-to-use format. Over 4000 U.S., Canadian, and Mexican medications are covered with up to 43 key points of information in each monograph. The handbook contains basic pharmacology concepts and nursing issues such as patient factors that influence drug therapy (ie, pregnancy, age, weight, etc) and general nursing issues (ie, assessment, administration, monitoring, and patient education). The Appendix contains over 230 pages of valuable information.

PHARMACOGENOMICS HANDBOOK

by Larisa M. Humma, PharmD, BCPS; Vicki L. Ellingrod, PharmD, BCPP; Jill M. Kolesar, PharmD, FCCP, BCPS

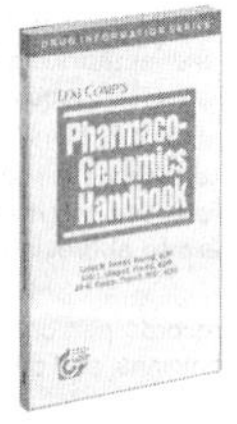

This exciting new title introduces Pharmacogenomics to the forward-thinking healthcare professional and student! It presents information concerning key genetic variations that may influence drug disposition and/or sensitivity. Brief introductions to fundamental concepts in genetics and genomics are provided in order to bring the reader up-to-date on these rapidly emerging sciences. This book provides a foundation for all clinicians who will be called on to integrate rapidly expanding genomic knowledge into the management of drug therapy. A great introduction to pharmacogenetic principles as well as a concise reference on key polymorphisms known to influence drug response!

To order call toll free anywhere in the U.S.: 1-866-EXP-DIFF (397-3433)
Outside of the U.S. call: 330-650-6506 or order online at www.lexi.com

Products offered by LEXI-COMP

INFECTIOUS DISEASES HANDBOOK

by Carlos M. Isada, MD; Bernard L. Kasten Jr., MD; Morton P. Goldman, PharmD; Larry D. Gray, PhD; and Judith A. Aberg, MD

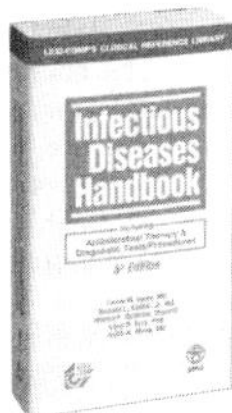

A four-in-one quick reference concerned with the identification and treatment of infectious diseases. Each of the four sections of the book contains related information and cross-referencing to one or more of the other three sections. The Disease Syndrome section provides the clinical presentation, differential diagnosis, diagnostic tests, and drug therapy recommended for treatment of more common infectious diseases. The Organism section presents the microbiology, epidemiology, diagnosis, and treatment of each organism. The Laboratory Diagnosis section describes performance of specific tests and procedures. The Antimicrobial Therapy section presents important facts and considerations regarding each drug recommended for specific diseases of organisms. Also contains an International Brand Name Index with names from 58 different countries.

DRUG INFORMATION HANDBOOK FOR ONCOLOGY

by Dominic A. Solimando, Jr, MA, BCOP

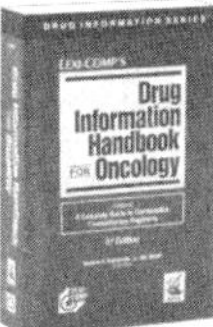

Presented in a concise and uniform format, this book contains the most comprehensive collection of oncology-related drug information available. Organized like a dictionary for ease of use, drugs can be found by looking up the brand or generic name!

This book contains individual monographs for both antineoplastic agents and ancillary medications.

The fields of information for each monograph include: Use, Investigational, Unlabeled/Labeled Contraindications, Vesicant, Emetic Potential. A Special Topics Section, Appendix, and Therapeutic Category & Key Word Index are valuable features of this book, as well.

ANESTHESIOLOGY & CRITICAL CARE DRUG HANDBOOK

by Andrew J. Donnelly, PharmD; Francesca E. Cunningham, PharmD; Verna L. Baughman, MD

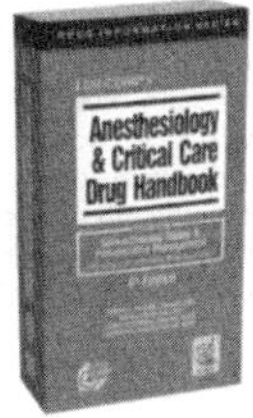

Contains the most common perioperative drugs in the critical care setting along with Special Issues and Topics including: Allergic Reaction, Cardiac Patients in Noncardiac Surgery, Obstetric Patients in Nonobstetric Surgery, Patients With Liver Disease, Chronic Pain Management, Chronic Renal Failure, Conscious Sedation, Perioperative Management of Patients on Antiseizure Medication, and more.

The Appendix includes Abbreviations & Measurements, Anesthesiology Information, Assessment of Liver & Renal Function, Comparative Drug Charts, Infectious Disease-Prophylaxis & Treatment, Laboratory Values, Therapy Recommendations, Toxicology Information, and much more.

International Brand Name Index with names from over 58 different countries is also included.

To order call toll free anywhere in the U.S.: 1-866-EXP-DIFF (397-3433)
Outside of the U.S. call: 330-650-6506 or order online at www.lexi.com

Products offered by LEXI-COMP

POISONING & TOXICOLOGY HANDBOOK

by Jerrold B. Leikin, MD and Frank P. Paloucek, PharmD

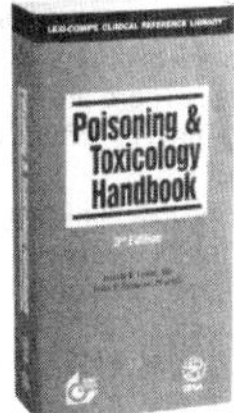

It's back by popular demand! The small size of our Poisoning & Toxicology Handbook is once again available. Better than ever, this comprehensive, portable reference contains 80 antidotes and drugs used in toxicology with 694 medicinal agents, 287 nonmedicinal agents, 291 biological agents, 57 herbal agents, and more than 200 laboratory tests. Monographs are extensively referenced and contain valuable information on overdose symptomatology and treatment considerations, as well as admission criteria and impairment potential of select agents. Designed for quick reference with monographs arranged alphabetically, plus a cross-referencing index. The authors have expanded current information on drugs of abuse and use of antidotes, while providing concise tables, graphics, and other pertinent toxicology text.

LABORATORY TEST HANDBOOK & LTH CONCISE version

by David S. Jacobs MD, FACP; Wayne R. DeMott, MD, FACP; and Dwight K. Oxley, MD, FACP

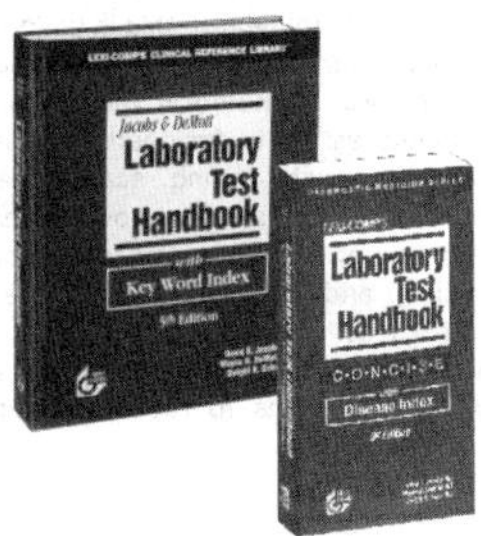

Contains over 900 clinical laboratory tests and is an excellent source of laboratory information for physicians of all specialties, nurses, laboratory professionals, students, medical personnel, or anyone who needs quick access to both routine and specialized testing procedures available in today's clinical laboratory. Each monograph contains test name, synonyms, patient care, specimen requirements, reference ranges, and interpretive information with footnotes, references, and selected web sites. The Laboratory Test Handbook Concise is a portable, abridged (800 tests) version and is an ideal, quick reference for anyone requiring information concerning patient preparation, specimen collection and handling, and test result interpretation.

DIAGNOSTIC PROCEDURES HANDBOOK by Frank Michota, MD

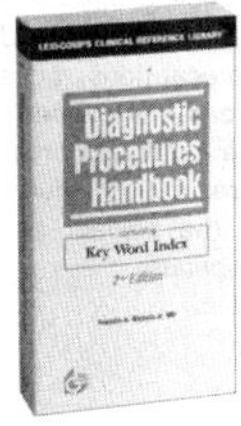

A comprehensive, yet concise, quick reference source for physicians, nurses, students, medical records personnel, or anyone needing access to diagnostic procedure information. This handbook is an excellent source for information in the following areas: allergy; rheumatology; infectious diseases; cardiology; computed tomography; diagnostic radiology; gastroenterology; invasive radiology; magnetic resonance imaging; nephrology, urology, and hematology; neurology; nuclear medicine; pulmonary function; pulmonary medicine and critical care; ultrasound; and women's health.

To order call toll free anywhere in the U.S.: 1-866-EXP-DIFF (397-3433)
Outside of the U.S. call: 330-650-6506 or order online at www.lexi.com

Products offered by LEXI-COMP

DRUG INFORMATION HANDBOOK FOR DENTISTRY

by Richard L. Wynn, BSPharm, PhD; Timothy F. Meiller, DDS, PhD; Harold L. Crossley, DDS, PhD

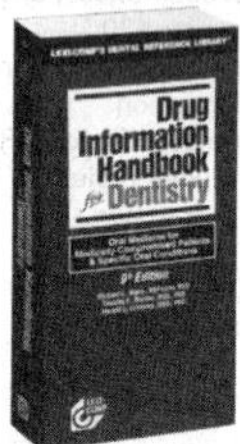

For all dental professionals requiring quick access to concisely-stated drug information pertaining to medications commonly prescribed by dentists and physicians.

Designed and written by dentists for all dental professionals as a portable, chair-side resource. Includes drugs commonly prescribed by dentists or being taken by dental patients and written in an easy-to-understand format. There are 24 key points of information for each drug including **Local Anesthetic/Vasoconstrictor Precautions, Effects on Dental Treatment,** and **Drug Interactions**. Includes information on dental treatment for medically-compromised patients and dental management of specific oral conditions.

Also contains Canadian & Mexican brand names.

ORAL SOFT TISSUE DISEASES

by J. Robert Newland, DDS, MS; Timothy F. Meiller, DDS, PhD; Richard L. Wynn, BSPharm, PhD; and Harold L.Crossley, DDS, PhD

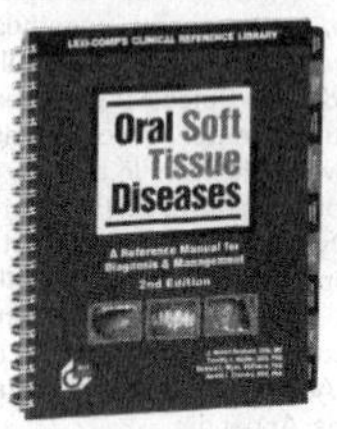

Designed for all dental professionals, this is a pictorial reference to assist in the diagnosis and management of oral soft tissue diseases (over 160 photos). Easy-to-use sections include: Diagnosis process: obtaining a history, examining the patient, establishing a differential diagnosis, selecting appropriate diagnostic tests, interpreting the results, etc.; white lesions; red lesions; blistering-sloughing lesions; ulcerated lesions; pigmented lesions; papillary lesions; soft tissue swelling (each lesion is illustrated with a color-representative photograph); specific medications to treat oral soft tissue diseases; sample prescriptions; and special topics.

ORAL HARD TISSUE DISEASES

by J. Robert Newland, DDS, MS

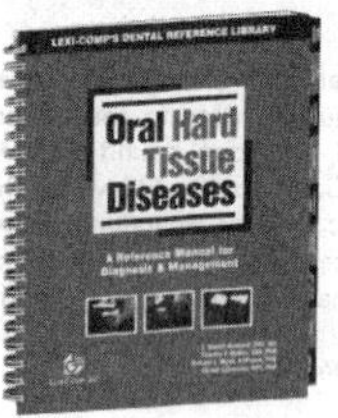

A reference manual for radiographic diagnosis, visually-cued with over 130 high quality radiographs, this book is designed to require little more than visual recognition to make an accurate diagnosis. Each lesion is illustrated by one or more photographs depicting the typical radiographic features and common variations. There are 12 chapters tabbed for easy access: 1) Periapical Radiolucent Lesions; 2) Pericoronal Radiolucent Lesions; 3) Inter-Radicular Radiolucent Lesions; 4) Periodontal Radiolucent Lesions; 5) Radiolucent Lesions Not Associated With Teeth; 6) Radiolucent Lesions With Irregular Margins; 7) Periapical Radiopaque Lesions; 8) Pericoronal Radiopaque Lesions; 9) Inter-Radicular Radiopaque Lesions; 10) Radiopaque Lesions Not Associated With Teeth; 11) Radiopaque Lesions With Irregular Margins; 12) Selected Readings / Alphabetical Index

To order call toll free anywhere in the U.S.: 1-866-EXP-DIFF (397-3433)
Outside of the U.S. call: 330-650-6506 or order online at www.lexi.com

LEXI-COMP ON-HAND™ SOFTWARE LIBRARY

For Palm OS® and
Windows™ Powered Pocket PC Devices

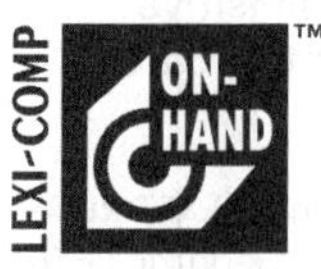

Lexi-Comp's handheld software solutions provide quick, portable access to clinical informationat the point-of-care. Whether you require laboratory test or diagnostic procedure information, to validate a dose, or to check multiple medications and natural products for potential interactions, Lexi-Comp has the information you need in the palm of your hand. Lexi-Comp also provides advanced linking technology to allow you to hyperlink to related information topics within a title, or to the same topic in another title for more extensive information. No longer will you have to exit one database (such as Griffith's 5-Minute Clinical Consult) to look up a drug dose in Lexi-Drugs® or lab test information in Lexi-Lab & Diagnostic Procedures™. Seamless linking between all databases **saves valuable time and helps to improve patient care.**

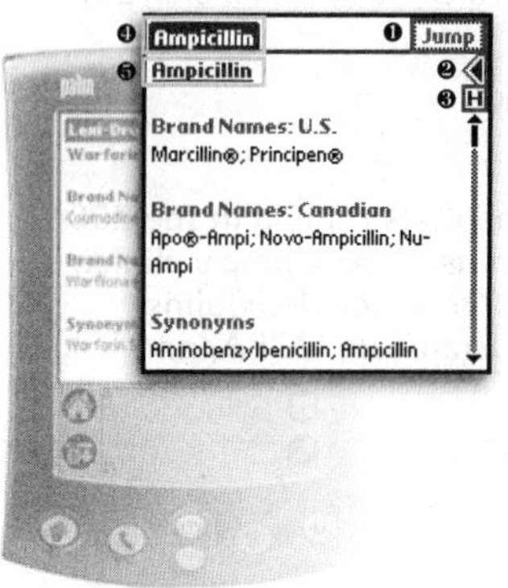

Palm OS® Device shown

Navigational Tools:

❶ **"Jump"** provides a drop down list of available fields to easily navigate through information.

❷ **Back arrow** returns to the index from a monograph or to the "Installed Books" menu from the Index.

❸ **"H"** provides a linkable History to return to any of the last 12 Topics viewed during your session.

❹ **Title bar:** Tap the monograph or topic title bar to activate a menu to "Edit a Note" or return to the list of "Installed Books".

❺ **Linking:** Link to another LEXI-COMP® database by clicking the topic or monograph title link or within a database, noted by various hyperlinked (colorized and underlined) text.